mental ray® Handbooks

Edited by
Rolf Herken

Vol. 2

SpringerWienNewYork

Th. Driemeyer and R. Herken (eds.)

Programming mental ray®

SpringerWienNewYork

Thomas Driemeyer
Rolf Herken

mental images
Gesellschaft für Computerfilm und Maschinenintelligenz mbH & Co. KG
Fasanenstraße 81
D-10623 Berlin

Printed in Austria

Printing A. Holzhausens Nfg., 1070 Wien
Printed on acid-free and chlorine-free bleached paper

SPIN: 10747531
CIP data applied for

ISSN 1438-9835
ISBN 3-211-83404-4 Springer-Verlag Wien New York

Table of Contents

Series Editor's Foreword

The mental ray series of handbooks is conceived to provide concise and up to date general and technical information about the commercially available rendering software mental ray. The series addresses the needs of professional and non-professional users of the software as well as of software developers who intend to integrate the stand-alone version of mental ray or the mental ray component software into applications that require interactive photorealistic and high image quality programmable rendering. In addition, the series provides comprehensive information to students and researchers in computer graphics. mental ray is a valuable tool for teaching and demonstrating the fundamental concepts of photorealistic and programmable rendering as well as a benchmark and catalyst for further research.

The rendering software mental ray and many of its unique underlying concepts are the result of ongoing research and development at the company mental images since its incorporation in 1986. Leading vendors of 3D digital content creation and 3D CAD and product design software have made mental ray their rendering software of choice for all purposes of high end visualization and image synthesis ranging from digital special effects and 3D animation for motion picture, video film, and games production to 3D mechanical and architectural CAD and to industrial product design and automotive styling.

The first three volumes of the series are written by staff members of the R&D team at mental images. Forthcoming volumes will be written by users and researchers and will focus on advanced topics such as the use of mental ray Phenomena for achieving any imaginable or physically correct visual effect.

The development of mental ray was funded in part by the European Commission in ESPRIT projects 6173 (DESIRE) and 22.765 (DESIRE II). The publication of this series faciliates the dissemination of widely accessible information about the resulting software in a timely manner and in more technical detail than it could be achieved otherwise.

It is a great pleasure for me to thank Rudolf Siegle, Director of Springer-Verlag Wien/New York, and Silvia Schilgerius, Planning Department Manager, for their interest in the project and for their willingness to publish the series at Springer-Verlag Wien/New York as part of its distinguished publication program in computer graphics.

Rolf Herken
Berlin, September 1999

Introduction

Organization of this Book

This book is the definitive reference manual for mental ray® version 2.0 and 2.1. It begins with a brief overview over the features of mental ray and continues with the specifications of the mental ray scene description language and the mental ray shader interface. All material is presented in reference form, organized by grammar elements and C function call, rather than by feature set. It is intended for translator writers and shader writers who are familiar with the C and C++ programming languages.

For a tutorial-style description of mental ray, refer to the book "Rendering with mental ray" [Driemeyer 99], which is intended for non-programmers who want to effectively use mental ray without concern for its internal structure and programming interfaces. The functionality of mental ray is presented in much greater detail there.

This book is organized in six chapters and an appendix:

Chapter 1	gives a brief overview over the functionality of mental ray.
Chapter 2	describes the scene language in detail. This chapter is organized by language unit.
Chapter 3	explains how custom shaders and Phenomena™ are written, and documents the shader call interface.
Chapter 4	describes the extended geometry shader interface.
Chapter 5	describes the command-line interface of mental ray.
Chapter 6	contains porting guidelines for users and shader writers upgrading from the previous generation of mental ray, 1.9.
Appendix A	contains the source code of mental ray's scene language parser.

At the time this book went into print, mental ray was at version 2.0.28.18 and 2.1.35.

Introduction to mental ray

mental ray is a general-purpose renderer which creates images of exceptional quality and achieves high performance through the exploitation of parallelism on both multiprocessor machines and across networks of machines.

The software uses advanced rendering acceleration techniques such as a scanline algorithm for primary visible surface determination and the BSP (binary space partitioning) algorithm for secondary rays. mental ray also supports ray classification for secondary rays, and separate shadow ray classification to accelerate the calculation of shadows, as well as grid acceleration. These algorithms can be fine-tuned by optional user-settable parameters to achieve even higher performance than normally achieved by the built-in automatic scene cost analysis.

mental ray supports caustics and global illumination[2.1] simulation using the Photon Map™ method. Caustics caused by multiple reflections and/or refractions, caustics that are themselves reflected or refracted, and volume caustics are supported. Complete, physically correct simulation of general global illumination is also supported: any combination of diffuse, glossy, and specular reflection and transmission can be simulated. For example color bleeding caused by diffuse interreflections, and multiple volume scattering.

mental ray has been designed to take full advantage of parallel hardware, including both thread parallelism on a single machine, and process level parallelism across networks of machines, and on massively parallel distributed-memory systems. mental ray takes advantage of thread parallelism automatically; the use of other machines on the network as render servers may be configured by the user. The renderer balances the computational load among the available processors using a distributed shared database that distributes parts of the scene in an optimal way based on demand.

mental ray can be combined with any suitable modeling and/or animation system via the `.mi` file format, or by integrating the library version into the modeling and animation system, or by combining the library with a translator that reads the modeling system's native file format. mental ray has been fully integrated into SOFTIMAGE|3D, and supports all rendering features of Version 3.x for SGI and Windows NT, as well as additional rendering functionality which is made easily accessible through corresponding enhancements to the user interface of SOFTIMAGE|3D. mental ray is also the rendering component of Dassault Système's CATIA system. Specifically, it is integrated into the CATIA Visualization Studio, supporting all geometric and nongeometric CATIA entities. mental ray is also available as a plug-in for Autodesk 3D Studio MAX 3.0, and Alias|Wavefront Maya. Finally, mental ray is available as a stand-alone program for batch-mode rendering.

In addition, translators are currently available for Alias|Wavefront's Advanced Visualizer, Alias|Wavefront Power Animator, RenderMan RIB, Side Effects' Prisms, IGES, and the DESIRE format.

mental ray is a library for integration into third-party software, as well as for integration in standalone versions that read a variety of scene formats. In the standard standalone version, input is via a scene file in ASCII format. The .mi format is the native scene description format of mental ray. Supported geometric primitives include polygons, and trimmed free-form surfaces.

Polygons may be concave or convex and may contain holes. Displacement maps may be built on top of them.

Free-form surfaces may be input in non-uniform rational B-spline (NURB), Bézier, Taylor monomial, or cardinal form, or through the use of basis matrices. Free-form surfaces may be of arbitrary degree. The geometry of free-form surfaces may be further modified by the application of trimming curves and displacement maps. Trimming curves need not have the same representation as the surface. Surfaces are triangulated internally using a variety of available approximation techniques which may be dependent on or independent of the distance from the surface to the camera.

Connectivity information between free-form surfaces can be given which will stitch surfaces together and close gaps. If the connectivity is unknown, it can be automatically determined at run-time.

mental ray supports incremental changes to the scene database. Only the parts of the scene that change from one frame to the next need to be redefined. This feature allows mental ray to optimize scene tessellation, preparation, acceleration data structure management, and network transfers, taking advantage of the time coherency of the animation.

The functionality of mental ray may be extended through runtime linking of user-supplied C or C++ subroutines, called shaders. This feature can be used to create geometric elements at runtime of the renderer, procedural textures, including bump and displacement maps, materials, atmosphere and other volume rendering effects, environments, camera lenses, and light sources. The user has access to a convenient environment of supporting functions and macros for use in writing shaders. The parameters of a user-provided shader can be freely chosen with name and type; user-defined shaders are not restricted to a list of predefined parameters. Available parameter types include integers, scalars, vectors, colors, textures, light sources, arrays, and nested structures. When a user-defined shader is called, mental ray will provide parameter values according to standard C calling conventions.

The built-in material shaders provide a rich variety of parameters for describing material properties, including ambient color, diffuse color, specular color, transmission and shadow colors, a specular exponent, reflectivity, and transparency coefficients, and an index of refraction. These parameters are interpreted by the shader specified for the material. All material parameters except the index of refraction may be mapped with one or more textures. Color textures include opacity information and if multiple textures are applied to a single parameter they are composited. In addition, one or more bump, displacement, and/or reflection maps may be associated with a material.

Light passing through the space surrounding objects, as well as light passing through solid objects, is modified according to volume shaders, which allow the creation of effects such as fog and non-homogeneous transparency effects and visible caustics beams. In addition to standard material environment maps, a global environment map can be specified that provides a solid background for rays leaving the scene.

mental ray can generate a variety of output formats, including common picture file formats and special-purpose formats for depth maps and label channels. Alpha channels and both 8 and 16 bits per component are supported, as well as a 32-bit floating-point component mode. User-supplied functions can be applied to the rendered image before it is written to disk.

Contour lines can be placed at discontinuities of depth or surface orientation, between different materials, or where the color contrast is high. The contour lines are anti-aliased, and there can be several levels of contours created by reflection or seen through semitransparent materials. The contours can be different for each material (and some materials can have no contours at all). The color and thickness of the contours can depend on geometry, position, illumination, material, frame number, and various other parameters. The resulting image may be output as a pure contour image, a contour image composited onto the regular image (in raster form in any of the supported formats), or as a PostScript file.

Phenomena consist of one or more cooperating shaders or shader trees (actually, shader DAGs; a DAG is a directed acyclic graph). A phenomenon consists of an "interface node" that looks exactly like a regular shader to the outside, and in fact may be a regular shader, but generally it will contain a link to a shader DAG. mental ray takes care of integrating all aspects of the phenomenon into the scene, which may include the introduction or modification of geometry, introduction of lenses, environments, and compile options, and other shaders and parameters.

The Phenomenon concept is conceived to unify — by packaging and hiding complexity — all those seemingly disparate approaches, techniques, and tricks, most notably (but not limited to) the concept of a shader, which are characteristic for today's state of the art in high-end 3D Animation and in Digital Special Effects production. The aim is to provide a comprehensive, coherent, and consistent foundation for the reproduction of all visual phenomena by means of rendering. The Phenomenon concept provides the missing framework for the completion of the definition of a scene for the purpose of rendering in a unified manner.

This book describes versions 2.0 and 2.1 of mental ray. Features that are available only in mental ray 2.1 but not in mental ray 2.0 are marked with "[2.1]".

WWW Resources

mental images' homepage is `http://www.mentalimages.com`. For errata and changes that were made after this book went into print, and downloadable .mi scene file examples, see `http://www.mentalimages.com/books.html`.

The source code for the base and physics shader libraries included with the mental ray distribution is available on `ftp://www.mentalimages.com/pub/`. See the README file at this location for the exact path.

mental images runs several discussion mailing lists; see `http://www.mentalimages.com` for details and instructions for subscribing and posting (follow the *Forum* link).

Acknowledgements

This book is the combined effort of many people at mental images over the past five years. We would like to thank Alexander Biersack, Per Christensen, Susanna Fishel, Martin Grabenstein, Simon Hardy-Francis, Henrik Wann Jensen, Kristjan Valur Jonsson, Alexander Keller, Jochen Kornitzky, Alexander Lobodzinski, Runa Loeber, Charlotte Manning, Bernd Raabe, Steffen Römer, Karl Johann Schmidt, Matthias Senz, Gunter Sprenger, Tom-Michael Thamm, Steffen Volz, and Barbara Wolfers. We would also like to thank these and the other members of the team at mental images for providing support in numerous ways and for maintaining the creative environment in which the software described in this book was, and continues to be, developed. Finally, we would like to thank Claude Benoit, Craig Hall, and Marc Petit at Softimage and Arnauld Lamorlette at BUF Compagnie for their technical contributions and valuable feedback.

Acknowledgements

Chapter 1

Functionality

mental ray offers all the features traditionally expected of photorealistic rendering, together with functionality not found in most rendering software. The following sections describe parallelism, free-form surface input geometry, edge merging and adjacency detection and various input entities such as materials, texture mapping and light sources, and global illumination features such as caustics.

1.1 Parallelism

mental ray has been designed to take full advantage of parallel hardware. On multiprocessor machines that provide the necessary facilities, it automatically exploits thread parallelism where multiple threads of execution access shared memory. No user intervention is required to take advantage of this type of parallelism. mental ray is also capable of exploiting thread and process level parallelism where multiple threads or processes cooperate in the rendering of a single image but do not share memory. This is done using a distributed shared database that provides demand-driven transparent sharing of database items on multiple systems.[1] This allows parallel execution across a network of computers, and on multiprocessor machines which do not support thread parallelism.

A queue of tasks to be executed in parallel is generated by subdividing the screen space. Each task consists of a rectangular portion of the screen to be rendered. A rendering process, whether on the machine where mental ray was started or on some remote host, requests tasks from this queue and renders the corresponding portion of the image. Faster processes will request and complete more tasks than slower processes during the course of rendering an image, thus balancing the load. The same task-based adaptive load distribution is also used for a variety of other parallel computations in mental ray, such as tessellation of free-form surfaces. mental ray keeps track of the actual distribution to ensure that related tasks, even if they are part of different computations,

[1]The parallel rendering technology which is required for the support of distributed shared databases has been developed by mental images as part of the ESPRIT Project 6173 *Design by Simulation and Rendering on Parallel Architectures* (DESIRE). See [Herken 94].

are performed on the same host to make optimal use of the distributed shared database with a minimum of network traffic.

The host that reads or translates the scene, or runs client application such as a front-end application software that mental ray is integrated in, is called the *client host*. The client host is responsible for connecting to all other hosts, called *server hosts*. A server host may also act as client host if an independent copy of mental ray is used by another user; systems do not become unavailable for other jobs if used as servers. However, running a mental ray server on a host may degrade the performance of independent interactive application programs such as modelers on that host significantly.

The list of hosts to connect to is stored in the `.rayhosts` file. The first existing file of `.ray2hosts`, `.rayhosts`, `$HOME/.ray2hosts`, `$HOME/.rayhosts` is used as `.rayhosts` file. Each line contains a hostname with an optional colon-separated port number of the service to connect to and an optional whitespace-separated parameter list that is passed to the host to supply additional command line parameters. Only the following parameters are supported here: `-threads`, `-c_compiler`, `-c_flags`, `-c_linker`, and `-ld_libs`. See the chapter on Command Line Options for a description of these parameters. The first line that literally matches the name of the host the client runs on is ignored; this allows all hosts on the network to share a single `.rayhosts` file, each ignoring the first reference to itself. Only clients ever access the host list. If the `-hosts` option is given to mental ray, the `.rayhosts` file is ignored, and the hosts are taken from the command line. In this case, no hosts are ignored. The library version of mental ray may get its host list directly from the application.

1.2 Free-Form Surfaces

mental ray supports free-form curves and surfaces in non-uniform rational B-spline (NURB), Bézier, Taylor (monomial), cardinal or basis matrix form. Any of these forms may be rational and may be of degree up to twenty-one.[2] Surfaces may be trimmed.

Internally, free-form surfaces are triangulated (approximated) before rendering. A variety of approximation techniques is available, including uniform and regular parametric, uniform spatial, curvature dependent, and combined methods.

The uniform parametric technique (referred to in the input file as `parametric`) subdivides the surface at equal intervals in parameter space. The input file specifies a factor which is multiplied by the surface degree to obtain the number of subdivisions in each parametric direction per patch.

The regular parametric technique (`regular parametric` in the input file) is a simpler variant of the previous technique. It subdivides the surface at equal intervals in parameter space. The number of subdivisions per surface is directly specified in the input file.

The uniform spatial technique (`spatial` in the input file) subdivides the surface at equal intervals in camera space (in the `mi1` format) or in object space (in the `mi2` format) — or, rather, the intervals will never exceed the given upper bound. Optionally, this bound may be specified in

[2] Although the user-settable degree is currently limited to 21, mental ray has no inherent limit.

raster space (in units of pixel diagonals) rather than camera or object space. If, for example, one wanted to approximate a surface with sub-pixel size triangles, one could use the uniform spatial approximation technique with a raster space accuracy of 0.5 pixel diagonals. Note that the apparent size of a subdivided portion of a surface is computed as if the surface was parallel to the screen. Thus, the triangulation does not become more coarse towards the edge of the object's silhouette. This has the advantage that the object will be well approximated even if seen in a mirror from a different angle, but such a definition can also result in an overly fine triangulation.

View-dependent subdivision means that objects that are instanced more than once must be triangulated in multiple ways. A tradeoff between the additional memory required to store multiple objects, and the reduced total number of instanced triangles must be evaluated to achieve optimal speed. Camera dependency works best if it is used for objects that are not instanced too many times.

The curvature dependent technique (known as `curvature` in the input file), subdivides a surface until two approximation criteria are satisfied simultaneously. The first is an upper bound on the maximum distance in the space the object is defined in between the actual surface and its polygonal approximation (known as the *distance tolerance*). The second is an upper bound on the maximum angle (in degrees) between any two normals on a subdivided portion of the surface (known as the *angle tolerance*). Note that the first criterion is scale dependent while the second is scale independent. That is, one must know the size of the object in order to choose a suitable tolerance in the first case but not the second. In spite of this apparent advantage of the angle criterion over the distance criterion, the angle criterion has the undesirable property of resolving small discontinuities ad infinitum, whereas the distance criterion will not resolve features whose scale is below the given tolerance. Either criterion can be disabled by setting the corresponding tolerance to zero. The distance criterion may be optionally given in raster space, again in units of pixel diagonals.

It is also possible to use an approximation technique which combines the bounds of the spatial technique and the curvature dependent technique.

Both the uniform spatial and curvature dependent approximation techniques use a recursive subdivision process that can also be controlled by two additional parameters, specifying the minimum and maximum number of recursion levels. The subdivision can be forced to proceed at least as far as the given minimum level, and refinement can be halted at the maximum level.

All subdivisions of a free-form surface apart from the regular parametric technique and the Delaunay technique[2.1] begin at the patch level. If, for example, a plane is modeled with ten by ten patches it will be approximated by at least two hundred triangles, although two triangles might be adequate. If mental ray seems to be producing a large number of triangles in spite of a low approximation accuracy, this is often due to the selected patch subdivision algorithm.

The curvature dependent approximation technique with the distance tolerance given in raster space and the angle tolerance set to zero has proved to be the most useful technique for high quality rendering.

For a quick rendering to examine materials or object positions, the uniform parametric technique may be used with a factor of zero.

Free-form curves (trimming curves) may also be approximated by any of the above described methods using a technique and tolerances which are distinct from those of the surface which the curve trims. The definitions are essentially the same if one considers a curve segment to correspond to a surface patch. An important difference is that the uniform spatial, curvature dependent, and combined approximation techniques will coalesce curve segments if possible. A straight line consisting of one hundred co-linear segments may be approximated by a single line segment.

1.3 Edge Merging and Adjacency Detection

Surfaces are generally approximated independently of each other and small cracks may be visible between them, especially if the approximation is coarse. It may be desirable to use a smaller tolerance for the trimming curves than for the surfaces themselves. If an object is well-modeled, if surfaces meet smoothly along their trimming curves and if the curves are approximated to a high accuracy, the gaps between surfaces become invisible. The ideal solution, however, is to triangulate surfaces consistently along shared edges.

mental ray provides the `connect` construct for specifying connectivity between surfaces. The two surfaces are named, along with the two trimming curves and the parameter ranges along which they meet. Along such a connection the surfaces will be triangulated consistently resulting in a seamless join.

If the system generating the input for mental ray cannot determine such connectivity, adjacency detection may be used to discover connectivity automatically. One may give a `merge` epsilon within a geometry group which will cause all surfaces in that group to be examined. If any two surfaces approach each other along a trimming curve (or the surface boundary, if the surface is not trimmed) to within the given epsilon, they will be considered adjacent and an appropriate connection will be generated.

Essential to the fast and correct determination of adjacency is the gathering of surfaces into appropriate groups. Obviously, the door of a car should not be considered connected to the body no matter how close the two surfaces approach each other. Moreover, the larger the groups, the more time will be required for adjacency detection.

1.4 Special Points and Curves

Special points and curves force the triangulation of a free-form surface to include specific features. A special point is given in the parameter space of the surface and will be included as a corresponding vertex in the triangulation. A special curve is similar to a trimming curve but does not cause portions of the surface to be trimmed. Rather, the curve is included as a polyline in the triangulation of the surface. Special curves are useful for introducing flexibility in the triangulation along specific features. For example, if letters were to be embossed on a planar surface using displacement mapping, a series of contour curves around the letters could be created with special curves.

1.5 Atmospheres and Volumes

The medium which surrounds all objects in a scene is known as the atmosphere. This is normally a transparent material with a refractive index of 1.0. A procedural atmosphere can be specified by naming a volume shader that determines the attenuation of light as it travels along a ray of a given length through the atmosphere. As with all other types of shaders, a user-written shader can be used in place of the standard volume shader. This capability can be used, for example, to create procedurally defined fog.

1.6 Materials

A material determines the response of a surface to illumination. Materials in mental ray consist of a material name and one mandatory and seven optional shaders, each of which can be a standard shader or a user-provided C function:

- The first function is the material shader itself. It may not be omitted. The material shader determines the color of a point on an object, based on its parameters which may include object colors, textures, lists of light sources, and other arbitrary parameters.
- An optional volume shader controls rays passing through the inside of the object. This is functionally equivalent to atmosphere calculations, but takes place inside objects, not outside.
- An optional photon shader determines how the material interacts with indirect illumination if caustics or global illumination are enabled, much like the main material shader determines how the material interacts with direct illumination.
- An optional photon volume shader determines how the inside of the object interacts with indirect illumination if caustics or global illumination are enabled, much like the volume shader determines how the volume interacts with direct illumination.
- An optional environment shader provides an environment map for non-raytraced reflections.
- An optional displacement shader can be named that displaces a free-form surface at each point in the direction of the local surface normal. Displacement maps affect the triangles resulting from the tessellation of free-form surfaces and polygonal meshes.
- An optional shadow shader determines the way shadow rays pass through the object. This can be used for calculating colored shadows.
- An optional contour shader specifies how contours should be drawn in and around the object that this material is applied to, if contour rendering is enabled.

The shading function may be either a user written function linked at run time, or it may be one of the standard functions. Shaders may define parameters that control their behavior. Shaders are completely free to define any set of parameters required for their function, but there is a set of commonly used terms and parameter names that will be found in many parameter lists.

Parameters have names and values. For example, a shader might have a parameter named `"diffuse"` with the value `1.0 1.0 0.0`, which specifies a yellow color. Parameters can be given in any order. Parameters can also be omitted; mental ray will substitute null values. Here is a list of commonly used parameters. Note that data types may vary: some shaders may accept a single scalar value for parameters such as transparency while others expect a color (three or four scalars) to specify the transparency of red, green, blue, and perhaps alpha separately. For a description of the parameters accepted by a specific shader, refer to the documentation of the shader library that the shader belongs to.

The *index of refraction* controls the bending of light as it passes through a transparent object. Although actually dependent on the ratio of indices between the transparent material being entered and that being left, in practice one may say that the higher the index of refraction, the more the light is bent. Typical values are 1.0 for air, 1.33 for water and 1.5 for glass.

The *shinyness* material parameter effectively controls the size of highlights on a surface. It is also known as the specular exponent. The higher the value, the smaller the highlight.

The *dissolve* parameter controls the fading transparency of a material independent of refractive effects. This is more accurately described as a blending operation between the surface and whatever lies beyond. If the transparency is 0.0, the surface is completely opaque. A value of 0.5 would cause an equal blend of the surface and the background. A value of 1.0 would result in an invisible surface. This parameter is used by the Wavefront-compatible shaders only.

The *transparency* parameter controls the refractive transparency of a material. Unlike dissolve, this parameter has a physically correct interpretation. The range is, as for transparency, from 0.0 for opaque to 1.0 for a completely transparent surface. The interpretation of transparency is left entirely to the material shader.

The *reflect* parameter controls the reflectivity of a material. If reflect is 0.0 no reflections would be visible on a surface. A perfect mirror would have a reflect value of 1.0.

The *ambient* component approximates the color of a light source which illuminates a surface from all directions without attenuation or shadowing.

The *diffuse* component is the color of the surface which is dependent on its angle to a light source but independent of the position of the viewer. A piece of felt is an example of a material with only a diffuse component.

The *specular* component is the color of the surface which is dependent both on the position of the light source and the position of the viewer. It is the color of highlights on the surface.

The *transmit* component (transmission filter) is a color which filters light refracted through an object. A piece of glass which imparts a green tint to the objects seen through it would have a green transmit component. This parameter is used by the Wavefront shader only.

Finally, the *shade* component (shadow filter) is a color which filters light as it passes through a transparent object which casts a shadow. A blue glass ball would have a blue shade component. This parameter is also used by the Wavefront shader only.

1.7 Light Sources

A light source illuminates the objects in a scene. Light sources in mental ray are programmable and consist of a light source name, a named light shader function, and an optional origin and direction (exactly one of the two must be present). All light shaders also accept shader parameters that depend on the shader. All standard shaders require a light color parameter.

The lights available to a scene are defined outside materials and referenced by name inside materials. Only those lights which a material references will illuminate surfaces which use that material.

The shading function for light sources may be either a user written function linked at run time, or it may be one of the standard functions. There are standard shader libraries for Alias, Alias Maya, Autodesk 3D Studio MAX, Dassault CATIA, SOFTIMAGE, SolidWorks, and Wavefront compatibility, as well as generic shader libraries such as mental images' base, physics, and Lume shader libraries.

Some shaders accept a boolean parameter `shadow` that turns shadow casting on or off for that light source, and a floating point `factor` that is the shadow factor. The shadow factor controls penetration of opaque objects.

For example, the `mib_light_spot` shader in the base shader library implements a spot light. It has a `color` parameter that must be set to the color of the light, as three scalars for the red, green, and blue components. It also allows a boolean `shadow` parameter that enables shadows cast from this light if its value is on, and a `factor` parameter that controls shadow penetration, ranging from `0.0` for black shadows to `1.0` for invisible shadows. The shader also accepts a boolean `atten` parameter that turns distance attenuation on or off, and two scalar parameters `start` and `stop` that specify the range over which the attenuation falls off if `atten` is on. The spot light mode requires an origin, a direction, and a spread value in the light definition in the scene description file. The spread value in the light definition and the `cone` parameter of the shader together define the spot characteristics of the light. The `cone` parameter specifies the angle of the inner solid cone and the spread statement specifies the outer falloff cone. The spot casts a cone of light with a softened edge where the intensity falls off to zero between the cone and spread angles. This and most other shaders specify angles not in degrees but in the cosine of one-half of the opening angle to improve performance: 1.0 is an opening angle of 0 degrees (a laser beam too narrow to see), 0.707 specifies an opening angle of approximately 90 degrees (because $cos \frac{90}{2} \approx 0.707$) and 0.0 specifies an opening angle of 180 degrees.

1.8 Area Light Sources

The main purpose of area light sources is to generate more realistic lighting, resulting in soft shadows. This is achieved by using one of four primitives (rectangles, discs, spheres, and cylinders) as light sources with nonzero area. This means that a point on an object may be illuminated by only a part of a light source. Area light sources are based on similar principles as motion blurring, and, like motion blur, may reduce rendering speed.

Area light sources are specified in the `.mi` file by naming a primitive in a standard light definition. Any of the standard spot and point lights can be turned into an area light source. The orientation of the disc and rectangle primitives may be chosen independently of the light direction of spot and directional light sources. Any type of light shading function can be used.

1.9 Shadow Maps

Shadow mapping is a technique that generates fast approximate shadows. It can be used for fast previewing of models or as an alternative to the more accurate (but also more costly) ray tracing based approach in scenes where accurate shadows are not required. Shadow maps are particularly efficient when a scene is rendered several times without changes in the shadows (for example an animation where only the camera is moving).

A shadow map is a fast depth buffer rendering of the model as seen from a light source. This means that each pixel in a shadow map contains information about the distance to the nearest object in the model in a particular direction from the light source. This information can be used to compute shadows without using shadow rays to test for occluding objects. The shadow computation is based only on the depth information available in the shadow maps. For fast previewing of scenes, shadow maps can be used in combination with scanline rendering to produce fast approximate renderings with shadows — without using any ray tracing.

Two different kind of shadows can be produced with shadow maps: sharp and soft (blurry) shadows. Sharp shadows are very fast, and depending on the resolution of the shadow map they will approximate the result produced with simple ray tracing. Soft shadows are produced by distributing one or more samples in a region of the shadow map. This technique produces soft shadows everywhere and is not as accurate as the ray tracing based approach for computing soft shadows but is much faster.

1.10 Texture, Bump, Displacement, and Reflection Mapping

mental ray supports texture, bump, displacement and reflection mapping, all of which may be derived from an image file or procedurally defined using user-supplied functions.

The following table lists the file formats accepted by mental ray:

format	description	comp	bits/comp	colormap	compress
rla/rlb	Wavefront image	3, 4	8	no	RLE
		3, 4	16	no	RLE
pic	SOFTIMAGE image	3, 4	8	no	RLE, no
alias	Alias image	3	8	no	RLE
rgb	SGI color	$3^{2.1}$, 4	8, $16^{2.1}$	no	RLE, no
jpg	JFIF image	3	8	no	JPEG*
tif	TIFF image	1	1, 4, 8	no	RLE, no
		1	4, 8	yes	RLE, no
		3, 4	8	no	RLE, no
		3, 4	16	no	RLE, no
picture	Dassault Systèmes picture	3	8	no	RLE
ppm	Portable pixmap	3	8, 16	no	no
tga	Targa image	1	8	no, yes	RLE, no
		3	5	no	RLE, no
		3/1	5/1	no	RLE, no
		3, 4	8	no	RLE, no
bmp	MS Windows/OS2 bitmap	1	1, 4, 8	yes	no
		3, 4	8	no	no
qnt	Quantel/Abekas YUV image	3	8	no	no
ct	mental images texture	4	8, 16, float	no	no
st	mental images alpha texture	1	8, 16	no	no
vt/wt	mental images basis vectors	2	16	no	no
zt	mental images depth channel	1	float	no	no
nt/mt	mental images vectors	3	float	no	no
tt	mental images tag channel	1	32	no	no
bit	mental images bit mask	1	1	no	no
map	memory mapped textures	any	any	no	no

In the table any combination of comma separated values determines a valid format subtype. For example, the SGI RGB image format will be read when the data type is 8 bits per component with or without alpha, either RLE compressed or uncompressed. The actual image format is determined by analyzing the file content, not just by checking the filename extension. This allows replacing texture files with memory-mapped textures without changing the name, for example.

Typical image types like black/white, grayscale, colormapped and truecolor images, optionally compressed, are supported. Some of them could be used to supply additional alpha channel information (number of components greater than 3). The collection covers most common platform independent formats like TIFF and JFIF/JPEG[3], special UNIX (PPM) or Windows bitmap (BMP) types and well known application formats. The mental images formats, normally created by mental ray itself, are mainly available to exchange data not storable with other formats.

The other way to define any sort of map is supplying user functions, which are linked to mental ray at run time without user intervention. The function may require parameters which could specify, for example, the turbulence of a procedural marble texture.

[3]The JPEG software is based in part on the work of the Independent JPEG Group.

Frequently, a function is used to apply texture coordinate transformations such as scaling, cropping, and repetitions. Such a function would have a sub-texture argument that refers to the actual image file texture.

A user-defined material shader is not restricted to the above applications for textures. It is free to evaluate any texture and any number of textures for a given point, and use the result for any purpose.

In the parameter list of the standard material shaders, a list of texture maps may be given in addition to, for example, a literal RGB value for the diffuse component of a material. The color of the diffuse component will then vary across a surface. To shade a given point on a surface, the coordinates in texture space are first determined for the point. The diffuse color used for shading calculations is then the value of the texture map at these coordinates. The SOFTIMAGE-compatible material shader uses a different approach; it accepts a single list of textures, with parameters attached to each texture that control the way the texture is applied to ambient, diffuse, and other parameters. The shader interface is extremely flexible and permits user-defined shaders to use either of these approaches, or completely different formats. The remainder of this section describes the standard shader parameters only.

The standard material shaders support texture mapping for all standard material parameters except the index of refraction. Shinyness, transparency, refraction transparency, and reflectivity are scalar values and may be mapped by a scalar map. Most shaders use color maps to implement bump mapping by sampling the color map three times, but some shaders such as the Wavefront material shader accept a vector map that requires only a single sample.

Determining the texture coordinates of a point on a surface to be shaded requires defining a mapping from points in camera space to points in texture space. Such a mapping is itself referred to as a texture space for the surface. Multiple texture spaces may be specified for a surface. If the geometry is a polygon, a texture space is created by associating texture vertices with the geometric vertices. If the geometry is a free-form surface, a texture space is created by associating a texture surface with the surface. A texture surface is a free-form surface which defines the mapping from the natural surface parameter space to texture space. Texture maps, and therefore texture spaces and texture vertices, may be one, two, or three dimensional.

Pyramid textures are a variant of mip-map textures. When loading a texture that is flagged with the `filter` keyword, mental ray builds a hierarchy of different-resolution texture images that allow elliptical filtering of texture samples. Without filtering, distant textures would be point-sampled at widely separated locations, missing the texture areas between the samples, which causes texture aliasing. Texture filtering attempts to project the screen pixel on the texture, which results in an elliptic area on the texture. Pyramid textures allow sampling this ellipse very efficiently, taking every pixel in the texture in the ellipse into account without sampling every pixel. Pyramid textures are not restricted to square and power-of-two resolutions, and work with any RGB or RGBA picture file format. The shader can either rely on mental ray's texture projection or specify its own. Filter blurriness can be adjusted per texture.

A procedural texture is free to use the texture space in any way it wants, but texture files are always defined to have unit size and to be repeated through all of texture space. That is, the lower-left corner of the file maps to (0.0, 0.0) in texture space, and again to (1.0, 0.0), (2.0, 0.0), and so on; the lower-right corner maps to (1.0, 0.0), (2.0, 0.0), ... and the upper right to (1.0, 1.0), (2.0, 2.0), ...

Just as a texture map can vary a parameter such as the diffuse color over every point on a surface, a bump map can be associated with a material, perturbing the normal at every point on a surface which uses the material. This will affect the shading, though not the geometry, giving the illusion of a pattern being embossed on the surface.

Bump maps, like texture maps, require a texture space. In addition, bump maps require a pair of *basis vectors* to define the coordinate system in which the normal is displaced. A bump map defines a scalar x and a scalar y displacement over the texture space. These components are used together with the respective basis vectors in order to calculate a perturbed surface normal. The basis vectors are automatically defined for free-form surfaces in a way which conforms to the texture space. For polygons, the basis vectors must be explicitly given along with the texture coordinates for every polygon vertex.

A displacement map is a scalar map which is used to displace a free-form surface or a polygon at each point in the direction of the local normal. Like texture, bump and reflection maps, a displacement map may be either a file or a user-defined function, or a combination of the two.

The surface must be triangulated fine enough to reveal the details of the displacement map. In general, the triangles must be smaller than the smallest feature of the displacement map which is to be resolved.

Displacement mapped polygons are at first triangulated as ordinary polygons. The initial triangulation is then further subdivided according to the specified approximation criteria. The parametric technique subdivides each triangle a given number of times. All the other techniques take the displacement into account. The length criterion, for example, limits the size of the edges of the triangles of the displaced polygons and ensures that at least all features of this size are resolved. As the displaced surface is not known analytically, the distance criterion compares the displacements of the vertices of a triangle with each other. The criterion is fulfilled only if they differ by less than the given threshold. Subdivision is finest in areas where the displacement changes. The angle criterion limits the angle under which two triangles meet in an edge contained in the triangulation. Subdivision stops as soon as the given criterion or combination of them is satisfied or the maximum subdivision level is reached. This does not preclude the possibility that at an even finer scale new details may show up which would again violate the approximation criteria.

For displacement mapped free-form surfaces approximation techniques can be specified either on the underlying geometric surface or for the surface resulting from the displacement. Before mental ray version 2.0, only the former method existed. This is still available, but it does not take into account variations in curvature imparted to the surface as a result of displacement mapping. If one wants to control the approximation from the geometric surface the most suitable technique for use with displacement mapping on free-from surfaces is usually the view dependent uniform spatial subdivision technique, which allows specification of triangle size in raster space. An alternative is to place special curves on the surface which follow the contours or isolines of the displacement map, thus creating flexibility in the surface tessellation at those points where it is most needed for displacement. This would also facilitate the approximation of the displacement map by the new adaptive triangulation method. In addition to or even instead of specifying the subdivision criteria for the base surface they can be given for the displaced surface itself. This approximation statement works exactly the same way as for polygons, i.e. an initial tessellation is subdivided until the criteria on the displaced surface are met.

The final type of map which may be associated with a material is an environment map. This is a color-mapped virtual sphere of usually infinite radius which surrounds any object referencing the given material. This sphere is also seen by refracted rays; the environment seen by first-generation (primary) rays can also be specified but is part of the `camera`, not of any particular material. In general, if a ray does not intersect any objects, or if casting such a ray would exceed the trace depth, the ray is considered to strike the sphere of the environment map of the last material visited, or the `camera` environment map in the case of first-generation rays that did not hit any material.

The environment map always covers the entire sphere exactly once. Rotations, translations, and repetitions are supported by special shader parameters or remapping shader nodes such as the ones found in the base shader library. There are also environment shaders that implement cubical instead of spherical environment maps, and cubical maps of finite instead of infinite size.

1.11 Texture Filtering

mental ray provides two methods for texture filtering: a fast filtered texture lookup using image pyramids (which are similar to mip-maps but have no restrictions on texture size), and a high-quality filtering method using elliptical projections. Both methods operate on image pyramids. There is a `.map` image format defined by mental ray that supporting filters.

When standard image files (such as `.rgb`) are used for filtered texture lookups (both methods), the pyramid must be created by mental ray when the image is accessed. For high-resolution images this can take a long time (sometimes up to a minute), so it is highly recommended to create this image pyramid "offline" by mental images' `imf_copy` utility. When called with the `-p` option on the command line, it down-filters the source texture image file and writes out the filtered images in memory-mapped image format. If such a file is read with a `local filter color texture` statement in .mi scene file, the pyramid is read almost instantaneously.

Also, it is recommended to make local copies of the texture files on the machines in order to speed up access. When machines with different byte order are used in the network, there is a performance penalty when using only one version of the pyramid .map file (it has to be byte swapped), so it is recommended to generate the `.map` file in the native byte order on the respective machines.

The prefiltered `.map` file containing the pyramid can also be used for standard nonfiltered texture lookups (using a simple `local color texture` statement), in this case only the first (finest) level of the image pyramid is used.

Now the two methods in detail:

1.11.1 Pyramid Filtering

This method can be used very easily with existing .mi files, it is only necessary to add a "`filter` *scale*" modifier to the texture load statements in the scene file. Here is an example:

```
local filter 0.8 color texture "tex_0" "mytexture.map"
```

The basic idea behind pyramid filtering is that when a pixel rectangle (the current sampling location) is projected into texture space, mental ray has to calculate the (weighted) average of all texture pixels (texels) inside this area and return it for the texture lookup. Using the average of the pixels, high frequencies which cause aliasing are eliminated. To speed up this averaging, the compression value is calculated for the current pixel location which is the inverse size of the pixel in texture space. For example, if the pixel has a projected size of four texels in texture space, then one texel is compressed to 1/4 in the focal plane (severe compression gives those aliasing artifacts).

It is very costly to project a rectangle to texture space, so usually the quadrilateral in texture space is approximated by a square and the length of one side is used for the compression value. The compression value is used as an index into the image pyramid, and since this value has a fractional part, the two levels that the value falls in between of are looked up using bilinear interpolation at each level, followed by a linear interpolation of the two colors from the level lookups. (mental ray uses also bilinear texture interpolation when no filtering is applied).

Just specifying "`filter` *scale* `color texture`" is not sufficient for an exact projection of the pixel to texture space. The texture shader modifies the UV texture coordinates (either from specified texture surfaces or generated by cylinder projections) according to remapping shader parameters etc. In *mi_lookup_color_texture*, mental ray only has the UV texture coordinates, and it is almost impossible to project the pixel corners to texture space since it is not known how to obtain additional UV coordinates or how to remap them. The remapping is done before *mi_lookup_color_texture* is called.

mental ray's implementation of pyramid mapping therefore adds a vector to the current intersection point in object space and transforms this point into raster space. The length of the offset vector is calculated by dividing the object extent by the texture resolution (the larger value of width and height is used). This approach assumes that texture space corresponds to object space (that is, if the object size is one object unit, the texture fully covers it). If a texture shader applies texture replications, the filter value should be set to the replication count or larger to adjust for this effect. The compression value is calculated as the distance between the raster position mentioned above and the current raster position ($state \rightarrow raster\_x$, $state \rightarrow raster\_y$).

Since this can not always attain satisfying results, mental ray allows multiplication of a "user scaling" value — the *scale* value in the `filter` statement. Using this value, it is possible to reduce blurring ($scale < 1$) or increase blurring ($scale > 1$). For example, if the texture is replicated 10 times, which makes it appear smaller in raster space and hence requires more blurring, the filter constant should be multiplied by 10. Since texture projections are handled by shaders and not by the mental ray core, this cannot be done automatically.

Pyramid filtering also works when reflection or refraction is used, but mathematical correctness cannot be guaranteed since mental ray cannot take reflection or refraction paths into account, for the same reason.

1.11.2 Elliptical Projection Filter Lookup

This method was implemented in mental ray in order to provide a very high quality texture filtering, far superior to the pyramid filtering explained above. It eliminates most if not all of the aliasing in high texture frequencies. When using checkerboard textures mapped onto a rectangle, for example, there is much less blurring at the horizon where the texture compression is severe. With mip-mapping as explained above, the blurring at such extreme compressions is sometimes still visible.

The main cause for the excessively blurry-looking images using mip-maps is the approximation of the pixel projection area by a square. With elliptical filtering a circle around the current sampling location is projected to texture space and will give either a circle or an ellipse as a projection shape. Instead of approximating this curve by simple shapes like squares, a direct convolution (averaging) of all texels which are inside the ellipse area is done. Averaging all texels in this area can take quite long, so mental ray uses pyramids of prefiltered textures to accelerate this. There are various parameters explained below which control modification of ellipse shape and level selection in the pyramid.

The most difficult part when elliptical projections are used is that a screen to texture space transformation matrix has to be provided. This matrix is used in the filtering code to transform the circle around the current sampling location to texture space. mental ray provides two helper functions for constructing this matrix when UV texture coordinates are available; see *mi_texture_filter_project* in the Writing Shaders chapter. If those are not available and (for example) direct cylinder projective mappings are used, it is much more easier to calculate this matrix.

The following filtering algorithm is applied: first, a circle in the current sampling location is transformed to the ellipse using the provided transformation matrix. Then the eccentricity of the ellipse is calculated (major radius divided by minor radius). If the eccentricity is larger than a specified maximum, the minor radius is adjusted (made larger) to make sure that this eccentricity maximum always holds. The reason for this enlargement is that the direct convolution is done in the pyramid level based on the minor axis length of the ellipse. There is another parameter which specifies the maximum allowed number of texels the minor radius may cover. If that number is exceeded in the finest level (zero), a higher level is used. In the second level, for example, the minor radius as half the size etc. Enlarging the minor radius when the eccentricity is exceeded, basically means that we are going up in the pyramid. So, for very large this ellipses, mental ray is making them "fatter" and uses a higher level in the pyramid. Referring to the checkerboard-mapped plane example above, the circle is projected to very large thin ellipses near the horizon, covering thousands of texels, and using the technique above mental ray just makes a few texture lookups in the higher pyramid levels.

There is another parameter which modifies the size of the circle to be projected, usually the radius is 0.5, making it larger introduces more blurring, making it less gives more aliasing.

The projection helper functions expect another parameter which is the maximum offset of the central sampling location to the two other points which have to be selected. The other two points should be inside the pixel, but since mental ray is using the current intersection primitive (the triangle) also for these points to determine the UV texture coordinates, a smaller value than 0.5 (pixel corners) is appropriate since mental ray might hit the triangle plane outside the triangle area. Usually 0.3 gives good results. When the UV coordinates are calculated using cylinder projections, it is possible to obtain the UV coordinates much faster and also much more accurately.

1.12 User-Defined Shaders

In addition to standard shaders, user-defined shaders written in standard C or C++ can be precompiled and linked at runtime, or can be both compiled and linked at runtime. User-defined shaders can be used in place of any standard shader, redefining materials, textures, lights, environments, volumes, displacements etc.

mental ray can link in user-defined shaders in either object, source, or dynamic shared object (DSO or DLL) form.

Every user-defined shader must be declared before it can be used. A declaration is a statement that names the shader, and lists the name and type of all its parameters.

Declarations may appear in the `.mi` scene description file, but are typically stored in an external file included at run time. Note that all `code` and `link` statements must precede the first declaration in the `.mi` file.

Available parameter types are boolean, integer, scalar, string, color (RGBA), vector, transform (4×4 matrix), scalar texture, color texture, vector texture, shader, material, geometry, and light. In addition to these primitive types, compound types may be built using struct and array declarations. Structs may be nested but arrays may not.

An instance of a shader can be created by creating a material, texture, light etc. that names a declared shader and associates a parameter list with values with it. Any parameter name that appeared in the declaration can be omitted or listed in any order, followed by a value that depends on the parameter type. Omitted parameters default to 0. Scalars accept floating point numbers, vectors accept one to three floating point numbers, and textures accept a texture name.

After a material, texture, light etc has been created, it can be used. Materials are used by giving its name in object geometry statements, and textures and lights are used by naming them as parameter values in other shaders, typically material shaders.

When the C function that implements a user-defined shader is called, it receives three pointers: one points to the result, one to global state, and one to a data structure that contains the parameter values. mental ray stores the parameter values in that data structure using a layout that corresponds exactly to the layout a C compiler would create, so that the C function can access parameters simply by dereferencing the pointer and accessing the data structure members by name. For this, it is necessary that a struct declaration is available in C syntax that corresponds exactly to the declaration in `.mi` syntax.

For details on user-defined shaders, refer to the "Writing Shaders" chapter.

1.13 The Camera

The camera is fixed at the origin, looking down the negative Z axis, with up being the positive Y axis. To view a scene from a given position and orientation, the scene must be transformed such that the camera is at this standard location.

By default, the camera is a pin-hole perspective camera for which the focal length, aperture and aspect ratio may be specified in either the `camera` construct of the input file or on the command line of mental ray. Optionally, lens effects such as depth of field can be achieved by specifying one or more lens shaders.

1.14 Lens Effects

Lens effects are distortions of the rendered image achieved by changing the light path through the camera lens. Because lens effects are applied to first-generation rays, there is no loss of quality that would be unavoidable if the distortion were applied in a post-processing stage after rendering.

Lens effects are introduced by specifying one or more lens shaders in the `camera` statement. If no lens shaders are present, the standard pinhole camera is used. Each lens shader is called with two state variables that specify the ray origin and the ray direction. The lens shader calculates a new origin and a new direction, and casts an eye ray using the *mi_trace_eye* function. The first lens shader always gets the position of the pinhole camera. All following lens shaders get the origin and direction that the previous lens shader used when calling *mi_trace_eye*.

Lens shaders imply ray tracing. If lens shaders change the origin or direction of a ray they only work correctly if scanline rendering is turned off. If scanline is turned on, a warning is printed. Then, the lens shaders must not change the origin or direction of a ray. Lens shaders have no effect on the trace depth limit, eye rays are not counted towards the ray trace depth.

1.15 Depth of Field

Depth of field is an effect that simulates a plane of maximum sharpness, and blurs objects closer or more distant than this plane. There are two methods for implementing depth of field: a lens shader can be used that takes multiple samples using different paths to reach the same point on the focus plane to interpolate the depth effect; or a combination of a volume shader and an output shader that collect depth information during rendering and then apply a blurring filter as a postprocessing step over the finished image using this depth information. Both methods are supported by standard shaders supplied with mental ray.

1.16 Animation

The input file consists of a list of frames, each of which is complete and self-contained. Animation is accomplished by specifying geometry, light sources and materials which change incrementally from one frame to the next.

1.17 Motion Blur

There are two different motion blur algorithms. One is completely general and computes motion blur of highlights, textures, shadows, reflections, refractions, transparency, and intersecting objects. The other algorithm is much faster, but cannot handle reflections and refractions (and shadows have to be approximated with shadow maps). However, motion blur of highlights, textures, transparency, and intersecting objects still work with the faster algorithm. The faster algorithm is used for scanline samples (first-generation non-raytraced).

The movement of objects is specified by associating linear motion vectors with polygon vertices and surface control points. These vectors give the direction and distance that the vertex or control point moves during one time unit. If a motion vector is not specified, the vertex is assumed to be stationary. Motion blurring computations may be expensive, but note that these computations are only done for those polygons in a scene which include motion information.

A shutter speed may be given for the camera with the `-shutter` option on the command line or `shutter` in the options statement, with the default speed of zero turning motion blurring off. The shutter opens instantaneously at time zero and closes after the shutter speed time has elapsed.

1.18 Sampling Algorithms

Jittering, motion blurring, area light sources, and the depth-of-field lens shader are based on multiple sampling that is based on varying the sample locations in time, 2D or 3D space. mental ray offers a proprietary implementation of the Quasi-Monte Carlo method for achieving these variations. Sample locations in time, 2D and 3D space are deterministically chosen on fixed points that ensure optimal coverage of the sample space. The algorithm is similar to fixed-raster algorithms, but avoids the regular lattice appearance of such algorithms. The resulting images are identical if the scene is re-rendered with the same options due to the deterministic nature of the algorithm.

Quasi-Monte Carlo methods can be succinctly described as strictly deterministic sampling methods. Determinism enters in two ways, namely, by working with deterministic points rather than random samples and by the availability of deterministic error bounds ([Niederreiter 92]).

1.19 OpenGL Acceleration

2.1By default, mental ray uses a scanline rendering algorithm for primary rays when no lens shaders are present that modify the ray direction. This algorithm can cope with both static and motion blurred scenes. In addition, mental ray supports OpenGL®[4] hardware to further accelerate scanline rendering of static scenes (without motion blurring). If the client host provides OpenGL acceleration with sufficient resolution, mental ray can use this to generate acceleration data that is subsequently used during regular rendering. This combines the speed of a hardware OpenGL accelerator with the full shading capabilities of mental ray, and is particularly effective for scenes with high polygon counts.

Shadow maps can also be rendering with OpenGL acceleration. This is particularly effective since shadow maps need no shading. Most of the computation involved is then performed by the OpenGL system, which greatly improves performance.

However, the accuracy of OpenGL acceleration is generally lower than that of the standard software scanline rendering algorithm.

1.20 Color Calculations

All colors in mental ray are given in the RGBA color space and all internal calculations are performed in RGBA. The alpha channel is used to determine transparency; `0` means fully transparent and 1 means fully opaque. mental ray uses premultiplied colors, which means that the R, G, and B components are scaled by A and may not exceed A. Optionally, RGBA colors may be stored in the output image in non-premultiplied form to increase the precision of highly transparent pixels, but internally mental ray and all shaders work with premultiplied colors. Premultiplication is used to simplify compositing operations.

Internally, colors are not restricted to the unit cube in RGB space. As a final step before output, colors are clipped using one of two methods. By default, the red, green and blue values are simply truncated. Optionally, colors may be clipped using a desaturation method which maintains intensity (if possible), but shifts the hue towards the white axis of the cube. Desaturation color clipping may be selected with either the `-desaturate on` option on the command line or `desaturate on` in the options block in the scene. The alpha channel is always truncated.

1.21 Output Shaders

mental ray can generate more than one type of image. There are up to five main frame buffers: for RGBA, depth, normal vectors, motion vectors, and labels. The depth, normal vector, motion vector, and label frame buffers store the Z coordinate, the normal vector, the motion vector, and the label of the frontmost object at each sample of the image. If multiple samples are taken for a pixel, the frame buffer value for that pixel may be either any one sample value, or a blend

[4]OpenGL is a registered trademark of Silicon Graphics, Inc.

of all samples. The number and type of frame buffers to be rendered is controlled by output statements. Output statements specify what is to be done with each frame buffer. If a frame buffer is not listed by any output statement, it is not rendered (except for RGBA, which always exists). There are two types of output statements, those specifying output shaders and those specifying files to write.

There are also up to eight user-defined frame buffers[2.1]that can be defined with any data type, using a frame buffer statement in the options block.

Output shaders are user-written functions that can be linked at runtime that have access to every pixel in all available frame buffers after rendering. They can be used to perform operations like post-filtering or compositing.

Files to write are specified with data type, file format and file name. If the data type is omitted a default data type is used that is assumed to be the "best" type for the given image format. The data type implies the frame buffer type. There are special file formats for depth, vector, and label files, in addition to a variety of standard color file formats. By listing the appropriate number and type of output statements, it is possible to write multiple files. For example, both a filtered file and the unfiltered version can be written to separate files by listing three output statements: one to write the unfiltered image, one that runs an output shader that does the filtering, and finally another one to write the filtered image. Output statements are executed in sequence.

The following file formats are supported:

Symbol	File format	Supported data types
"rla"	Wavefront image	rgba
"pic"	SOFTIMAGE image	rgba
"alias"	Alias Research image	rgb
"rgb"	SGI color	rgba
"jpg"	JFIF image	rgb
"tif"	compressed TIFF image	rgba, rgba_16, rgb, rgb_16
"tifu"	uncompressed TIFF image	rgba, rgba_16, rgb, rgb_16
"picture"	Dassault Systèmes PICTURE	rgb
"ppm"	Portable pixmap	rgb
"targa"	Targa image	rgba
"bmp"	MS Windows BMP bitmap	rgba
"qntpal"	Quantel/Abekas YUV image, 720x576	rgb
"qntntsc"	Quantel/Abekas YUV image, 720x486	rgb
"ct"	mental images color texture	rgba, rgba_16, rgba_fp
"st"	mental images alpha texture	s, s_16
"nt"	mental images normal vectors	n
"mt"	mental images motion vectors	m
"zt"	mental images depth (-Z) channel	z
"tt"	mental images tag channel	tag
"bit"	mental images bit mask	bit
"Zpic"	SOFTIMAGE depth (-Z) channel	z
"map"	for memory mapped textures	any

Each of these file formats implies a particular default data type (the first entry in column "Supported data types"); for example, "rgb" implies 8-bit RGBA, and "zt" implies Z. The default data type may be overridden by explicitly specifying another data type, such as a 16-bit type, in the output statement, as long as it is supported and appears in the above table. mental ray will adjust its frame buffer list to compute the requested types. For example, the standard RGBA frame buffer stores 8 bits per component by default, but if any output statement references a 16-bit type, the RGBA frame buffer also switches to 16 bits.

The available data types are:

Symbol	Data type
"rgb"	8-bit RGB color
"rgb_16"	16-bit RGB color
"rgba"	8-bit RGBA color and alpha
"rgba_16"	16-bit RGBA color and alpha
"rgba_fp"	floating-point RGBA color and alpha
"a"	8-bit alpha channel
"a_16"	16-bit alpha channel
"vta"	vector texture derived from alpha, 2 floats per pixel
"vts"	vector texture derived from intensity, 2 floats per pixel
"z"	depth information, 1 float per pixel
"n"	normal vectors, 3 floats per pixel (X,Y,Z)
"m"	motion vectors, 3 floats per pixel (X,Y,Z)
"tag"	object labels, 1 32-bit unsigned integer per pixel
"bit"	bit mask, 1 bit per pixel
"contour"	contour lines

The difference between "vta" and "vts", and between n and m, is significant only when automatic conversions are done. The file contents are identical except for the magic number in the file header.

The floating-point RGBA data type "rgba_fp" allows color and alpha values outside the normal range (0, . . . 1), and no dithering is applied even if explicitly enabled. In contrast, any conversion to the 8-bit or 16-bit formats will clamp values outside this interval. Note that dithering reduces the effectivity of RLE compression.

All mental images file formats contain a header followed by simple uncompressed image data, pixel by pixel beginning in the lower left corner. Each pixel consists of one to four 8-bit, 16-bit, or 32-bit component values, in RGBA, XYZ, or UV order. The header consists of a magic number byte identifying the format, a null byte, width and height as unsigned shorts, and two unused null bytes reserved for future use. All shorts, integers, and floats are big-endian (most significant byte first).

mental ray can combine samples within a pixel in different ways. The combination of existing samples can also pad the frame buffers to "bridge" unsampled pixels. Interpolation of colors, depths, normals, and motion vectors means that they are averaged, while interpolation of the labels means that the maximum label is used (taking the average label is not a good idea). Interpolation of depths only takes the average of non-infinite depths, and interpolation of normals and motion vectors only takes the average of vectors different from the null vector. Interpolation is turned on by writing a "+" in the beginning of the output type and turned off by writing a "–" there. For example, to interpolate the depth samples, write "+z" in the output statement. If interpolation is turned off for a frame buffer, the last sample value (color, normal, motion vector, or label) within each pixel is stored, and pixels without samples get a copy from one of the neighbor pixels. Interpolation off for depth images is an exception: rather than using the last sample depth, the min depth is used — this can be useful for compositing. Interpolation is on by default for color frame buffers (including alpha and intensity frame buffers) and off by default for depth, normal, motion vector, and label frame buffers.

1.22 Contours

Contour lines can be an important visual cue to distinguish objects and accentuate their forms and spatial relationship. Contour lines are especially useful for cartoon animation production.

Contours can be placed at discontinuities of depth or surface orientation, between different materials, or where the color contrast is high. The contour lines are anti-aliased, and there can be several levels of contours created by reflection or seen through semitransparent materials.

The contours can be different for each material, and some materials can have no contours at all. The color and thickness of the contours can depend on geometry, position, illumination, material, frame number, and various other parameters.

The resulting image may be output as a pure contour image, a contour image composited onto the regular image (in raster form in any of the supported formats), or as a PostScript file.

It is not possible to render contours in a scene with motion blur.

Contour shaders are called while the normal color image is created. Contours are computed using information stored by a *contour store shader*. The contour store shader is called once for each intersection of a ray with a material. The position of contours are determined by a *contour contrast shader*. It compares the two sets of information for a pair of points, and decides whether there should be a contour between the points. The color and thickness of the contours are determined by *contour shaders*.

1.23 Memory-mapped Textures

mental ray supports memory mapping of textures in UNIX environments. Memory mapping means that the texture is not loaded into memory, but is accessed directly from disk when a shader accesses it. There is no special keyword or option for this; if a texture is memory-mappable, mental ray will recognize it and memory-map it automatically. Only the map image file format (extension `.map`) can be mapped. See the Output Shaders chapter for a list of supported file formats.

Note that memory mapping is based on the concept that the image data on disk does not require decoding or data type conversion, but is available in the exact format that mental ray uses internally during rendering. Normally mental ray will attempt to auto-convert image data formats; for example if a color image file is given in a `scalar texture` construct, mental ray will silently convert the color pixels to scalars as the texture is read in. Most data types are auto-converted to most other data types. This does not work for memory-mapped textures.

Memory mapping requires several preparation steps:

- The texture must be converted to `.map` format using a utility like mental images' *imf_copy*. The scene file must be changed to reference this texture. Note that mental ray recognizes `.map` textures even if they have an extension other than `.map`; this can be exploited by continuing to use the old file name with the "wrong" extension.
- Memory-mapped textures are automatically considered `local` by mental ray, as if the `local` keyword had been used in the scene file. This means that if the scene is rendered on multiple hosts, each will try to access the given path instead of transferring the texture across the network, which would defeat memory mapping. The given path must be valid on every host participating in the render.
- The texture should not be on an NFS-mounted file system (one that is imported across the network from another host). Although this simplifies the requirement that the texture must exist on all hosts, the necessary network transfers reduce the effectiveness and can easily make memory-mapping slower than regular textures.
- Memory-mapping works best if there are extremely large textures containing many tens of megabytes that are sampled infrequently because then most of the large texture file is never loaded into memory.

If the textures and the scene are so large that they do not fit into physical memory, loading a texture is equivalent to loading the file into memory, decompressing it, and copying it out to swap. (The swap is a disk partition that acts as a low-speed extension of the physical memory that exists as RAM chips in the computer). From then on, accessing a texture means accessing the swap. Memory mapping eliminates the read-decompress-write step and accesses the texture from the file system instead of from swap. This has the side effect that less swap space is needed. If the texture and scene are not large and fit into memory, and if the texture is accessed frequently, memory-mapped textures are slower than regular textures because the swap would not have been used.

1.24 Caustics

Caustics are light patterns that are created when light from a light source illuminates a diffuse surface via one or more specular reflections or transmissions. Examples are:

- The light patterns created on the bottom of a swimming pool as light is refracted by the water surface and reflected by the diffuse pool bottom.
- Light being focused by a glass of water onto a diffuse table cloth.
- The light emanating from the headlights of a car: the light is emitted by the filament of a light bulb, reflected by a parabolic mirror reflector (thereby being focused in the forward direction), and reflected by the diffuse road surface.

Caustics cannot be simulated efficiently using standard ray tracing since predicting the potential specular paths to a light source from any given surface is a difficult (and in many situations impossible) task. To overcome this problem mental ray uses a photon map.[5] The photon map is generated in a preprocessing step in which photons are emitted from the light sources and traced through the scene using photon tracing.

The emission of photons is controlled using either one of the standard photon emitters for point lights, spot lights, directional lights, and area lights, or by using a user defined photon emitting shader.

A photon leaving the light source can be reflected or transmitted specularly by objects. The photon is traced through the scene until it either hits a diffuse surface or until it has been reflected or transmitted a maximum number of times as indicated by the photon trace depth. When a caustic photon hits a diffuse object it is stored in a caustic photon map and not traced any further.

To control the behavior of photons as they hit objects in the scene, it is necessary to attach photon material shaders to these objects. Photon material shaders are similar to normal material shaders with the main difference being that they trace the light in the opposite direction. Also, a photon shader distributes energy (flux) instead of collecting a color (radiance). Another important difference is the fact that photon material shaders do not need to send light rays to sample the contribution from the light sources in the scene.

In order to use the photon shaders, it is necessary to include the appropriate shader declaration file, such as `physics.mi` for physics-based material shaders and photon shaders from the physics shader library in the standard distribution.

To turn caustics on, specify `caustic on` in the `options` or use the command-line option `-caustic on`.

1.24.1 Light Sources

Photons are emitted from the light sources in the scene. It is necessary to attach some extra information to each light source to control the energy being distributed into the scene (and/or the number of photons emitted).

[5] The concept was introduced by H. Wann Jensen in "Global Illumination using Photon Maps", *Rendering Techniques '96*, Springer-Verlag, Wien, 1996, pp. 21-30.

To generate caustics from a particular light source, one must specify the energy emitted by the light source. This is given by the *energy* keyword. The energy is the flux distributed by the light source and it will be distributed into the scene by each photon which will carry a fraction of the light source energy. If the energy is zero (the default), no photons will be emitted.

Another important factor is the number of photons to be generated by this light source. This can optionally be specified using the *caustic photons* keyword (10000 photons is the default). This will be the number of photons stored in the photon map and thus a good indication of the quality of the generated caustics. It is also a direct indication of the memory usage which will be proportional to the number of photons in the photon map. For quick, low-quality caustics, `caustic photons 10000` is adequate, for medium quality 100000 is typically needed, and for highly accurate effects, `caustic photons 1000000` can be necessary. It is also possible to specify a second integer, which is the maximum number[2.1] of photons to be emitted from the light source, or *only* the number of emitted photons by setting the first integer to zero (mental ray 2.1.37 and up). By default there is no upper limit (indicated by the value 0), in which case emission will continue until the specified number of photons have been stored. Notice that the emitted number of photons and the preprocessing time is most often proportional to the number of photons generated in the photon map.

For most light sources, the distribution of energy using photons will give the natural inverse square fall-off of the energy. This might be an unwanted effect since some light shaders implement a linear fall-off. It can be avoided by using the *exponent* keyword. If the exponent is p, the fall-off is $1/r^p$, where r is the distance to the light source. Exponent values between 1 and 2 make the indirect light less dependent on distance. Exponents of less than 1 is not advisable, as it often gives visible noise. Exponent 2 is the default.

The following is an example of a light that uses the `soft_point` light shader and is capable of generating caustics:

```
light "caustic-light1" "soft_point" (
      "color"        1.0 1.0 0.95,
      "shadow"       on,
      "factor"       0.6,
      "atten"        on,
      "start"        16.0,
      "stop"         200.0
   )
   origin            20.0 30.0 -40.0
   energy            700 700 700
   caustic photons   100000
   exponent          1.5
end light
```

An example of a light source which uses the inverse square fall-off to compute illumination (and the default 10000 photons) is:

```
light "point1" "physical_light" (
      "color"        700.0 700.0 700.0
```

```
    )
    origin          20.0 30.0 -40.0
    energy          700 700 700
end light
```

It is important to note the difference between `color` and `energy`. `color` is the power of the direct illumination, while `energy` will be the power of the caustic. It is therefore possible to tune the brightness of caustics to make them more or less visible.

If area light source information, such as a `rectangle` statement, is added to the light source definition, both the direct and global illumination will be emitted from an area light source. This tends to make caustics more fuzzy.

To emphasize caustics, the energy of the light sources can be higher than their colors (that determine the direct illumination). If, for whatever reason, the user wants to have the sources of caustics to be at different positions than the sources of direct illumination, this is possible too. It might also be that a single light source is sufficient for the caustics, while several light sources are needed to fine-tune the direct illumination.

1.24.2 Objects

By default, all objects can cast and receive caustics, that is, photons are emitted in all directions from a point light source (and with all possible origins for a directional light source). For some scenes, this is fine – for example if a point light source is surrounded by specular surfaces. But for some scenes, it is very inefficient – for example a point light far away from a single small specular object.

To generate caustics more efficiently in such scenes, objects can be flagged such that the photons are only emitted towards certain objects and stored only on selected objects. Objects are then divided into caustic-casting (`caustic 1` flag) and caustic-receiving (`caustic 2` flag), or both (`caustic 3` flag), or neither (`caustic 0` flag). For example, caustics on the bottom of a swimming pool require a caustic-casting water surface and a caustic-receiving pool bottom. Objects can also be flagged `caustic off`, which means that caustic photons will not hit them at all (the objects will be "invisible" to caustic photons), or flagged `caustic on` which is the same as `caustic 3`. The caustic mode is an object attribute. Photons are emitted only in the direction of caustic-casting objects, and only stored on caustic-receiving objects.

To use this optimization requires that the default object caustic flag (specified in the options) is set to something different than 3 (which is the default value, enabling all objects to cast and receive caustics).

For example, the options can contain

```
caustic on
caustic 0
```

The definition of a caustic-casting object can for example begin as

```
object "revol4"   caustic 1   visible   shadow   trace   tag 13
```

The material of a caustic-casting object has to be mainly specular (little or no diffuse reflection), and for most materials, the sum of reflection and transparency should be close to or larger than 1. For caustics generated by refraction, the index of refraction has to be different from 1. For example, the index of refraction for water is 1.33, for glass 1.5 to 1.7, and for diamond 2.42.

1.24.3 Material Shaders and Photon Shaders for Caustics

mental ray comes with three material shaders that support caustics (and global illumination[2.1]) *soft_material*, *dgs_material* and *dielectric_material*. Their photon shader equivalents are *soft_material_photon*, *dgs_material_photon* and *dielectric_material_photon*. When defining a material it is necessary to specify both the regular material shader and the photon shader. Most often, however, the photon shader can inherit the parameter setting from the regular material shader. In addition to these six shaders, users can write new material and photon material shaders.

1.24.3.1 Physically Plausible Material Shaders

A pair of material shaders that emphasize physical accuracy are `dgs_material` and `dgs_material_photon`. They simulate three types of reflection:

- diffuse (Lambert's cosine law),
- glossy (isotropic or anisotropic),
- specular (mirror),

as well as the corresponding types of refraction and translucency, and any combination of these. Therefore, they can simulate mirrors, glossy paint or plastic, anisotropic glossy materials such as brushed metal, diffuse materials such as paper, translucent materials such as frosted glass, and any combination of these.

Each material declaration using `dgs_material` has to have a `photon "dgs_material_photon" ()` statement. These two shaders should be used together for physical accuracy. An example is:

```
material "mirror"  opaque    # ideal mirror material
   "dgs_material" (
      "specular"      1.0 1.0 1.0,
      "lights" ["arealight-i"]
   )
   shadow "dgs_material" ()
   photon "dgs_material_photon" ()
end material
```

Another pair of physically based shaders is `dielectric_material` and `dielectric_material_-photon`.

For further details on `dgs_material`, `dielectric_material`, and their photon shaders, see the documentation of the Physics Shader Library.

1.24.4 Shader Functions

There are two functions that are especially important to writers of photon shaders.

The shader interface function *mi_choose_scatter_type* chooses a scatter type for a photon based on the probabilities for diffuse, glossy, and specular reflection and refraction. It can also choose absorption, that is, that the photon should be traced no further. The function also ensures a correct energy level in the scene by altering the reflection coefficients according to the scatter choice.

During regular ray tracing, material shaders of caustic-receiving objects should call the *mi_-compute_irradiance* function to "pick up" the illumination caused by photons reaching the object during preprocessing.

1.24.5 Fine-tuning Caustics

The number of photons used to estimate the caustic brightness can be changed with the global option `caustic accuracy`. The accuracy controls how many photons are considered during rendering. The default is 100; larger numbers make the caustic smoother. There is also an optional radius parameter. The radius controls the maximum distance at which mental ray considers photons. For example, to specify that at most 200 photons should be used to compute the caustic brightness, and that only photons within 1 scene unit away should be used, specify:

```
caustic accuracy 200 1.0
```

in the `options`. (Similar accuracy parameters are available for global illumination, volume caustics and global illumination, and final gathering.)

Accuracy parameters can be used to select two fundamentally different sampling policies. If R is relatively large (as is the default) the overall limiting factor becomes N and R only catches runaway situations with very few photons. Since darker areas have fewer photons than brighter areas, the effective radius within which the N photons are found is larger in dark areas. The effect is that low intensity areas will have less detail than high intensity areas. Also, increasing the number of photons in the scene will result in the effective radius becoming smaller, so if N is not adjusted to compensate the same amount of noise will be seen, only on a smaller scale.

The other policy is to select R small, on the scale of the detail the user wishes to see. N is then kept high, or even set to 0 (unlimited). In this case, a constant radius is examined which results in the scale of the detail remaining constant between light and dark areas. Increasing the number of photons in the map will have the effect of reducing the error noise. In practice, one will often use a combination of the two, with a small radius to get detail in dark areas, and N set at a moderate value to speed up rendering. Irrespective of the chosen policy, a large effective radius gives less noise, but a more blurred result. To decrease the noise without blurring detail, it is necessary to increase the number of photons in the photon map. It is very instructive to explore the effect of setting these options with the aid of the `diagnostic photon`[2.1] option since the false color image it generates shows the difference in estimated density more clearly. For fast previewing of caustics it can be useful to use N=20.

1.25 Global Illumination[2.1]

Global illumination[2.1] is the simulation of all light interreflection effects in a scene (except caustics). This includes effects such as color bleeding: if a red table is next to a white wall, the white wall gets a slightly pink tint. This effect is not possible with ordinary ray tracing algorithms. But if the pink tint is lacking in an image, the image looks fake, even though it might be hard to point out precisely why. Global illumination effects are subtle but add realism to a scene.

Simulation of global illumination has at least two distinct uses:

- Physically accurate simulation of the illumination in an environment. For example the light distribution inside an office building.
- Visually pleasing lighting effects for applications in the entertainment industry. Here physical accuracy is not the most important aspect, the images just have to look believable.

The computation of global illumination requires photon tracing, just like computation of caustics. In fact, the same photon material shaders can be used. Since caustics are treated separately in mental ray, the global illumination simulation does not include caustics. So if *all* light interreflections should be simulated, both global illumination and caustics must be enabled.

The photons stored during global illumination simulation are stored in a separate photon map, the global illumination photon map. When the material shader calls *mi_compute_irradiance*, the irradiance from both the caustics photon map and the global illumination photon map are computed.

To turn global illumination on, specify `globillum on` in the `options` or give command-line option `-globillum on`.

1.25.1 Light Sources

Each light source that should emit global illumination should have an `energy` statement (just as for caustics). Each light source can also optionally have a `globillum photons` statement to specify how many photons should be emitted, or specify emitted photons only by setting the first number to zero (similar to `caustic photons` for caustics). The default value is 100000 globillum photons. For example:

```
light "globillum-light" "physical_light" (
      "color"        700.0 700.0 700.0
   )
   origin             20.0 30.0 -40.0
   energy             700 700 700
   globillum photons  100000
end light
```

1.25.2 Objects

By default, all objects can participate in global illumination computations. This is necessary for simulation of real global illumination. However, sometimes one might just be interested in color bleeding from one object to another, and the rest of the scene does not need to participate in the global illumination simulation.

To simulate global illumination more efficiently in such cases, objects can be flagged such that the photons are only emitted towards certain objects and stored only on selected objects. Objects are then divided into globillum-casting (`globillum 1` flag) and globillum-receiving (`globillum 2` flag), or both (`globillum 3` flag), or neither (`globillum 0` flag). For example, color bleeding from a red diffuse table onto a diffuse white wall requires a globillum-casting table and a globillum-receiving wall. Objects can also be flagged `globillum off`, which means that globillum photons will not hit them at all (the objects will be "invisible" to globillum photons), or flagged `globillum on` which is the same as `globillum 3`. The globillum mode is an object attribute. Photons are emitted only in the direction of globillum-casting objects, and only stored on globillum-receiving objects.

To use this optimization requires that the default object globillum flag (specified in the options) is set to something different than 3 (which is the default value, enabling all objects to cast and receive global illumination).

1.25.3 Fine-tuning Global Illumination

To change the number of photons used to compute the local intensity of global illumination, specify a `globillum accuracy` (and optionally a maximum radius) in the `options`. For example,

```
globillum accuracy 300 2.0
```

The default number is 500; larger numbers make the global illumination smoother but increases render time. The default radius depends on the scene extent.

1.26 Final Gathering[2.1]

For diffuse scenes, final gathering[2.1] can improve the quality of the global illumination solution. Without final gathering, the global illumination on a diffuse surface is computed by estimating the photon density (and energy) near that point. With final gathering, many new rays are sent out to sample the hemisphere above the point to determine the incident illumination. Some of these rays hit diffuse surfaces, and the global illumination at those points is then computed by the material shaders at these point, using illumination from the globillum photon map if available and other material properties. Other rays hit specular surfaces and do not contribute to the final gather color (since that type of light transport is a secondary caustic). Tracing many rays (each with a photon map lookup) is very time-consuming, so it is only done when necessary — in most cases, interpolation and extrapolation from previous nearby final gathers is sufficient.

Final gathering is useful in scenes with slow variation in the indirect illumination. For example purely diffuse scenes. For such scenes, final gathering eliminates photon map artifacts such as low frequency noise and dark corners. With final gathering, fewer photons are needed in the globillum photon map and lower globillum accuracy is sufficient since each final gather averages over many values of indirect illumination.

Final gathering is `off` by default, but can be turned `on` in the options.

To change the number of rays shot in each final gather (and optionally the max distance at which a final gathering result can be used for interpolation and the min distance at which is must be used), specify a `finalgather accuracy` in the options. For example,

```
finalgather accuracy 1000 1.5 0.25
```

Increasing the number of rays reduces noise in scenes with complex illumination and geometry; the default number of rays is 1000. The default maximum distance depends on the scene extent; decreasing it will reduce noise but increase render time. The default minimum distance is 10% of the maximum distance.

1.27 Volume Caustics

Volume caustics are caused by light that has been specularly reflected or refracted by one or more surfaces and is then scattered by a participating medium in a volume. Examples are:

- Sunlight refracted by a wavy water surface and then scattered by little silt particles in the water.
- Car fog lamps: light emitted by a bulb filament, reflected by a parabolic reflector, and scattered by fog.

In order to create volume caustics, the same light sources, material shaders, photon shaders, and caustic tags as for caustics are needed. But in addition, volume shaders and volume photon shaders are needed. For example:

```
material "volsurf"  opaque    # material for surfaces of volume
   "transmat" ()
   shadow "transmat" ()
   photon "transmat_photon" ()
   volume "parti_volume" (
      "scatter" 0.05 0.05 0.05,
      "extinction" 0.05,
      "lights" ["arealight-i"]
   )
   photonvol "parti_volume_photon" (
      "scatter" 0.05 0.05 0.05,
      "extinction" 0.05
   )
end material
```

Photons that get scattered multiple times in the volume are stored in a volume photon map. During rendering, volume shaders can call the function *mi_compute_volume_irradiance* to get irradiance from the photons stored in the volume photon map.

In order to fine-tune the volume caustic, it is possible to change the number of photons that is used to compute the indirect light in the volume caustic. This is done with a `photonvol accuracy` statement in the options. The default is 30 photons and a radius that depends on the scene extent.

1.28 Global Illumination in Participating Media[2.1]

Global illumination in volumes[2.1] can be used to simulate for example:

- Color bleeding from a colored wall onto gray smoke.
- Multiple light scattering in clouds or other participating media.

Global illumination in participating media is computed much the same way as global illumination on surfaces, except that volume shaders and volume photon shaders are needed.

To change the number of photons used to compute the local intensity of global illumination in volumes, specify a `photonvol accuracy` (and optionally a radius) in the `options` (similar to volume caustics).

1.29 Diagnostic modes[2.1]

mental ray supports a number of diagnostic modes that help visualizing and optimizing the rendering process. They modify the output image to include grid lines or dot patterns that indicate coordinate spaces or sampling or photon densities. These graphs allow simple detection of insufficient or excessive sampling densities, and help to tune parameters such as numbers of photons or sampling and contrast limits.

Grid Mode This mode renders a grid on top of all objects in the scene, in object, camera, or world space. It's useful to get an idea of the scene scale and to enable rough estimates of distances and areas.

Photon Density ModeThis mode replaces shows a false color rendering of photon density on all materials. This is useful when tuning the number of photons to trace in a scene, and to select the optimum accuracy settings for estimation of global illumination or caustics. It also works well in combination with the Grid Mode described above.

Samples modeThis mode shows how spatial supersamples were placed in the rendered image, by producing a grayscale image signifying sample density. This is useful when tuning the level and the contrast threshold for spatial supersampling.

Diagnostic modes are enabled with the `-diagnostic` option on the command line, or the `diagnostic` statement in the options block in the scene description file.

Chapter 2

Scene Description Language

The mental images scene description language allows reading a scene from an ASCII or binary file called the `.mi` file. It contains a list of commands and scene entities. Commands are instructions that set options such as verbosity or external shaders to be linked. Scene entities describe geometrical objects and shaders and other components. Animations are rendered by setting up the first frame and rendering it, followed by scene modifications and another render command for every successive frame. These scene modifications are called incremental changes.

This book describes version 2 of the .mi format, abbreviated as .mi2. Although mental ray 2.x still supports the frame-based scene definition method supported by version 1.x of mental ray, this is not recommended for future designs and not described here. Both versions of the format can easily be distinguished: .mi1 files contain `frame` statements while .mi2 files contain `instance` statements. The recommended file extension is `.mi` regardless of the version.

This section discusses the parts that make up an `.mi` file. A less formal syntax is used for the syntax description: a bar "|" denotes alternatives, items enclosed in tall square brackets "[ ]" are optional, and the ellipsis "..." denotes omission, as in "zero or more repetitions of the preceding construct." Literal text is set in `teletype`, while variable metasymbols are set in *italics*. All other punctuation characters are literals. Strings are quoted with double quotes; this includes all names. Names, such as material, light, or object names, need not be quoted, but it is highly recommended to avoid conflicts with reserved words[1], and to allow non-alphabetic characters. Without quotes, only lowercase and uppercase letters, underscores, and digits may be used; a digit may not be the first character of an unquoted name. No such restrictions apply to quoted names.

Integers are distinguished from floating point numbers by appending the suffix **int**, as in $degree_{int}$. Integers are an optional "+" or "–" sign followed by a sequence of digits "0" through "9". Floating-point numbers follow the same rules, but may optionally contain a decimal point "." and an optional exponent. If the number begins with a decimal point, a leading zero is assumed. Exponential notation has the form *n*e*m*, which is interpreted as $n \cdot 10^m$. Strings can be distinguished from numbers because the grammar always requires them to be enclosed in double quotes.

[1]Future versions may reserve more words than described here

The "#" character introduces comments, unless quoted, except between `$code` and `$end code`. Comments extend to the end of the line.

Unquoted whitespace acts as a separator but is otherwise ignored. Line breaks and indentation have no syntactical relevance, except where otherwise noted (commands beginning with a dollar sign, for example, must appear at the beginning of the line).

By convention, the first line of any .mi file should begin with the three characters `#mi`, followed by a blank (not a tab), followed by the partial or full version number of the earliest required mental ray version number. For the syntax described in this book this is `2.0.28` or `2.1.30`. This comment serves as a "magic number" that helps interactive programs or utilities like `file` to decide whether this is a .mi file or something else. It is not parsed by mental ray itself.

2.1 Shader Declarations

Shaders are procedural elements that are implemented in C or C++. They are typically, but not necessarily, precompiled and stored in shared libraries. They are linked by mental ray at runtime and perform a variety of functions, such as determining the surface characteristics of an object. The term "shader" originally referred to "surface shading" (color and illumination computation) but has expanded and now refers to any custom function, regardless of its use.

All shading functions linked with a code or link statement, and all shading functions built into mental ray, must be declared. When called, shaders accept a pointer to an arbitrary parameter structure as their third argument, and mental ray must know the structure declaration in order to put together the parameter block according to C/C++ structure layout conventions. Usually, declarations are included from a separate file using the `$include` statement. For a detailed description of shader declarations, see the chapter on writing shaders.

A declaration is a top-level statement that informs mental ray about the shader name (which is identical to the C/C++ function name), the return type, and the types and names of all the parameters. Certain options can also be specified.

```
declare shader
    [type] "shader_name" (
        type "parameter_name",
        type "parameter_name",
        ...
        type "parameter_name"
    )
    [ version version_int ]
    [ apply shader_type_list ]
    [ options ]
end declare
```

It is recommended that *shader_name* and *parameter_name* are enclosed in double quotes to disambiguate them from reserved keywords and to allow special characters such as punctuation marks. Note that old-style declarations of the form

`declare` [*type*] "*shader_name*" `(...)`

are also still supported for backwards compatibility, but they should not be used because they do not support versioning, apply masks, and options. The optional (but highly recommended) *version* is an arbitrary integer that identifies the shader version. The default is `0`. See the discussion of shader versioning in section 3.7.

2.1.1 Parameter Types

The declaration gives the type and name of the shader to declare, which is the name of the C function and the name used when the shader is called, followed by a list of parameters with types. Names are normally quoted to disambiguate them from keywords reserved by mental ray. Commas separate parameter declarations. The following types are supported:

`boolean` — A boolean is either true or false. Possible values are `on`, `off`, `true`, and `false`.

`integer` — Integers are in the range $-2^{31} \ldots 2^{31} - 1$.

`scalar` — Scalars are floating-point numbers, defined as an optional minus sign, a sequence of digits containing an optional decimal point at any place, followed by an optional decimal exponent. A decimal exponent is the letter `e` or `E` followed by a positive or negative integer. Examples are `1.0`, `.5`, `2.`, `1.e4`, or `-2.3e-6`.

`vector` — A vector is a sequence of three scalars as defined above, describing the x, y, and z components of the vector.

`transform` — A transformation is a 4×4 matrix of scalars, with the translation in the last row. The data structure consists of an array of 16 `miScalars` in row-major order.

`color` — A color is a sequence of three or four scalars as defined above, describing the red, blue, green, and alpha components of the color, in this order. If alpha is omitted, it defaults to `0.0`.

`shader` — Shader names defined with the `shader` statement (not to be confused with the shader declaration statement) can be passed to other shaders that have parameters of this type. The shader receives a tag that it can call using *mi_call_shader* and similar shader interface functions.

`color texture`	Color textures name a texture as defined by a `color texture` statement in the .mi file. The `color texture` statement names either a texture file, or a texture shader followed by a user parameter list. Note that a color texture does not name the texture shader directly. When a color texture is evaluated, it returns an RGBA color.
`scalar texture`	Scalar textures are equivalent to color textures, except that they name a `scalar texture` statement in the .mi file. When a scalar texture is evaluated, it returns a scalar (a single floating-point number). This is most often used to apply a texture map to a scalar material parameter such as transparency.
`vector texture`	Vector textures are another variation. They name a `vector texture` statement in the .mi file, which returns a vector when evaluated. Bump map bases on materials are typical applications for vector textures. Vector textures are rarely used.
`light`	Lights specify a light instance as defined by an `instance` statement in the .mi file, which in turn names a light. Despite the name, shader parameters of type `light` do not name the light directly because only the light's instance provides the necessary position and orientation information. Like textures, light parameters do not name light shaders directly.
`string`	Strings are quoted character strings of arbitrary length. The data type is a tag, which can be converted by the shader to a character pointer using the *mi_db_access* and *mi_db_unpin* shader interface functions.
`geometry`	Geometry references objects or instances. They are allowed for all types of shaders but are primarily useful for geometry shaders, which can introduce geometric scene entities. Geometry shaders have a different shader API than other shaders. They are described in chapter 4.3. Shaders and phenomena whose return type is `geometry` can be used in instance definition statements (see page 118).
`material`	Material references. Their purpose is to operate on materials in phenomenon definitions, which may contain materials in addition to shaders. Shaders and phenomena whose return type is `material` can be used in material definition statements (see page 80).
`struct { ... }`	Structures define sub-lists of parameters. This is normally used to build arrays of structures, for example to declare an array of textures, each of which comes with a blending factor and other sub-parameters. The ellipsis ... stands for another comma-separated sequence of type/parameter_name pairs.
`array` *type*	Arrays are different from all other types in that they are not named. The `array` keyword is a prefix to any of the above types that turns

a single value into a one-dimensional array of values. For example, `array scalar "terms"` declares a parameter named `terms` that is an array of scalars. The number of elements in the array size is dynamic and unlimited. Arrays of arrays are not supported but arrays of structs containing arrays can be used.

When choosing names, avoid double colons and periods, which have a special meaning when accessing interface parameters in phenomenon subshaders.

The return type of the shader must either be a simple type (any type except `struct` or `array`), or an unnamed `struct` containing only simple types. Unnamed means that there is no name between the `struct` keyword and the opening brace.

2.1.2 Shader Apply Flags

The `apply` statement allows specification of possible uses for the shader. The *shader_type_list* consists of a comma-separated list of one or more of the following keywords:

keyword	*shader application*
`lens`	lens shader in a camera
`material`	material shader in a material
`light`	light shader
`shadow`	shadow shader in a material
`environment`	environment shader in a material or camera
`volume`	volume shader in a material or camera
`texture`	texture shader
`photon`	photon shader in a material
`geometry`	geometry shader
`displace`	displacement shader in a material
`emitter`	photon emitter shader in a light
`output`	output shader in a camera

If the apply statement is missing, the applicability of a shader is unknown. This will commonly be the case for base shaders, for example, which can be used for any purpose. Apply lists help user interfaces to categorize shaders. mental ray performs no checks to make sure that shaders are used only in legal contexts. (Future versions may use a material shader as shadow or photon shader if its applicability list allows it and there is no other shadow or photon shader listed in the material.)

2.1.3 Declaration Options

Declarations of shaders (and phenomena, see page 51) allow a number of options to be specified in the declaration block. These options specify *requirements* of the shader or phenomenon, specifying conditions that must be met before the shader or phenomenon can run correctly, or information about the shader that tells mental ray how to call it. They should be used only if it is impossible for the shader to do its job without this option, but not to second-guess the user, assuming that if this shader is used, then the user "probably" wants this option. Shader requirements take away control from the user and should be used with care. Before rendering, mental ray collects the requirements of all shaders defined in the scene, checks for conflicts, and adjusts global options and camera parameters to suit the shaders. Shaders should not assume that an option specified in the declaration has an effect because mental ray may choose to ignore it if there is a conflict with another declaration.

For example, if a shader specifies that it can operate only if ray tracing is enabled, it should specify the `trace on` option to tell mental ray to enable ray tracing even if no ray tracing was specified in the global `options` statement.

Here is the complete list of available options. If an option is not present, the default is "don't care" unless otherwise noted. If specified, these options are equivalent to the corresponding options given in the `options` top-level statement; refer to the description of option blocks for more details on the operation of these options.

`scanline on|off`	The scanline rendering algorithm must be turned on or off, respectively.
`trace on|off`	Ray tracingray tracing must be turned on or off. For example, lens shaders that modify the ray direction should set this to on.
`shadow off`	Shadowsshadow must be turned off for this shader to function.
`shadow on`	Shadowing must be enabled, either regular, sorted, or segmented.
`shadow sort`	Shadowing must be enabled, either sorted or segmented. Regular is not sufficient.
`shadow segments`	Segmented shadows must be enabled. Regular or sorted shadows are not sufficient.
`face front|back|both`	Intersection testing should consider at least front-facing, back-facing, or both front-facing and back-facing geometry, respectively. "At least" means that a request for either front-facing or back-facing geometry is met of "both" is enabled.
`derivative [1] [2]`	The object that this shader or phenomenon is attached to (by being named in its material, for example) must have first or second derivatives, respectively, or both. This option has an effect only on free-form surface geometry because mental ray cannot compute derivatives for polygons.
`object space`	The shader functions only if all geometry is defined in object coordinates.

`camera space` — The shader functions only if all geometry is defined in camera coordinates.

`mixed space` — The shader functions only if all geometry is defined in camera coordinates, but it is ok if the camera is defined in object coordinates. This is done for certain kinds of walkthrough scenes and is not recommended for general shaders.

2.2 Shader Definitions

After a shader has been declared, it can be used in a definition. While a shader is made known to mental ray using a declaration only once, it may be used any number of times. Each use is called a *definition*shader definition. A definition supplies numerical or other values for shader parameters, and is attached to some other scene element.

In this book, shader definitions will be used in many places, denoted by the *shader* metasymbol. A shader is defined as a shading function name followed by parameters:

```
"shader_name" (parameters)
```

This sequence can be inserted for every instance of *shader* in the rest of this book. (There are other forms, lists and named references, that can also be used in place of *shader*. They are described later.)

The shader name must have been previously declared with a `declare` command; see above. Normally shader libraries containing compiled C/C++ shaders come with a `$include` file that contains all declarations for the shaders in the library. The library itself is typically linked into mental ray with a `link` command. There are usually many shader references for every declaration, each with a unique set of parameters. The syntax of shader calls is described in the chapter on shaders; they are basically a comma-separated sequence of quoted parameter names, each followed by a parameter value.

The parenthesized *parameters* list is a comma-separated list of shader parameter assignments that have one of the following three forms:

```
"parameter_name" value
"parameter_name" = "shader_name"
"parameter_name" = interface "ifname"
```

The first form assigns a constant value to the parameter. The format of constant values depends on the parameter type:

type	*value*
boolean	true
	false
integer	$value_{int}$
scalar	*value*
vector	*x y z*
transform	$a_{00}\ a_{01}\ a_{02}\ a_{03}\ a_{10}\ a_{11}\ a_{12}\ a_{13}\ a_{20}\ a_{21}\ a_{22}\ a_{23}\ a_{30}\ a_{31}\ a_{32}\ a_{33}$
color	*red green blue*
	red green blue alpha
shader	"*shader_name*"
color texture	"*texture_name*"
scalar texture	"*texture_name*"
vector texture	"*texture_name*"
light	"*light_instance_name*"
struct	{*parameters*}
array	[*comma-separated value list*]

Integer values must be signed 32-bit values. All other numerical values are floating-point numbers that may contain a decimal point and/or a decimal exponent introduced by the letter `e`, as in `1.6e-27`. The *shader_name* must be the name of a named shader from a preceding `shader` statement; the *texture_name* must be the name of a previously defined `color texture`, `scalar texture`, or `vector texture` statement, respectively.

The special value keyword `null` can be used to replace any number, symbol, string, `true`, or `false`. It stores the numerical value 0 in the parameter. Its main purpose is to create "holes" in arrays by listing `null`s between the square brackets.

The two non-constant forms of parameter assignment are explained later.

The above shader definition form is also called an anonymous shader because the shader name/parameter pair is formed on the fly and used in place. Sometimes it is useful to give a name to a shader/parameters pair using a `shader` statement and use it more than once:

```
shader "named_shader"
    "shader_name" (parameters)
```

Such pairs are called named shaders. After the pair was set up with a `shader` statement, it can be used in any place where a *shader* can be used, as an alternative to the anonymous shader statement listed above:

```
= "named_shader"
```

This is especially useful if the same shader/parameters pair is used in many different places in the scene, and it changes for every frame. Since `shader` statements allow incremental changes, an incremental change to a named shader affects all places that reference it (with the exception of displacement shaders — once an object is tessellated it remains unchanged until explicitly modified). Without named shaders it would be necessary to incrementally change every scene element containing the shader.

2.3 Shader Lists

In most constructs accepting a shader, shader lists are also accepted. A shader list consist of one or more *shader* items like one of the two above in sequence. For example, suppose that a named shader has been defined with the following command:

```
shader "named_shader2" "shader2" (parameters)
```

then the following shader list can be written:

```
"shader1" (parameters)
= "named_shader2"
"shader3" (parameters)
```

This shader list will call three shaders in sequence, `shader1`, `shader2`, and `shader3`, in this order, each with its parameters. All shaders get the same *result* pointer, so each operates on the results of the previous. A shader list like this can be substituted for all instances of the metasymbol *shader_list* in this chapter.

Shader lists are maintained by storing a link to the next shader in the previous shader. In the above example, the anonymous shader `shader1` contains a link to `name_shader2`, which contains a link to `shader3`. This means that once this list is set up, any reference to `named_shader2` will implicitly also call `shader3` because the link in `named_shader2` will remain in the shader until changed in another shader list. This can have surprising results. This is not a problem in anonymous shaders because, not having a name, they cannot be referenced in more than one place. In general it is a good idea to avoid putting named shaders in shader lists.

2.4 Shader Graphs

Instead of assigning a constant value to a parameter in a shader definition, it is possible to assign a shader:

"*parameter_name*" = "*shader_name*"

For parameters assigned in this way, no value is stored in the shader definition. It is obtained by calling *shader_name* at runtime. For example, if the *ambient* parameter of a material shader has the constant value `1 0 0`, it is always red, but if another shader is assigned to it that other shader is called when the material shader asks for the value using the *mi_eval* function or one of its derivatives. The other shader could be a texture shader, for example, resulting in a textured ambient value.

The return type of the assigned shader must agree with the parameter type. If the return type of the assigned shader is `struct`, it is possible to select a structure member by appending a period and the name of the struct member to the shader name. Consider the following assignment:

```
declare shader
   color "phong" (color "ambient",
                  color "diffuse",
                  color "specular")
   version 1
end declare

declare shader
   struct {color "a", color "b"}
         "texture" (color texture "picture")
   version 1
end declare

color texture "fluffy" "/tmp/image.rgb"

shader "map" "texture" (
   "picture"   "fluffy")

shader "mtlsh" "phong" (
   "ambient"   0.3 0.3 0.3,
   "diffuse"   = "map.a",
   "specular"  = "map.b")
```

This defines a material shader that does not support texturing in any way because it has no parameters of type `shader` or `color texture`. Yet, shader assignments allow its diffuse and specular components to be textured without the phong shader being aware of it. Whenever phong accesses its ambient parameter value by calling *mi_eval*, it gets a constant color 0.3 0.3 0.3, but when it accesses its diffuse or specular colors a call to the named shader `map` results (which actually calls shader `texture`), whose result is then returned to the `phong` shader.

In this example, the `map` shader returns two colors `a` and `b`, which are selected in the shader assignment by appending `.a` and `.b` to `map`. (For this reason periods should be avoided in parameter names.) If the shader had returned only a single color, only `"map"` would have been assigned, without appending a period and a structure member name.

In the example, `map` is assigned twice. Obviously it is not desirable to actually call it twice, because the first call will already have set both its `a` and `b` return values. After the first call from a shader, mental ray caches the return value to avoid further calls. As soon as the shader `phong` returns, the cache is discarded to ensure that the next call to `phong`, most likely with a different state, calls `map` instead of using a stale cache.

Note that shaders that support shader graphs must use the *mi_eval* function to access their parameters. This was done to ensure that only those assigned shaders whose values are actually used are evaluated. For example, a material shader that has two color parameters, one for the front and one for the back side of the surface, will access only one of its parameters by using *mi_eval* only once.

To see how the *phong* shader is implemented as a C shader, see the section "Parameter Assignments and *mi_eval*" in chapter 3.

The advantage of shader assignment is that it is not necessary to write shaders to accept procedural values. Without shader assignments, a simple Phong material shader would need parameters of type `shader` or *color texture* in addition to the standard ambient, diffuse, and specular parameters. Shader assignment allows writing small, reusable "base shaders" that can be easily combined into powerful shader graphs, instead of writing large monolithic shaders that are hard to modify and inflexible to use.

The third form of parameter assigning using the `interface` keyword is available only inside phenomena, which will be discussed next.

2.5 Phenomena

This section only describes the representation of phenomena in the .mi language. The declaration of a phenomenon is very similar to the declaration of a shader, except that the keyword `shader` is replaced with `phenomenon`, and the addition of new optional statements in the declaration block:

```
declare phenomenon
    [type] "phenomenon_name" (
        type "parameter_name",
        type "parameter_name",
        ...
        type "parameter_name"
    )
```

```
    [ version version_int ]
    [ shader "name" ...
    [ material "name" ... end material
    [ light "name" ... end light
    [ instance "name" ... end instance
    [ roots ]
    [ options ]
end declare
```

For a description of version, shader, material, light, and instance definitions, see the corresponding section above; the syntax is identical to the one described there. The *options* are identical to the options described in the shader declaration section above. The *roots* are described below.

The phenomenon *phenomenon_name* declared with this statement is available for the definition of shaders just like a shader declared with a `declare shader` statement. Named and anonymous shader definitions can be derived from either type of declaration. Phenomena were designed to extend the concept of shaders, not replace it.

2.5.1 Phenomenon Interface Parameters

Phenomena, like shaders, have parameters. In the phenomenon case they are called "interface parameters" because they form the gateway between the rest of the scene and the internal implementation of the phenomenon. Interface parameters are what makes the phenomenon look like a simple shader to the named and anonymous shader definitions. Phenomena are implemented in terms of subshader nodes, each with their own parameters. Subshader parameters can be assigned from the interface using an assignment of the following form:

```
"parameter_name" = interface "ifname"
```

This looks similar to the shader assignments described above, but when the shader calls *mi_eval* on a parameter assigned to the interface of the phenomenon it is defined in, no shader is called but the value is obtained from the phenomenon interface. For example:

```
declare shader
   color "phong" (color "ambient",
                  color "diffuse",
                  color "specular")
   version 1
end declare

declare phenomenon
   color "phong_phen" (color "col")
   version 1
```

```
    shader "sub" "phong" (
        "ambient"   0.3 0.3 0.3,
        "diffuse"   = interface "col",
        "specular"  1.0 1.0 1.0)

    root = "sub"
end declare

shader "mtlsh" "phong_phen" (
    "col"   1.0 0.5 0.0)
```

For the shader definition, the phenomenon *phong_phen* looks like a shader with a single color parameter *col*. Internally, it contains the definition of a simple shader *sub* with three parameters, two of which have constant values and one which takes its value from the interface. When the shader definition *mtlsh* is called from a material or elsewhere in the scene, it calls the phenomenon *phong_phen* with the value 1.0 0.5 0.0 for the interface parameter *col*. This value is propagated to the *diffuse* parameter of the shader *sub* during evaluation of the phenomenon.

It is important to distinguish parameter *values*, such as 1.0 1.0 1.0 for `specular`, from shader *assignments*, which begin with an "=" sign. In particular, consider the shader parameter type `shader`: if a shader name is given as the value without "=" sign, the named shader will be returned but not called by *mi_eval*. With an "=" sign, *mi_eval* will call the shader and expect it to return another shader (so its return value must have type `shader`) which is then returned by *mi_eval*. The latter involves an indirection, and is not often used for parameters of type `shader`. This is a common mistake, and return type mismatches will result in mental ray warning messages.

When calling a phenomenon, all its parameters must pass through the interface. The shader *sub* and everything else defined inside the phenomenon block is visible only inside the phenomenon, and no names defined outside the phenomenon are visible to definitions inside the phenomenon. The interface is the only connection point between the inner and outer world. This encapsulation ensures the integrity and completeness of phenomena independently of the scene they are used in.

Phenomena may also contain material, light, and instance definitions in addition to shader definitions.

By convention, anonymous shader definitions should not be used in phenomenon declarations. There is no functional disadvantage in using anonymous shader definitions but it makes life difficult for graphical phenomenon editing tools like mental images' Phenomenon Creator™, which uses shader names to label the icons and boxes that represent subshaders in its graph and browser views.

The return type of a phenomenon may be any type that is a valid return type for a shader.

2.5.2 Phenomenon Roots

The above example also illustrates a new option allowed in phenomenon but not shader definitions, the phenomenon root. There are several types of root statements:

`root`	*shader*
`root material`	"*material_name*"
`geometry`	*shader*
`volume`	*shader*
`environment`	*shader*
`lens`	*shader*
`output`	*shader*
`output`	["*type*"] "*format*" [*opt*] "*filename*"
`contour store`	*shader*
`contour contrast`	*shader*
`volume priority`	$priority_{int}$
`environment priority`	$priority_{int}$
`lens priority`	$priority_{int}$
`output priority`	$priority_{int}$

All of these except one of the first two are optional. The first `root` statement specifies the primary root shader of a phenomenon that is called when the phenomenon is called. In the above example, the *mtlsh* shader, when called, calls the phenomenon *phong_phen*, which immediately calls its subshader *sub* because *sub* is specified in its `root` statement.

The `root material` variant creates a material phenomenon. This type of phenomenon must be declared with the return type `material`. It is instanced normally with a `shader` statement, which provides the interface parameter values. The resulting shader is different from regular shaders; its name can be used everywhere where a material name is valid. A regular phenomenon that does not have type `material` and no `root material` statement, when instanced using a `shader` statement, becomes a shader, not a material. Material phenomena should be used instead of regular phenomena if the phenomenon depends on not only assigning a single shader, such as a material shader, but other material components such as shadow shader, photon shader, volume shader etc. as well. See page 82 for an example of a material phenomenon.

In addition to the main `root` statement, other roots may be defined that reference shaders of other types:

`geometry` The geometry shader or shader list is evaluated before rendering starts. This allows the phenomenon to introduce procedural geometry into the scene. For example, a light beam phenomenon might install a transparent cone in the scene that bounds the volume effect.

`volume` The volume shader or shader list is added to the camera before rendering starts. This allows the phenomenon to specify a global atmosphere that should be installed if the phenomenon is defined.

`environment` The environment shader or shader list is added to the camera before rendering starts. This allows the phenomenon to specify a global environment shader that should be installed if the phenomenon is defined. Environment shaders are called when a ray does not intersect any object.

`lens` This root is doing the same thing for lens shaders that should be added to the camera before rendering starts.

`output` The list of output shaders and file output statement is added to the camera before rendering starts. This allows the phenomenon to specify output shaders that should be installed if the phenomenon is defined. For example, the phenomenon might write a label frame buffer whose values are picked up by the output shader after rendering completes.

`contour store` The contour store shader is used for contour rendering.

`contour contrast` The contour contrast shader is used for contour rendering.

Note that during rendering, only `root` (or `root material` in the material phenomenon case) has any significance because the others have been removed and added to the camera or the scene before rendering started. After rendering and output shading completes, all these changes are undone. Note that if the phenomenon is defined several times (using multiple `shader` statements or anonymous shader definitions that reference it), the roots other than the main `root` are added to the scene more than once. [2]

The shader priority statements provide control over the the placing of the specified shaders or shader lists in the corresponding shader list in the camera. Shaders with greater priority numbers are appended to shaders with smaller priority numbers, and hence execute later. Shaders with no priority number have priority `0`, so they get executed before shaders with positive priority numbers.

2.6 Commands

Commands are instructions to mental ray that are executed the moment they are read from the input scene file. They do not add elements to the scene database. Since the scene file is only read by the client host in a network configuration, commands are never seen by server hosts.

`$include "`*filename*`"`

[2]Shaders attached directly or indirectly to the `output`, `contour store`, and `contour contrast` roots may not use interface or shader parameter assignments.

`$include` <*filename*>

The $ sign must appear in the first column of the line. The named file is included (pasted into) the `.mi` file in place of the $include statement. Includes can be nested. The main purpose is to include declarations (see below), but materials, light sources, even objects can be included. The only place where $include cannot be used is between $code and $end code; use the standard C #include statement there. The included file is read on the client host only. If the *filename* is enclosed in angle brackets, the standard include path is prepended, by default `/usr/include`. The standard path can be changed with the `-I` command-line option.

`set` "*name*" ["*value*"]

Assign the value *value* to the variable *name*. Variables are not used by mental ray but provide a general syntax for passing parameters from translators to interactive programs that read scene files without actually parsing any geometric data. For example, translators can store the translator version and name, source scene name, frame range, and other useful information in variables.

[`min`] `version` "*string*"
`max version` "*string*"

This commands informs mental ray that this .mi file requires the given mental ray version. `min` means "at least" and `max` means "at most". Version strings consist of numbers separated with dots, such as "`1.2.3.4`". The string can underspecify the version, as in "`2.1`". Missing numbers are implicitly assumed to be `0` so "`2.1`" becomes "`2.1.0.0`". Each number, beginning with the first, is checked in turn. If the number in the *string* is greater (`min`) or less than (`max`) than the version number built into mental ray, an error message is printed and mental ray aborts; otherwise the next number is considered. If all given numbers pass the test, mental ray continues. This command is recommended for declaration files included with `$include`[3]

`verbose on|off|` $level_{int}$

This command controls verbose messages. There are seven levels: fatal errors (0), errors (1), warnings (2), progress reports (3), informational messages (4), debugging messages (5), and verbose debugging messages (6). All message categories numerically less than *level* are printed. Verbose `off` is equivalent to level 2 (fatal errors and errors); verbose on is equivalent to level 5 (everything except debugging messages). Verbose messages can slow down mental ray while parsing, especially on systems with poor I/O systems such as Windows NT because of slow scrolling. The verbose command can be overridden with the `-verbose` command-line option.

[3]Some versions of mental ray *require* that included files contain version limits because incorrect declarations can have severe consequences. However, shader versioning (see page 168) provides an alternate and more flexible way of shader version verification.

```
echo "message"
```

The named *message*, which must be enclosed in double quotes, is printed to stdout. The echo command is executed synchronously during parsing the .mi file. Echoing requires verbosity level 1 or higher.

```
call shader_list [, "camera_inst" "options"]
```

The given shader is called immediately, and parsing stops until the shader completes. Since the shader is called during parsing and not during tessellation or rendering, the entire state passed to the shader is filled with nulls, which limits what the shader can do (it cannot cast rays, for example). If the name of a camera instance element and the name of an options element is given, *state* $\rightarrow$ *options* and *state* $\rightarrow$ *camera* are set up for the shader. The return value is ignored. The call statement is intended for early initialization of shader packages, or even to start interactive front-end packages. Shader init and exit functions are not called by the `call` statement. For shader initialization, shader init functions are more useful because they are called with a full state, and only if the corresponding shader is actually needed.

```
system "shell_command"
```

This command starts a shell, which executes the named *shell_command*. The shell command must be enclosed in double quotes. mental ray waits until the shell command has completed; this can be defeated by ending the command with a shell & command. The system command, like echo, is executed while parsing, not during rendering. Its main purpose is writing finished pictures to an output device such as a film recorder.

```
code "filename"
```

The named *filename* is interpreted as a C source file, ending with the extension ".c", is compiled and linked into mental ray. From this point on, the shaders it defines are available in mental ray as shading functions. For example, if the source defines a C function *myshader*, with the usual three parameters *result*, *state*, and *paras* (see chapter 3 for details), the name *myshader* may be used in materials, lights, textures and so on as the quoted shader name. The command-line option `-code` provides an alternative way of compiling and linking C source. Multiple code commands are possible. This is intended mainly for debugging because linking precompiled shader libraries is much more efficient. Note that every shading function must also be declared; see section 2.1.

```
$code
```

```
C source text
$end code
```

The $ signs must appear in column 1 of the line. This command also compiles and links C source code, but the code is read directly from the `.mi` file rather than from a separate source file. The *C source text* follows standard C syntax. In fact, it is written out to a temporary file, which is then compiled as if a `code` command had been used. Multiple $code commands are allowed. Note that every shading function must also be declared; see below.

```
link "filename"
```

Like the code command, the link command attaches external shaders to mental ray, which can then be used as shading functions. While the code command accepts ".c" files as *filename*, the link command expects either object files ending in ".o", or dynamic shared object (DSO on Unix, DLL on Windows NT) files ending in ".so". Object files are linked, while DSOs are just attached without any preprocessing. DSOs are the fastest way of attaching an external shader, and require no compilers or development options, which are sometimes sold separately by system vendors[4]. However, certain old systems do not support DSOs. The `-link` command-line option provides an alternative way of linking object files and DSOs. Any number of files can be linked. Note that every shading function must also be declared; see section 2.1. If Dynamical Shared Objects are to be linked on Unix machines, the `LD_LIBRARY_PATH` or `LD_LIBRARYN32_PATH` (SGI) environment variable must include the path of the DSO file to be linked; see section 3.1.

```
delete "element_name"
```

Delete a named scene element, such as objects, materials, lights, textures, instances, and instance groups. Declarations and shaders cannot be deleted. It is possible to delete an element and recreate it with the same name, but this breaks all links. For example, if a light is created and then an instance is created for it, naming the light, the link between instance and light is broken when the light is deleted and recreated. The instance retains a *dangling link* that will cause havoc during later processing. The `delete` command should be used only for entities that disappear permanently. All instances and instance groups that contained the name must be updated *before* the name is deleted.

Instead of deleting and recreating an element, an incremental change should be used by prefixing the element definition with the `incremental` modifier. This has the additional advantage that the element retains all contents that are not modified during the new incremental definition. For example, an incremental change to a camera containing nothing but a new frame number specification will leave the camera unchanged except for the frame number. As an exception, objects and instgroups are cleared first because merging is not generally useful in these cases.

[4]For system and development software requirements, see the Release and Installation Notes.

```
render "root_instgroup_name" "camera_inst_name" "options_name"
```

This statement renders the scene. The name of an options element, a camera instance element (which must also have been attached to the root instance group), and the root instance group must be given.

2.7 Scene Entities

A .mi file contains commands and scene entities in any order, with the restriction that an element must be defined before it can be referenced. All entities are named; all references are done by name. The following entities can be defined:

options	global options
camera	camera: output files, aperture, resolution, etc.
material	shading, shadows, volumes, environments, contour, etc.
texture	procedural texture or texture image
light	light
object	polygonal or free-form surface geometry
instance	places objects, lights, cameras, and groups in 3D space
instgroup	for grouping instances; the nodes of the scene DAG
shader	optional named shaders

All of these can be defined at any place, as long as they are not nested (the definition of an element must be completed before the next element can be defined). All these entities can also be incrementally changed by introducing the definition with the `incremental` keyword, which tells mental ray to re-define an existing element instead of starting a new one. The contents of the existing element become the defaults for the new one.

`options` This element contains rendering options such as the shadow mode, tracing depth, sampling algorithm and its parameters, acceleration algorithm and its parameters, dithering and other modes.

`camera` The camera is a description of the camera characteristics such as focal length and aperture that determine the field of view.

`texture` Textures to apply 2D or 3D color, bump, transparency, displacement and other maps to objects. Textures are referenced by other shaders that include the texture in their color or other computation. Textures may appear verbatim in the file, or may be read from a texture file, or may be fully procedural, or a combination of these.

`material` Materials describe the surface properties of objects, volumic properties of the space enclosed by objects, transparent shadow casting, environment mapping, and displacement mapping, as well as a number of property flags.

`light` — Lights illuminate objects and volumes. Lights are referenced in materials only (through the light instance), they are not applied directly to objects. All lights name a shading function; there are predefined shaders for points, spots, and directional lights, optionally in combination with various types of area light sources.

`object` — Objects describe the actual geometry. Objects may reference materials to determine the visual appearance of the surface. Various types of geometry descriptions are supported, such as polygonal objects and free-form surfaces. By default, all objects are defined in a local coordinate space (object space), usually with the origin at the center of the object. Options exist to switch to camera space instead.

`instance` — When an object, light, camera, or instance group is defined, it does not become part of the scene. It must be placed in 3D space with an instance, which contains a transformation matrix, inherited parameters, and several flags. It is possible to have more than one instance reference the same object, light, camera, or instance group; this is called "multiple instancing". The instanced entity then appears several times in the final processed scene. It is possible to specify a "geometry shader" as the instanced item instead of an object. The "geometry shader" is expected to create a scene element which is defined in the local coordinate space of the instance.

`instgroup` — Instance groups are used to group instances so they can be instanced as a unit. Instance groups form the nodes of the scene DAG (Directed Acyclic Graph), which contains all entities used during processing. The instance group at the root of the DAG is called the "root instance group." Since instance groups can themselves be instanced the scene DAG can be built with any number of levels and sub-DAGs, each with its own local coordinate space.

`shader` — Shaders are user-provided functions used for a variety of purposes. They are not normally named; they are defined where they are needed, like in a material. An unnamed shader is also called an "anonymous shader." The `shader` statement allows giving a name to a shader; a named shader can be used in any place where an anonymous shader is expected by giving its name, introduced by an equals sign.

All scene entities are described in more detail in the following subsections.

2.7.1 Options

```
options "name"
    option_statements
end options
```

Options contain rendering modes. An options element must be specified to render a scene. There is a variety of *option_statements* that can be listed in the options. Most of them can be overridden with an appropriate command-line option; see appendix 5. The following *option_statements* are supported:

2.7.1.1 Sampling Quality

`contrast` *r g b* [*a*]

The contrast controls supersampling. If neighboring samples differ by more than the color *r*, *g*, *b*, *a*, supersampling is done as specified by the sampling parameters (see below). Default for *a* is the average of *r*, *g*, and *b*. The recursive supersampling algorithm controlled by `samples` modifies the contrast based on the recursion level: at sample level 0, the contrast is used directly; at sample level 1, the contrast is doubled (effectively requiring a higher contrast to force another subdivision), and so on. Negative levels divide the contrast, i.e. use a fraction $\frac{1}{2}$, $\frac{1}{4}$, and so on. In general, the contrast is multiplied by 2^{level} at the supersampling level *level*, which is bounded by `samples`. The default is 0.1 0.1 0.1 0.1.

This is the primary means of image quality control. Typically values are 0.1 for *r*, *g*, *b*, and *a*. Values such as 0.2 or 0.3 reduce quality; lower values increase quality. Values less than 0.05 do not further increase quality in most cases. r, g, b, a can be specified separately to allow physiologically correct contrast values; the human eye is much more sensitive to different shades of green than blue and red, and can only poorly distinguish shades of blue. The *a* value should be set to 1.0 if the matte (alpha) channel is not needed; it is also possible to set *a* lower than r, g, b to generate matte channels with a higher quality than the color image. If the *a* value is missing, it is set to the average of r, g, b. Note that for high-quality rendering, the `samples` parameters must be adjusted.

`time contrast` *r g b* [*a*]

The time contrast controls temporal supersampling for motion blurred scenes. It works similar to the spatial contrast parameter explained above: If neighboring samples in time differ by more than the color *r*, *g*, *b*, *a*, supersampling is done. Default for *a* is the average of *r*, *g*, and *b*. Using values for `time contrast` that are higher than `contrast` can speed up motion blur rendering at the price of more grainy images without degrading the quality of spatial antialiasing. The default is 0.2 0.2 0.2 0.2; much higher than the spatial contrast.

`samples` [min_{int}] max_{int} [`view`]

This statement determines the minimum and maximum sample rate. Each pixel is sampled at least $2^{2 \cdot min}$ times and at most $2^{2 \cdot max}$ times in each direction. If *min* is 0, each pixel is sampled at least once. Positive values increase the sample rate; negative numbers reduce the sample rate to less than one initial sample per pixel (infrasampling). *min* defaults to -2, which means that at least one sample per 4 × 4 pixels is taken. If *min* is chosen too small, small features may be lost if all samples happen to miss it (if it is found just once in any pixel of a task, mental ray will analyze the feature and render it correctly).

If `view` is specified, sample view mode[2.1] is turned on. In this mode, the rgb image will be replaced with an image that shows where samples were collected during rendering. This is useful for tuning the *min* and *max* values, and the `contrast` option and identifying troublesome areas in the image. A pixel's intensity reflects the number of samples collected within the pixel and on its bottom and left edges. It is normalized to the maximum number of samples per pixel. In addition, task boundaries are shown in red in the image.

If no *min* value is given, $max - 2$ is used by default. The defaults for *min* and *max* are −2 and 0, respectively. It is recommended to use *max* values larger than or equal to $min + 2$; the difference should not be higher than 3. Typical values for *min* and *max* are −20 for low-quality preview rendering, −11 for medium-quality rendering, and 02 or 13 for high-quality renders. Note that while this option offers simple control of rendering quality, it is recommended to control quality with the `contrast` option, which allows much finer control and deals more gracefully with high-contrast cases where the `samples` option can leave aliasing due to the hard cutoff. The `samples` statement should be used **only** as a hard sampling limit.

If a `filter` camera statement is used to set a filter other than `box 1 1`, *min* and *max* must be set to at least 1 1 for mental ray 2.0, or at least -1 0 for mental ray 2.1 or later.

`filter box|triangle|gauss|mitchell|lanczos` [*width* [*height*]]

The filter statement specifies how multiple samples are to be combined into a single pixel value. The filter defaults to a box filter of width and height 1.0, which is the fastest of the filters. This option allows changing the filter kernel or the filter size. The available kernels are: box, triangle, Gauss, Mitchell[2.1], and Lanczos[2.1]. The size of the filter is specified in pixel units. If no height is given it is taken to be equal to the width. Filters must be larger than 0.0. If the size of the filter is not specified, default values are used. These are 1.0 for box, 2.0 for triangle, 3.0 for Gauss and 4.0 for Mitchell and Lanczos. The default height is the same as the default width. Larger filter sizes result in softer images and may reduce rendering speed slightly, while values smaller than the defaults can introduce artifacts. Filters must be larger than 0.0 but sizes smaller than 1.0 are generally wasteful since they will discard some samples.

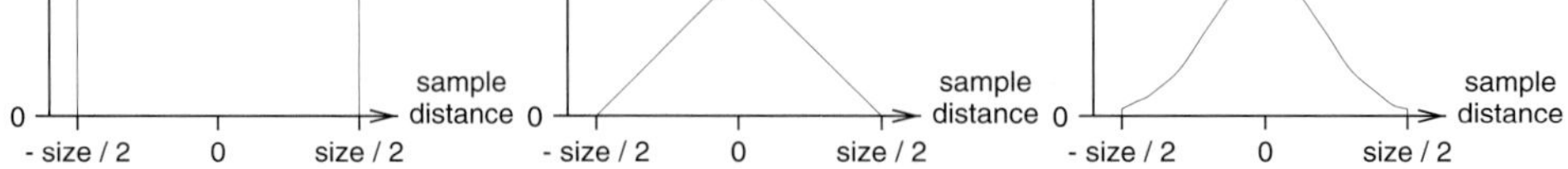

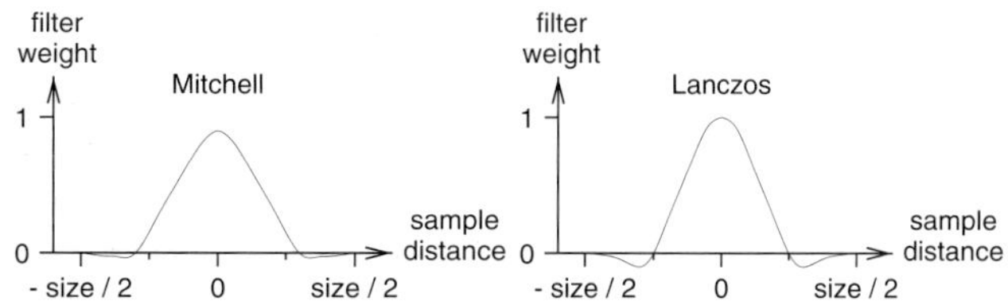

The box filter sums all samples in the filter area with an equal weight. The triangle filter functions has the shape of a pyramid centered on the pixel, which means that samples at the center of a rendered image pixel contribute more than more distant samples. The Gauss filter weights the samples using a Gauss curve that is cut off at an ellipse centered on the pixel. The Mitchell and Lanczos filters are both approximations of the theoretically ideal sinc filtering function, cut off after its second lobe. In most cases, the Mitchell filter gives better results. For these two, a filter width of 4.0 corresponds to a frequency cutoff of 2.0 pixels, the Nyquist frequency. In order to use non-default filters, the limits for the `samples` statement must specify $min = -1$ or greater, and $max = 0$ or greater (mental ray 2.0: 1 1 or greater). Otherwise a warning will be printed and the `filter` statement ignored.

`jitter` *jitter*

The jittering factor introduces systematic variations into sample locations. Without jittering, samples are taken at the corners of pixels or subpixels. Jittering displaces the samples by an amount calculated by lighting analysis. This is used to reduce artifacts. Jittering is turned off by default, or by specifying a *jitter* of 0.0. To turn jittering on, use a *jitter* value of 1.0. Jittering works best in ray tracing mode.

2.7.1.2 Tessellation Quality

`approximate` *technique* [min_{int} max_{int}] `all`

This statement overrides all approximations for base surfaces (i.e. the surface before applying displacement), free-form surfaces or polygons, in geometric objects. See section 2.7.8.8 for a more detailed description of approximations. Here is a brief summary of *technique*, which is a list of one or more of the following:

`view`
`tree`
`grid`
`[regular] parametric` *u_subdiv* [*v_subdiv*]
`length` *edge*
`distance` *dist*
`angle` *angle*
`spatial` *edge*
`curvature` *dist angle*

Like in object approximation statements, the subdivision limits *min* and max can be specified how often a triangle can be subdivided. The defaults for *min* and *max* are 0 and 5, respectively; 5 is a very high value because every increment of 1 can quadruple the number off triangles in the extreme case. In objects, the approximation technique is followed by the surface or curve it applies to; in the options the keyword `all` indicates that an option approximation overrides all object approximations.

`approximate displace` *technique* [min_{int} max_{int}] `all`

This statement overrides all approximations for displacement maps in geometric objects. Both kinds of approximation overrides are useful for temporarily reducing tessellation quality for previews to reduce tessellation and rendering time without redefining all objects, for example by specifying

```
approximate regular parametric 1.0 1.0 0 2 all
approximate displace regular parametric 1.0 1.0 0 2 all
```

2.7.1.3 Motion Blur

`shutter` *shutter*

This statement specifies the shutter open time. A *shutter* value of 0.0 turns motion blurring off, and values greater than 0.0 turn motion blurring on. The *shutter* value scales the motion vectors attached to object vertices or computed from motion transformations. If *shutter* is 1.0, each vertex moves the distance given by its motion vector, and is blurred in the image over this distance. Values less than 1.0 reduce the length of this path.

2.7.1.4 Trace Depth

`trace depth` $reflect_{int}$ [$refract_{int}$ [sum_{int}]]

The *reflect* parameter limits the number of recursive reflection rays. If it is set to 0, no reflection rays will be cast; if it is set to 1, one level is allowed but a reflection ray can not be reflected again, and so on. Similarly, *refract* controls the maximum depth of refraction and transparency rays (which implement transparency with and without index of refraction). Additionally, it is possible to limit the sum of reflection and refraction rays with *sum*. For example, if 3 3 4 is given, an eye ray may be reflected 3 times, or refracted 3 times, or reflected twice and then refracted twice, or any other combination that sums up to at most 4. The defaults are 2 2 4. Note that custom shaders may override these values.

2.7.1.5 Shadows

`shadow off`

This statement disables all shadows.

`shadow on`

Simple shadows are enabled. This is the most efficient and least flexible of the three shadow modes. If shadows overlap because multiple objects obscure the light source, the order in which these objects are considered (and their shadow shaders are called) is undefined. If one object is found to completely obscure the light, no other obscuring objects are considered. This statement turns off shadow sorting and shadow segments. Also see `shadowmap motion` below.

`shadow sort`

This shadow mode enables shadow sorting. It is similar to the preceding shadow mode, but ensures that the shadow shaders of obscuring objects are called in the correct order, object closest to the illuminated point first. This mode is slightly slower but allows specialized shaders to record information about obscuring objects. If no such special shader is used, this mode offers no advantage over simple `shadow on`.

`shadow segments`

Like with `shadow sort`, the shadow shaders are called in order. Additionally, shadow rays are traced much like regular rays, passing from one obscuring object to the next, from the light source to the illuminated point. Each such ray is called a shadow segment. This slows down rendering, but is required if volume effects should cast shadows (such as certain complex shaders like fur and smoke volume shaders). This mode requires support from the shadow shader, which must use the *mi_trace_shadow_seg* function to cast the next shadow ray segment.

`shadowmap on|off|opengl`

This flag turns shadow maps on or off for the entire rendering. Shadow map parameters are specified for each light source. The default is off because shadow maps, while often significantly faster, always assume opaque objects. *opengl*[2.1] mode causes mental ray to use OpenGL acceleration if available when rendering shadow maps. The same limitations apply as mentioned with the `scanline` option. Additionally, because of the difference of the rendering algorithm, shadow maps rendered with this option contain slightly different information from those generated with the regular algorithm, and the resulting shadows may look different. In particular, soft areas of shadows tend to be smaller and some areas may incorrectly be determined to be not in shadow. When OpenGL rendering of shadow maps is enabled, only the client host will participate, since the computation cost of the map is so small that the network transfer costs could not be recovered.

`shadowmap rebuild on|off`

Determines whether all shadow maps should be recomputed. If this option is off (the default) shadow maps are loaded from files or reused from previously rendered frames if possible. If this option is on, no shadow map is reused – everything is recomputed. The default is off.

`shadowmap motion on|off`
Determines whether shadow maps should be motion blurred such that moving objects will cast shadows along the path of motion. Turning this option off can improve performance of rendering shadow maps slightly faster. The default is on. Note that since shadow maps do not deal with transparent objects and motion blurring introduces a form of transparency at the edges, shadow map shadows can appear too large in the direction of motion if the object moves quickly.

2.7.1.6 Rendering Algorithms

`trace on|off`
Normally, mental ray will use a combination of a scanline algorithm and ray tracing to calculate samples of the scene. If `trace off` is specified, ray tracing is disabled, and mental ray will rely exclusively on the scanline algorithm. Since the scanline algorithm can only compute straight rays from the pinhole camera, reflection rays cannot be cast and refraction rays are computed like transparent rays, which do not allow control over the ray direction based on the index of refraction of the material. Lens shaders cannot alter the ray origin and direction. However, reflections onto environment maps do work. Motion blurring and shadows are also affected if ray tracing is turned off. Ray tracing is turned on by default.

`scanline on|off|opengl`
This statement allows turning off the scanline algorithm. By default, mental ray tries to use a scanline algorithm for straight rays from the pinhole camera, such as primary rays. In most cases this gives better performance than pure ray tracing. Turning scanline off forces mental ray to rely entirely on ray tracing. This will generally slow down rendering but in some cases, for example when the `task size` is very small, the overhead of initializing the scanline algorithm may outweigh its benefit and turning it off can result in an improvement in speed. The *opengl*[2.1] option will cause mental ray to use OpenGL hardware if present to further accelerate rendering. If possible, the master host will use OpenGL to generate acceleration data that the scanline algorithm then uses for intersection testing. Also see `task size` below.

`acceleration bsp`
Selects the binary space partitioning (BSP) ray tracing algorithm. This algorithm is often, but not always, faster. It is controlled by the `bsp size` and `bsp depth` statements. The BSP algorithm is the default.

`acceleration grid`
Selects the grid rendering algorithm. It provides faster preprocessing especially on multiprocessor systems. Memory usage is more conservative and much easier to control than with the BSP algorithm. Speed is comparable to BSP but more scene-dependent. It is controlled by the `grid size` statement.

`acceleration raycl`

Selects the ray classification ray tracing algorithm. Like the grid algorithm, this algorithm operates with a constant acceleration memory size. This size is controlled by the `raycl memory` and `raycl subdivision` statements. It only works in camera space scenes and exists mainly for backwards compatibility with mental ray 1.x.

`bsp size` $size_{int}$

The maximum number of primitives in a leaf of the BSP tree. This statement is used only if binary space partitioning is enabled. It has no effect on the other algorithms. Larger leaf sizes reduce memory consumption but increase rendering time. The default is 4.

`bsp depth` $depth_{int}$

The maximum number of levels in the BSP tree. This statement is used only if binary space partitioning is enabled. Larger tree depths reduce rendering time but increase memory consumption, and also slightly increase preprocessing time. The default is 24. If there are too many triangles in the scene to fit into the BSP tree with the size specified by `bsp size` and `bsp depth`, the `bsp size` value is disregarded and larger leaves are created. This slows down rendering significantly. Larger `bsp depth` values of 30, 40, or even 50 often massively improve rendering speed in BSP mode for larger scenes. The mental ray User's Manual discusses how to choose good parameters in detail.

`bsp memory` $memory_{int}$

The maximum memory in megabytes used in the BSP preprocessing. A value of zero indicates that there is no limit on the memory consumption, this is the default. This flag is useful only on multiprocessor machines since the memory consumption increases with the number of rendering threads. When the specified amount of allocated memory is reached, mental ray will prevent threads from being scheduled for preprocessing, thus reducing the memory requirements. The BSP tree itself is unaffected.

`raycl subdivision` $subdiv_{int}$ $subdiv\_2d_{int}$

If ray classification is enabled, mental ray uses a ray tracing algorithm that subdivides the space of all rays. The optimal subdivision is determined automatically by a built-in scene analysis. The `raycl subdivision` statement can be used to modify the result of this analysis: arguments of 0 leave the calculated subdivision unchanged, positive numbers increase and negative numbers reduce the subdivision. *subdiv* controls general subdivision; *subdiv_2d* controls primary (eye) and shadow rays. This option has no effect if the BSP or grid algorithms are used.

`raycl memory` $memory_{int}$

In ray classification mode, this statement sets the amount of memory to be used for acceleration data structures to *memory* megabytes on each CPU. It has no effect if the BSP or grid algorithms are used. mental ray allows presetting the amount of rendering acceleration memory independently of scene complexity without sacrificing speed. The default is set to 6 megabytes, which is sufficient for most scenes. Even for extremely large scenes, little can be gained from memory sizes greater than 12 megabytes. Note that this statement does not affect the amount of memory used for the scene description, which depends on the complexity of the geometry in the current frame.

`grid size` *size*$_{int}$

If the grid algorithm is used, this option adjusts the scene-dependent default grid voxel size. The default is 1.0. Larger values increase the number of voxels and shrink each voxel accordingly. Smaller voxels are faster to render because they contain fewer triangles to be tested, but larger numbers of voxels require more memory and long rays pass through more voxels that need to be tested.

2.7.1.7 Feature Disabling

`lens on|off`

Ignore all lens shaders if set to `off`. The default is `on`.

`volume on|off`

Ignore all volume shaders if set to `off`. The default is `on`.

`geometry on|off`

Ignore all geometry shaders if set to `off`. The default is `on`.

`displace on|off`

Ignore all displacement shaders if set to `off`. The default is `on`.

`output on|off`

Ignore all output shaders if set to `off`. The default is `on`. File output statements are not affected. Note that all five disable options also affect shaders installed by phenomena. This means that the phenomenon can fail if it installs cooperating shaders that rely on each other's existence, and one of them is disabled with these options. Phenomenon writers must allow for this case. The purpose of these options is fast preview rendering.

`merge on|off`

Ignore all merge epsilons and all connections in the scene.

2.7.1.8 Caustics

`caustic on|off`

Caustics are turned on or off. They are off by default. Caustics are lighting effects caused by specular focusing of light rays, such as the irregular light patterns on the floor of a swimming pool. Note that caustics are only computed for light sources that specify an energy explicitly. The material shader that receives the caustics must also cooperate, and either the options block or the object to receive caustics must have appropriate `caustic` flag set.

`caustic accuracy` *N* [*R*]

This option controls how caustics are estimated from the photon maps during rendering. The photon map is searched outwards from the intersection point and the photons that are encountered are examined. *N* specifies the maximum number of photons that should be examined, and *R* specifies the maximum radius that is searched for photons. If *N* is zero, the number of photons is only limited by *R*. The default for *N* is 100. If *R* is zero, a scene-size dependent radius is used instead. This is the default.

`caustic filter box|cone` [*filter_const*]

Filtering controls the sharpness of the caustics. Specifying a cone filter with the default *filter_const* of 1.1 generally has the effect that the caustics in the model looks sharper. Increasing the *filter_const* makes the caustics more blurry and decreasing makes it even sharper but also slightly more noisy. The *filter_const* must be larger than 1.0.

`photon trace depth` $reflect_{int}$ [$refract_{int}$ [sum_{int}]]

This option is similar to the `trace depth` option except that it applies to photons, not rays. The *reflect* parameter limits the number of recursive reflection photons. If it is set to 0, no photons will be reflected, if it is set to 1, one level is allowed but a photon cannot be reflected again, and so on. Similarly, *refract* controls the maximum depth of refracted photons. Additionally, it is possible to limit the sum of reflected and refracted photon levels with *sum*. Note that custom shaders may override these values.

`photonmap file "`*filename*`"`

Tells mental ray to use the file *filename* for the photon map. If the photon map file does not exist, it is created and the photon map is saved. If it exists, it is loaded and used without computing a new photon map.

`photonmap rebuild on|off`

If a filename is specified for the photon map (using the `photonmap` *filename* option) it is normally loaded and used if the file exists. If the `photonmap rebuild` option is turned on, any existing file will be ignored, and the photon map will be recomputed and an existing file will be overwritten. The default is off.

2.7.1.9 Global illumination[2.1]

`globillum on|off`

Global illumination[2.1] is turned on or off. The default is off. Global illumination permits effects such as indirect lighting, color bleeding, etc. See the mental ray User's Manual for details. Note that global illumination is computed only for light sources that have an energy specified explicitly; see section 2.7.5 for details. The material shader that receives global illumination must also cooperate.

`globillum accuracy` N $[R]$
: This option controls how the photon map is used to estimate the intensity of global illumination. For a more detailed discussion of how this works, see the `caustic accuracy` option above. The default values are $N = 500$ and $R = 0.0$. For fast previews of global illumination, it can be useful to set N to 100.

`photonvol accuracy` N
: This option controls how the photon map is used to estimate the intensity of caustics or global illumination within a participating medium. It applies to photon volume shaders, which compute light patterns in 3D space, such as volume caustics created by focused shafts of light cast by objects acting as lenses. The details are similar to what is described for the `caustic accuracy` option above. The default values are $N = 30$ and $R = 0.0$.

`photon trace depth`, `photonmap`, and `photonmap rebuild on|off` have the same meaning as for caustics.

`finalgather on|off`
: Final gathering[2.1] for global illumination is turned on or off. The default is off. Final gathering means that when the illumination is computed at a diffuse point, the hemisphere above the point is sampled for indirect illumination. The illumination at those points is then computed as direct illumination plus a contribution from the photon map if global illumination is on. Final gathering is best suited for scenes with slow variation in indirect illumination, for example purely diffuse scenes. Final gathering eliminates the low-frequency variation in the global illumination that can often be seen if too few photons are used. Performance is kept acceptable by reusing and interpolating nearby final gathers. (Without final gathering, global illumination is computed by direct lookup in the photon map at the point — similar to the way caustics are computed.)

`finalgather accuracy` N $[R_1$ $[R_2]]$
: N controls how many rays should be used in each final gathering step to compute the indirect illumination. The default is 1000. Increasing this number makes the indirect illumination less noisy but also increases the rendering time. R_1 is the maximum radius in which a final gather result can be interpolated or extrapolated. The default maximum radius is computed based on the scene extent. R_2 is the distance within a final gather result must be used for interpolation or extrapolation. The default is 10% of the maximum radius.

2.7.1.10 Frame Buffer Control

`colorclip rgb|alpha|raw`[2.1]

This option controls how colors are clipped into a valid range [0, 1] before being written to a non-floating point frame buffer or file. The `rgb` mode is the default. In this mode, RGB is first clipped to [0, 1] and alpha subsequently to $[max(R, G, B), 1]$. In `alpha` mode, alpha is first clipped to [0, 1] and RGB subsequently to $[0, A]$. In `raw` mode, RGB and A are both clipped to [0, 1] independently of each other. In all modes, the RGB components are clipped as specified by the `desaturate` option. The `rgb` and `alpha` modes ensure that the resulting color is a valid premultiplied color. `rgb` should be used if the alpha channel is considered less important than preserving the RGB color and intensity. `alpha` mode is intended for alpha compositing, where the alpha channel is more important than the absolute color value to preserve correct transparencies. `raw` mode should only be used if no layering based on alpha is going to take place. This mode also forces the `premultiply` mode to `on`. It should be used with care because shaders might receive "illegal" colors (colors that cannot be composited in standard ways).

`desaturate on|off`

If a color is output to a frame buffer that does not have 32-bit (floating-point) precision, and its RGB components are outside the range $[0, max]$, mental ray will clip the color to this legal range. If desaturation is turned off, the individual components are simply clipped into range. Otherwise, mental ray tries to maintain the brightness of the color by moving it towards the grayscale axis of the color cube, until the RGB components are in the legal range. *max* is determined by the `colorclip`[2.1] mode. Desaturation is turned off by default.

`premultiply on|off`

Premultiplication means that colors are stored with alpha multiplied to R, G, and B. For example, white at 10% opacity is not stored as (1, 1, 1, 0.1) but as (0.1, 0.1, 0.1, 0.1). This is the standard method in computer graphics to represent colors; mental ray always uses it internally and in all shaders. One implication is that R, G, and B can never exceed A. mental ray normally enforces this when storing color values into frame buffers. The `premultiply off` option instructs mental ray to always store colors *unpremultiplied* into frame buffers and files. It does this by undoing the internally applied premultiplication. (mental ray internally always works with premultiplied colors to present a uniform interface to shaders; since this is done with floating-point values there is no precision penalty.) This option is ignored if the `colorclip raw`[2.1] mode is in effect.

`dither on|off`

mental ray supports 8, 16, or 32 bits per color component. In some cases, 8 bits per pixel, as supported by all popular picture file formats, can cause visible banding when the floating-point color values calculated by the material shader are quantized to the 8-bit values used in the picture file.

Dithering mitigates the problem by introducing noise into the pixel such that the round-off errors are evened out. Note that this can cause run-length encoded picture files to be larger than without dithering. Dithering is turned off by default.

`gamma` *gamma_factor*

Gamma correction can be applied to rendered color pixels to compensate for output devices with a nonlinear color response. All R, G, B, and alpha component values are raised to 1*overgamma_factor*. The default gamma factor is 1.0, which turns gamma correction off.

`frame buffer` *n* ["*type*"]

Define or delete user-defined frame buffer[2.1]*n*. Up to eight user frame buffers are supported, numbered 0 through 7. The frame buffer type *type* may be any standard image type allowed in an output statement, such as rgba or `z`. If the type is prefixed with a "+" sign, samples are interpolated; if prefixed with a "-" sign, it is padded. Padding is the default for all types. For example, `+rgba_fp` is an interpolated floating-point color frame buffer. After a frame buffer is defined, it may be used as the type `fb`*n*, with *n* in the range 0...7, in output statements in cameras. The frame buffer is created in memory during rendering only if it is referenced by at least one output statement.

2.7.1.11 Scene Geometry

`camera space`

All geometry is expected to be defined in camera space. Camera space assumes that the camera is at the coordinate origin (0, 0, 0) and looks down the negative Z axis. This means that geometry will typically have negative Z coordinates. This is the default. In camera space mode, instance transformations have no effect.

`object space`

All geometry is expected to be defined in object space. Each object, light, and camera has its own coordinate space, typically but not necessarily with the coordinate origin (0, 0, 0) in the center of the object. The object coordinate coordinate space is positioned and oriented in world space with the instance transformation matrix (every object, light, and camera requires an instance). Object space allows multiple instancing where the object is placed in the scene more than once using multiple instance entities.

2.7.1.12 Contours

`contour store` *shader*

If the camera contains a contour output statement (see the mental ray User's manual, contour rendering is enabled and a contour store shader must be defined. This function stores information about the future contour edge, such as color, depth, normal, and other local information that is later used by the contour contrast shader to decide where the contour lines should be drawn, and by contour shaders to decide which colors and thicknesses the contours should have. Shader lists are not allowed here.

`contour contrast` *shader*

If contour rendering is enabled, a contour contrast shader must also be defined. It decides where the contour lines should be drawn based on values stored by contour store shaders. The contrast shader compares two such value sets at a time. See the mental ray User's Manual for details. Shader lists are not allowed here.

2.7.1.13 Diagnostic Modes[2.1]

`diagnostic grid off|object|world|camera` S[2.1]

Draws a colored grid on all objects in the scene visualizing the coordinate space given. The distance between grid lines is S units. This is useful to estimate the size and distances between objects and to visualize the object space of objects. The `off` argument turns this mode off.

`diagnostic photon off|density|irradiance` N[2.1]

When using photon maps, this mode replaces all material shaders in a scene with an internal shader that produces a false-color rendering of photon density, or the average of the red, green, and blue irradiance components. Photon density is the number of photons per unit surface area. N is the density (or irradiance) that is assigned to 100%, or red. The colors are, from 0% to 100%: blue, cyan, green, yellow, and red. Higher values fade to white. N can be given as zero in which case the appropriate maximum is automatically found. This mode is useful when tuning the number of photons in a photon map and setting the various `accuracy` options, since the density (or irradiance) is estimated using those settings. The `off` argument turns this mode off.

`diagnostic samples on|off`[2.1]

This mode replaces the rendered image with a grayscale image showing the number of image samples made for each pixel. A black pixel has had no samples, whereas a white pixel has had the maximum amount as specified with the `-samples` option. In addition, a red grid is drawn indicating task boundaries. Samples that lie exactly on pixel boundaries are considered to belong to the lower and/or left pixel. This mode is useful when tuning the `samples` and the `contrast` options for optimal effect.

2.7.1.14 Miscellaneous

`face front|back|both`

The *front* side of a geometric object in the scene is defined to be the side its normal vector points away from. By specifying that only front-facing triangles are to be rendered, speed can be improved because fewer triangles need to be tested for a ray. This works well unless there are objects whose back side is seen by refracted or reflected rays – with `face front`, the back side would not be visible. The default is `face both`, and works best if volume effects are used, which usually depend on closed volumes.

`task size` $size_{int}$

This option specifies the size of the image tasks during rendering. Smaller task sizes are convenient for previewing, but also increase the overall rendering time. This option can also be used in order to optimize load balancing for parallel rendering. If the `task_size` is not specified, an appropriate default value is used. Note that very small task sizes can cause the scanline algorithm to perform poorly and in such cases it may be desirable to turn it off. See `scanline` above.

`inheritance "`*function_name*`"`

To use parameter inheritance, a user-provided inheritance shader must be specified. The *function_name* is the name of a C function linked to mental ray using a `link` command. No user-defined parameters are passed. The inheritance shader is called for every pair of instances of which one is the parent (one level higher up in the scene DAG) of the other. The inheritance shader must compute a set of inherited parameters from the parameters stored in these two instances. It is called even for the instances that contain no parameters and for top-level instances; in this case the corresponding parameter argument pointer is zero. Inheritance shaders are not regular shaders; they are usually written by translator writers who need to emulate the inheritance methods used by the language to be translated.

2.7.2 Cameras

```
camera "name"
    camera_statements
end camera
```

A camera describes a view of the scene, including the list of files to write, the lens shaders to use, volume shaders to be used as the global atmosphere or fog, global environment shaders that control what happens to rays that leave the scene, and other parameters. Cameras are scene entities that need to be placed in the scene with an instance element. In object space mode (see `options` element above), the location of the camera in world space is determined by the camera instance transformation. Note that the camera instance must be attached to the root instance group of the scene. See below for information on instance groups.

Cameras contain output statements that specify output shaders and output files to write to disk, and control which frame buffers mental ray creates and maintains during rendering. More than one output file can be created, and output shaders such as filters can be listed that operate on the final rendered image, before it is written to a picture file. *outputs* is one or more output statements. Output statements are very similar to shader lists, like lens shader statements, but the syntax is different to allow type specifications and output file names:

```
output ["datatype"] "filetype" [options] "filename"
output "datatype" "shader_name" (parameters)
```

The first kind writes a picture to a file named *filename*, using the file format *filetype*. Normally, file formats imply a data type, but the defaults can be overridden by naming an explicit *datatype*. For example, the file type `"rgb"`, which stands for a SGI RGBA image file, implies the data type `"rgba"`.

The *options* specify additional format related parameters. Currently, the `"jpg"` file format supports one option `quality`[2.1] *q*, where *q* is an integer value between 0 and 100. Lower values force higher lossy compression resulting in lower image quality. A quality value of 0 will cause the use of the default quality 75.

The second kind of output statement calls an output shader, such as a filter, that may operate on all available frame buffers. Here, the *datatype* may be a comma-separated list of types if the shader requires multiple frame buffers. Each type can be prefixed with a "+" or "-" to turn interpolation on or off. Interpolation is averaging for color, depth, and normal images and max'ing for label images. Interpolation is on by default for the standard color frame buffer and off by default for all others. For example, a shader that filters the standard RGBA image with a filter whose size depends on the distance of objects needs both the interpolated RGBA buffer and the interpolated depth buffer, and would have a data type `"rgba,+z"`. mental ray creates all types of frame buffers requested by at least one output statement of either kind.

The data types `"fb0"` through `"fb7"` refer to user frame buffers[2.1] 0...7. User frame buffers are defined in the options statement using `frame buffer` statements. The actual data type of `fb`*n* is the type of frame buffer *n*. For example, the output statements

```
output "+rgba" "rgb"  "file1.rgb"
output "fb0"   "ctfp" "file2.ct"
```

write the standard frame buffer to the image file `file1.rgb`, and then write the contents of user frame buffer 0 to the image file `file2.ct`. This assumes that the options block contains a statement that defines user frame buffer 0, such as:

```
frame buffer 0 "+rgba_fp"
```

User frame buffers are empty unless some shader writes to them during rendering. Their purpose is to collect nonstandard image data during rendering, and making the data available for output shading and image file writing.

A special data type `"contour"` can be specified that enables contour rendering. Special contour output shaders must be specified that pick up the contour information from the contour cell frame buffer and compute a color image, which it can either put into the regular color frame buffer, or composite on top of the color frame buffer. In the latter case, one rendering phase creates a color image with contours. The color frame buffer can then be written to an image file using a regular image output statement. There is also a built-in contour output shader that creates a PostScript file instead of a color image. See the Contour chapter in this manual for details and examples.

There is a variety of *camera_statements* that can be listed in the camera. Some of them can be overridden by specifying an appropriate command-line option; see appendix 5.

There are four camera statements that accept shader lists: `output`, `lens`, `volume`, and `environment`. As with all types of shaders, more than one shader can be listed, or more than one such statement can be given, to attach multiple shaders (or output files in the case of the `output` statement) to each type. In an incremental change (the `incremental` keyword is used before the `camera` keyword), each of the four first resets the list from the previous incremental change and does not add to the existing list, as multiple statements inside the same `camera` ... `end camera` block would.

The following *camera_statements* are supported:

`focal` *distance* | `infinity`

The focal distance is set to *distance*. The focal distance is the distance from the camera to the viewing plane. The viewing plane is the plane that the rendered scene is projected onto; its edges correspond to the edges of the rendered image. A common approach is to set the focal distance to the middle distance of the interesting objects in the scene and then set the aperture such that it is a bit larger than the horizontal extent of the objects in camera space. If `infinity` is used in place of the *distance*, an orthographic view is rendered. An orthographic view turns off perspective, all camera rays are parallel. View-dependent surface tessellation is not possible in orthogonal mode.

`aperture` *aperture*

The aperture is the width of the viewing plane. The height of the viewing plane is *aperture* divided by *aspect*. Together with the `focal` and `aspect` *viewdefs*, `aperture` defines the lens of the standard pinhole camera.

`aspect` *aspect*

This is the aspect ratio of the camera. The default is 1.33. In camera space, *aperture* is the width of the viewing plane and *aperture* divided by *aspect* is the height. The viewing plane is divided into pixels as specified by the `resolution` *viewdef*, so the aspect will result in nonsquare pixels if it is not equal to the X resolution divided by the Y resolution. For example, to render a PAL image at a resolution of 720×576 pixels, at an image ratio of 3:4 as defined by the PAL standard, pixels are slightly wider than tall, by a factor of $\frac{576}{720} \cdot \frac{4}{3} = 1.0667$. If the aspect ratio is corrected by this number, objects will appear undistorted on a PAL video display (but not on a computer display with square pixels).

`resolution` x_{int} y_{int}
: Specifies the width and height of the output image in pixels.

`offset` *x y*
: Specifies an offset[2.1] for the rendered image. The default is 0.0 for both values, which means that the image will be centered on the camera's Z axis. Positive values translate the image up and to the right. The *offset* is measured in pixel units.

`window` x_low_{int} y_low_{int} x_high_{int} y_high_{int}
: Only the sub-rectangle of the image specified by the four bounds will be rendered. All pixels that fall outside the rectangle will be left black.

`clip` *hither yon*
: The *hither* (near) and *yon* (far) planes are planes parallel to the viewing plane that delimit the rendered scene. Points outside the space between the hither and yon planes will not be rendered (this does not apply to the infinite-radius environment maps because they are not geometric objects). The `clip` statement specifies the distance of the hither and yon planes from the camera. The defaults are 0.0001 for the hither distance and 1000000.0 for the yon plane.

`volume` [*shader_list*]
: This statement specifies volume (atmosphere) shaders. The atmosphere affects all rays passing through the space outside objects by attenuating the color of the ray. It is possible to specify a volume shader for the inside of objects too, by naming a volume shader in the `material` statement (see above). If no *shader_list* is specified, the existing volume shader list is deleted; this is useful in incremental changes. If a list is given, it replaces the current list if this is the first `volume` statement in the camera block, or it is appended to the current list otherwise.

`environment` [*shader_list*]
: This statement specifies environment shaders. Environment shaders control the color returned by primary rays that, after leaving the camera, never strike any object in the scene. They are similar to environment shaders named in materials, which control reflection rays cast by the material shader that leave the scene without striking another object (or exceeding the trace depth). If no *shader_list* is specified, the existing volume shader list is deleted; this is useful for incremental changes. If a list is given, it replaces the current list if this is the first `volume` statement in the camera block, or it is appended to the current list otherwise.

`lens` [*shader_list*]
: Lens shaders simulate lenses by changing the camera. If no lens shader is

present, the camera is a pinhole camera that casts rays from the origin in all directions that strike the viewing plane, or an orthographic camera that casts parallel rays if `focal infinity` is specified. A lens shader accepts the origin and direction of the camera ray, modifies them, and casts a new primary ray. Examples for lens shaders includes fish-eye lenses that exaggerate the direction vector in a nonlinear way (there is a code example in the Shader section). Multiple lenses can be specified in the camera; the n-th lens shader receives the origin and direction computed by the $n-1$st lens shader. If no *shader_list* is specified, the existing volume shader list is deleted; this is useful in incremental changes. If a list is given, it replaces the current list if this is the first `volume` statement in the camera block, or it is appended to the current list otherwise.

`frame` $frame_{int}$ [*time*] [`field` $field_{int}$]

Every camera should contain the current frame number *frame*. The time in seconds can optionally be specified as *time*. Optionally, a field number *field* can be specified; by convention, *field* should be `0` when rendering frames, 1 when rendering the first (odd) field, and 2 when rendering the second (even) field. If the `field` modifier is missing, the *field* number defaults to `0`. mental ray currently does not use any of these values but makes them available to shaders.

2.7.3 Textures

`scalar texture "`*texture_name*`"` `[`$width_{int}$ $height_{int}$ [$depth_{int}$] `]` *bytes* ...
[`local`] [`filter` [*scale_const*]] `scalar texture "`*texture_name*`" "`*filename*`"`
`scalar texture "`*texture_name*`"` *shader_list*

`color texture "`*texture_name*`"` `[`$width_{int}$ $height_{int}$ [$depth_{int}$] `]` *bytes* ...
[`local`] [`filter` [*scale_const*]] `color texture "`*texture_name*`" "`*filename*`"`
`color texture "`*texture_name*`"` *shader_list*

`vector texture "`*texture_name*`"` `[`$width_{int}$ $height_{int}$ `]` *bytes* ...
[`local`] `vector texture "`*texture_name*`" "`*filename*`"`
`vector texture "`*texture_name*`"` *shader_list*

Textures are lookup functions. They come in two flavors: lookups of two-dimensional texture or picture files or literal bytes, and procedural lookups. File textures require a file name parameter or a byte list; procedural textures require a shading function parameter. There are three types of texture functions: textures computing scalars, colors, and vectors. Which one is chosen depends on what the texture is used for. Textures are used as parameters to other shaders, typically material shaders. A material shader could, for example, use a color texture to wrap a picture around an object, or a scalar texture as a transparency or displacement map, or a vector texture as a bump map. The actual use of the texture result is entirely up to the shader that uses the texture.

All of the above syntax variations define a texture *texture_name*. The *texture_name* should be quoted to avoid reserved words and to allow non-alphabetic characters. This is the name that the texture will later be referenced as.

Non-procedural textures can be defined by specifying the *width* and *height* of the texture and an optional *depth* (bytes per component, 1 or 2, default is 1), followed by a list of *width* × *height* × *depth* hexadecimal two-digit bytes, most significant digit first if *depth* is 2, in RGBA order for colors and UV order for vectors. Note that the brackets around the sizes are literally part of the `.mi` file, while the skinny brackets around *depth* denote that the depth is optional and are not part of the `.mi` file.

Non-procedural textures can also be defined by naming a texture or picture file. For a list of allowed file formats, see the section on Available Output File Formats. In this case, the sizes (width, height, and depth) are read from the file. If the `local` keyword is not present, the file is read once on the client host and then transmitted over the network to all server hosts that participate in the rendering. With the `local` keyword, only the file name is transmitted to the server hosts; this requires the file exists locally on all server hosts but reduces network transfer times drastically if many texture files or very large texture files are used. Filename rewriting is available for interpreting the remote filename locally, for example to translate between Unix and Windows NT paths. Maximum speed improvements are achieved if local files reside on physical disks and not on NFS-mounted file systems (NFS stands for Network File System, distinguishable by the `nfs` type in the output of the Unix `df` command).

The `filter` keyword, if present, enables texture filtering based on texture pyramids, a technique comparable to mip-map textures. during rendering. Filtered textures are preprocessed before rendering begins and use approximately 30% more memory. Filtering should be used when the texture is large and seen at a distance, such that every sample covers many texture pixels. Without filtering, widely spaced samples "overlook" the areas between the samples; filtered textures perform a filter operation to take the skipped areas into account. The compression of the texture on the viewing plane can be scaled by the optional *scale* value if necessary.

When loading a texture image, it is checked whether the texture is memory-mappable. This is the case if the texture file has the special uncompressed `.map` format. If this is the case, the texture is not loaded into memory but mapped into virtual memory. Memory-mapped textures use far less physical RAM and no swap space, but they use virtual memory. Memory mapping is especially useful for large textures that are not used often (i.e., many or most of its pixels are not sampled or the textured object is small or far away from the camera), but is recommended for all nontrivial texture images. Memory-mapped textures are implicitly also local textures.

Procedural textures are defined by naming a shading function with parameters; the shading function can either be one of the built-in functions or an external function from a `code` or `link` command.

When the material shader (or any other shader) evaluates a texture by calling a texture evaluation function, the program either looks up non-procedural shaders by looking up the texture in the range [0, 1) in each dimension, or it calls the named shader in the procedural case. The shader is free to interpret the point for which it evaluates the texture in any way it wants, two-dimensional or three-dimensional.

2.7.4 Materials

```
material "material_name"
    [opaque]
    shader_list
    [displace [shader_list]]
    [shadow [shader_list]]
    [volume [shader_list]]
    [environment [shader_list]]
    [contour [shader_list]]
    [photon [shader_list]]
    [photonvol [shader_list]]
end material
```

Materials determine the look of geometric objects. They are referenced by *material_name* in the geometry definition in `object` statements (see below). Lights and textures cannot be referenced by objects; they are referenced by the material which uses them to compute the color of a point on the object's surface. All built-in material shaders accept textures and light instances as shader parameters.

When a primary ray cast from the camera hits an object, that object's material shader (the first, mandatory, *shader_list*) is called. The material shader then calculates a color (and certain other optional values such as labels, depths, and normals that can be written to special output files). This color may then be modified by the optional volume shader if present. The resulting color is stored in the output frame buffer, which is written to the output picture file when rendering has finished. In order to calculate the color, the material shader may cast secondary reflection, refraction, or transparency rays, which in turn may hit objects and cause other (or the same; multiple objects may share a material) material shaders to be called. The material shader bases the decision whether to cast secondary rays on its parameters, which are part of the scene description and may contain parameters such as the material's diffuse color or its reflectivity and transparency, light instances, and textures. The parameters depend entirely on the material shader. In this sense, material shaders are "primary" shaders that get help from "secondary" texture and light shaders.

It is possible to specify a shader type such as `shadow` without following it with a *shader_list*. This is useful if an incremental change is done to the material. The incremental change leaves the contents of the material undisturbed except where explicitly rewritten, so the shadow shader list remains intact. It can be replaced by specifying a new one, but it can only be deleted with a `shadow` keyword not followed by any shaders. In an incremental change, the first statement (say, `volume`) first resets the old volume list; every subsequent `volume` statement in the same material block adds to the list.

The *material_name* should be quoted to avoid conflicts with reserved names and non-alphabetic characters. The `opaque` flag, if present, informs mental ray that this material is not transparent (i.e., it does not cast refraction or transparency rays and always sets its alpha result value to 1); this allows certain optimizations that improve rendering speed. The material shader and its parameters are the only mandatory part of a material.

There are several optional functions that can be listed in a material. The displacement shader is a function returning a scalar that displaces the object's surface in the direction of its normal, or in arbitrary directions. Displacement shaders can be applied to both free-form surface objects and polygonal objects.

The shadow shader is called when a shadow calculation is done, and the shadow ray from the light source towards the point in shadow intersects with this material. The shadow shader then changes the color of the ray, which is initially the (possibly attenuated) color of the light to another color, typically a darker or tinted color if the material is colored glass. It returns black if the material is totally opaque, which is also the default if no shadow shader is present. Shadow shaders are usually reduced versions of the material shaders; they evaluate transparencies and colors but cast no secondary rays. Shadow shaders are only required for transparent objects. If global illumination is enabled, no shadow shaders should be used because global illumination provides a more powerful way to compute light transmission, and using two "competing" methods at the same time for the same object may produce incorrect results. This is explained in more detail in the mental ray User's Guide.

It is possible to use the material shader as a shadow shader; material shaders can find out whether they are called as material or shadow shaders and do only the required subset in the latter case. This is done by naming the material shader after the `shadow` keyword, and giving no parameters (i.e., giving `()`). mental ray will notice the absence of parameters and pass the material parameters instead. If the shadow shader has no parameters of its own, it is not defined whether it receives a pointer to the material shader parameters, or a pointer to a copy of the material shader parameters.

A volume shader affects rays traveling inside an object. Volume shaders are conceptually similar to fog or atmosphere shaders of other rendering programs. When a ray (either from the eye or from a light source) hits this material, the volume shader, if present, is called to change the color returned by the ray based on the distance the ray has traveled, and atmospheric or material parameters. A volume shader can also be named in the `camera` (see above); that shader is used for rays traveling outside objects. It is the material shader's responsibility to determine inside and outside of objects.

The environment shader is called when a reflection or refraction ray cast by the material shader leaves the scene entirely without striking another object. For example, the environment shader may map a texture on a sphere with an infinite radius surrounding the scene. (This is another example for an application of a texture; a texture name must be used as a parameter for the environment shader for this to work.) The `camera` statement also allows naming an environment shader; that shader is used when the ray leaves the scene without ever striking any object (or exceeding the trace depth).

If a contour shader is given, it is called when contours are enabled with an appropriate output statement in the camera element, and certain contour store and contour contrast shaders are specified in the options element. For more information on contour rendering see chapter 2.8.

If caustics or global illumination[2.1] computation is enabled, the photon shader is called during a preprocessing stage (before rendering) to determine the light distribution in the scene. Like shadow shaders, photon shaders without parameter lists are called with the material shader parameter lists. See the mental ray User's Guide for details.

A volume photon shader affects photons traveling inside an object. When a photon hits this material, the volume photon shader, if present, is called to trace the photon through the volume. Volume photon shaders are to volume shaders what photon shaders are to material shaders.

Materials can be replaced with phenomena. In all places where the name of a material may be given, the name of a shader that references a phenomenon declaration of type `material` is legal. Given the following scene fragment:

```
declare phenomenon
     material "phen_mtl" (color "param")
     material "mtl" opaque
          "shader" ("diffuse" = interface "param")
     end material
     root material "mtl"
end declare

shader "mtl_sh" "phen_mtl" ("param" 1.0 0.7 0.3)
```

the name `mtl_sh` can be used like a *material_name*, for example in polygon or free-form surface definitions in objects. For more information on material phenomena, see section 2.5.

Note that there are three ways to use material shaders in a scene:

- Every polygon and surface in an object specifies a material. They can be omitted but default to the previous polygon or surface in the object, but this is only a syntactical simplification. Effectively, every polygon and surface brings its own material, and no material inheritance takes place.
- If the object is marked `tagged`, polygons and surfaces do not specify materials but integer labels. In this case the inherited material in the instance is used. That material can use *mi_query* to obtain the label and modify its behavior based on the label.
- As a variation of the previous method, the instance may specify not a single material but a list of materials. In this case, mental ray will use the n-th material in the list if the label of the intersected primitive is n (or the first material if the label is greater than or equal to the number of materials in the list).

See section 2.7.9 for more details on material lists and material inheritance.

2.7.5 Lights

Lights have a large number of optional parameters that are used if global illumination, caustics or shadow maps are enabled. These techniques use a preprocessing step that analyzes how light travels through the scene. Lights that participate in this preprocessing stage must specify a number of extra parameters. For clarity, regular lights and more specialized lights are shown separately:

```
light "light_name"
    shader_list
    [ area_light_primitive ]
    [ origin x y z ]
    [ direction dx dy dz ]
    [ spread spread ]
    [ visible ]
end light
```

```
light "light_name"
    shader_list
    [ emitter shader_list ]
    [ area_light_primitive ]
    [ origin x y z ]
    [ direction dx dy dz ]
    [ spread spread ]
    [ visible ]
    [ tag label_int ]

    [ energy r g b ]
    [ exponent exp ]
    [ caustic photons store_int [ emit_int ]]
    [ globillum photons store_int [ emit_int ]]

    [ shadowmap [ on|off ]]
    [ shadowmap resolution res_int ]
    [ shadowmap samples num_int ]
    [ shadowmap softness size ]
    [ shadowmap file "filename" ]
end light
```

This statement defines a light source. All light sources need a light shader, such as the *mib_light_point* shader in the base shader library, or another shader linked with a `code` or `link` command (see above). "*shader*" above stands for the quoted name of the shader. Like any other shader, a parameter list enclosed in parentheses must be given. The parameters depend on the particular shader; they include the light color, attenuations, and spot light directions. The declaration of the shader determines which parameters are available in the *parameters* list; see chapter 2.1 for details on shader parameters. mental ray distinguishes three kinds of light shaders: point lights, giving off light in all directions; directional (infinite) lights, whose light rays are all parallel in a particular direction, and spot lights which emit light from a point along a certain direction. Point lights must define an `origin` but no `direction`, while directional lights must define a `direction` but no `origin`. Spot lights must define an `origin`, a `direction`, and a `spread`. The spread defines the maximum angle of the cone defined along the direction in which the spot produces illumination. The value of *spread* is the cosine of this maximum angle; it must be between 0 (infinitely thin) and 1 (hemisphere). Spot lights often use a directional attenuation, but this is purely a function of the shader that is independent of the `spread` and `direction` keywords in the light definition. All types of lights can be turned into area light sources.

After the definition, the light source can be instanced with an `instance` statement that references *light_name*. The instance can then be referenced in parameter lists of shaders (such as a material shader) by listing the light instance name. Material shaders normally have an array parameter accepting one or more light instances, which they loop over to accumulate the contribution by each light (unless they rely solely on the global light list). Light instances are one of the standard data types that are available for shader parameters. The *light_name* should be quoted to avoid clashes with predefined words, and to allow non-alphabetic characters.

Any point or spot light may be turned into an area light source by naming an *area_light_primitive*. Area light sources generate soft shadows because shadow-casting objects may partially obscure the light source. Four types of area light primitives are supported:

`rectangle` [x_0 y_0 z_0 x_1 y_1 z_1 *sampling*]
`disc` [*x y z radius sampling*]
`sphere` [*radius sampling*]
`cylinder` [*axis radius sampling*]

The common *sampling* substatement is optional:

[*u_samples v_samples* [*level* [*low_u_samples low_v_samples*]]]

All three area light types are centered at the *origin* position in the light definition. A rectangular area light is specified by two vectors from the center to two edges; a disc area light is specified by its normal vector and a radius; a sphere area light is specified only by its radius; and a cylinder area light is specified by its axis and radius. Note that the orientation of the rectangle, disc, or cylinder are independent of the *direction* and any directional attenuation the shader applies, although both will generally be similar. Also note that the end caps of the cylinder are not sampled.

The *u_samples* and *v_samples* parameters subdivide the area light source primitive. For discs and spheres, *u_samples* subdivides the radius and *v_samples* subdivides the angle. For a cylinder, *u_samples* subdivides the height and *v_samples* subdivides the angle. When sampling the area light source, mental ray samples one point in each subdivision at a location precisely determined by the sample parameters and a predefined lighting distribution, and then combines the results. The default is 3 for each sample parameter, so an area light source without explicitly given *samples* parameters is sampled 9 times.

If the optional *level* exists and is greater than 0, then mental ray will use *low_u_samples* and *low_v_samples* instead of *u_samples* and *v_samples*, respectively, if the sum of the reflection and refraction trace level exceeds *level*. The defaults for the low levels are 2. The effect is that reflections and refractions of soft shadows are sampled at lower precision, which can improve performance significantly. Since shaders have control over the trace level in the state, they can influence the switching depth, which can be used to sample soft volume shadows less precisely, for example.

If the rectangle, disc, sphere, or cylinder keyword is specified without any of the following arguments, then the light source reverts to a non-area light source. This is useful for incremental changes.

Light sources are by default invisible. However, area lights can be made visible by adding a `visible` flag to the light. Any `visible` flags on non-area lights are ignored since they have zero size. Light visibility cannot be inherited from the instance.

A label integer can be attached to a light using the `tag` statement. Labels are not used by mental ray in any way, but a shader can use the *mi_query* function to obtain the label of a light and perform light-specific operations.

The second light form is for caustics and global illumination[2.1]. It requires specification of the light energy. The light energy is given as an RGB triple to allow colors, but the RGB values are typically much higher than the usual 0...1 range for colors. The number of photons emitted from this light source in the preprocessing step is determined by *store*, and the number of emitted photons is determined by *emit*, if specified. When either limit is reached, photon emission stops. If *store* is 0, *emit* must be specified and storing is unlimited (this requires mental ray 2.1.37 or later). Physical correctness demands an $\frac{1}{r^2}$ power law for energy falloff, causing the energy received from a light source to fall off with the square of the distance to the light source. However, the `exponent` parameter allows modification of the power law to $\frac{1}{r^{exp}}$. For any *exp* other than 2, physical correctness is lost, but for achieving certain looks it is often useful to use *exp* values between 1 and 2 to reduce the falloff, and better approximate classical local illumination non-physically correct lights.

For caustics, one can specify a *caustics photons* value that controls the number of caustic photons stored during caustics preprocessing. Similarly, a *globillum photons* value can be specified for global illumination. Typical values range from 10,000 to 100,000; larger values improve accuracy and reduce blurriness.

Shadow maps are controlled per light source using the information about the light source type and the information provided by the shadow map keywords. Shadow maps are supported for spot lights with a cone-angle less than 90 degrees (i.e. *spread* > 0), for directional lights, and for point lights. A shadow map is activated for a light source by specifying the `shadowmap` keyword. The resolution of the shadow map which controls the quality and also the amount of memory used is specified with the `shadowmap resolution` keyword, which specifies the width and height of the shadowmap depth buffer in pixels. The `shadowmap softness` and `shadowmap samples` keywords determine the type of shadow produced with the shadow map; if the softness is zero a sharp shadow is generated. If softness is larger than zero, `shadowmap samples` different samples will be taken from the shadowmap, on a square region the size of `shadowmap softness`. This will make the boundaries of the shadows appear softer.

The softness is specified in internal space units on the shadow map projection plane. For directional lights, an orthographic projection is used, so the softness will be constant in the scene, the soft region having roughly the given softness value in size. For other lights, because of the projective projection used, apparent softness will increase with distance from the light. This means that much smaller softness values are usually required for spot lights than directional lights. If an excessively high softness value is specified, a warning will be given during rendering. Very high values tend to blur the shadow out of existence. The number of samples determines the quality of the soft shadow and in general the number of samples should be increased when the softness is increased.

The `shadowmap file` statement can be used to specify a shadow map file in which the shadow map will be saved the first time it is rendered, and subsequently loaded every times it is used. In the case of point lights, six different files will be saved, each for a different direction (the resolution of each file will be lower so that the total number of pixels rendered will be approximately *resolution* × *resolution*). If objects in the scene move, the old shadow map files should be deleted to prevent loading and re-using outdated shadow maps. If the filename contains the `#` character, it will be expanded by mental ray into a hash code number identifying the transformation of the light instance. This is useful when a light is multiply instanced, because it allows distinguishing between files representing multiple instances of the same light. However, the user must take care to remove obsolete files or they will eventually fill all available disk space.

For spot light sources, the extent of the shadow map is determined by the *spread* parameter. For directional light sources, the extent of the shadow map is determined by the extent of the parts of the scene that cast shadows. For example, in a scene with small objects on a large background polygon, the small objects casting shadows should have a `shadow` flag, while the background polygon should not. Then the extent of the shadow map will only cover the small objects that cast shadows. If the large background polygon also has the `shadow` flag, the extent of the shadow map will be larger, and the shadow map will lack detail at the small objects where detailed shadows are needed.

2.7.6 Objects

All geometry is specified in either camera space or object space, depending on the corresponding statement in the options statement (see section 2.7.1). In camera space mode, the camera is assumed to sit at the coordinate origin and point down the negative Z axis, and objects are defined using camera space coordinates. In object space mode, the camera location is determined by its instance, and objects are defined in local object coordinates that are positioned in the scene with its object instance. Every object, camera, and light requires an instance.

The appearance of the object, such as color and transparency, is determined by naming materials in the object definition. Before a material can be used in an object, it must be defined. Naming the material determines all aspects of the object's appearance. No further parameters, textures, or lights need to be specified; they are all part of the material definition.

The two most common approaches to materials and objects are to name all materials first and then all objects, which may simplify the implementation of material editors because all materials may be put in a separate file and then included in the `.mi` file using a `$include` command; or materials and objects may be interspersed. Either way, each material definition precedes its first use.

All polygonal and free-form surface objects have the same common format in the `.mi` file:

```
object "object_name"
    [ visible   [on|off] ]
    [ shadow    [on|off] ]
    [ trace     [on|off] ]
    [ tagged    [on|off] ]
    [ caustic   [on|off] ]
    [ globillum [on|off] ]
    [ caustic   [mode] ]
    [ globillum [mode] ]
    [ tag label_number_int ]
    [ basis list ]
    group
        [ merge epsilon ]
        vector list
        vertex list
        geometry list
        approximation list
    end group
    ...  # more groups
end object
```

The individual parameters are:

- The `object` name *object_name* serves to uniquely identify the object. The name is not used by mental ray in any form except to give meaningful progress reports and error messages. Object names should be enclosed in double quotes to disambiguate them from reserved words.
- The `visible` flag causes the object to be visible. Most objects will have this flag set. Not setting it will make the object invisible to primary rays (those originating from the camera), which means it will disappear from the image. The optional boolean argument defaults to 'on'.
- The `shadow` flag causes the object to cast shadows. The standard case is specifying both the `visible` and `shadow` flags. If an object is very complex, it may be desirable to set only the

visible flag but not the shadow flag, and create a second object that resembles the first one but is much simpler and set the shadow but not the visible flag on it. The effect is that the object appears unchanged, but shadow calculations see a much simpler shadow object that casts approximately the same shadow as the primary visible object would.

- The trace flag serves a similar purpose as the shadow flag. Normally, it is always set along with the visible and shadow flags. It controls whether the object is visible to secondary (reflected or refracted) rays. If the reflecting or refracting objects are fuzzy or only slightly reflective or refractive, it may result in a considerable speedup to make the reflection and refraction rays see a much simpler object than primary rays would. Like with the shadow flag, this is achieved by not setting the trace flag in the primary, high-definition object, and create a second one that roughly resembles the primary object that has the trace flag (and perhaps the shadow flag) but not the visible flag set.

- The tagged flag changes the way geometry is stored. Normally, every polygon, surface, and triangle comes with its own optional material. If an object specifies no materials, the material is inherited from the instance. Objects marked tagged do not store materials at all and always rely on the inherited instance material, and permit specifying a non-optional label integer in place of the material in polygon and surface definitions. (Non-optional means that a tagged object *must* contain one label integer for every polygon and surface.) This label can be accessed by shaders during rendering (i.e. not in displacement or output shaders) using the miQ_GEO_LABEL mode of the *mi_query* function. The idea is that a shared material distinguishes parts of the object by label integer, instead of attaching a different material to each polygon or surface.

- The caustic flag[2.1] lets the object participate in optimized generation of caustics. A caustic is an illumination effect caused by light that undergoes specular reflections or refractions before it hits a diffuse object. For example a water surface casts irregular light patterns on the floor of a swimming pool. To simulate this effect, the material shader of the floor object must be written to pick up caustic light, and the light source must contain a caustic photon statement and contain appropriate photon energy settings. For optimized caustic generation, the options should specify caustic 0 and the water surface and floor objects must have the caustic flag set. Refer to the Caustics chapter in this manual for details.

  The *mode* argument controls the caustic operation: 1 enables caustic casting, 2 enables caustic receiving, 3 enables both, and 0 neither. off means that the object is invisible to caustic photons, and 'on' is the same as 3. In the pool example, the water surface should have mode 1 and the floor should have mode 2. If the caustic keyword is given without *mode* argument, the mode defaults to on (that is, 3). If no caustic keyword is given, caustics default to mode 0.

- The globillum flag[2.1] lets the object participate in optimized generation of global illumination. Global illumination is an illumination effect caused by diffuse interreflection, such as a red table bleeding red color onto an adjacent white wall. To simulate this effect, the material shader of both the table and the wall must specify photon shaders, the wall object material shader must be written to pick up global illumination light, and the light source must contain appropriate photon energy settings. For optimized global illumination simulation, the options should specify globillum 0 and the red table and white wall must have the globillum flag set. Refer to the mental ray User's guide for details.

  The *mode* argument controls the global illumination mode: 1 enables global illumination casting, 2 enables global illumination receiving, 3 enables both, and 0 neither. The default is specified by the options. `off` means that the object is invisible to global illumination photons, and `on` (the default) enables global illumination interactions with this object. In the table example, the red table should have (at least) mode 1 and the white wall should have (at least) mode 2. If the `globillum` keyword is given without *mode* argument, the mode defaults to 3).

If an object is very complex, it may be desirable to set only the `visible` flag but not the `globillum` flag, and create a second object that resembles the first one but is much simpler and set the `globillum` but not the `visible` flag on it. The effect is that the object appears unchanged, but simulation of global illumination is faster since a simpler object is used.

- The `tag` specifies an arbitrary 32-bit number that identifies the object. mental ray normally uses the term *label*, but the keyword `tag` is retained for backwards compatibility. The term *tag* is used by mental ray to identify entries in the scene database; this is of concern only to shader writers. By specifying an appropriate `output` statement in the `camera` (see above), it is possible to cause mental ray to write a label file that, for each pixel, contains the label code of the object that the camera ray hits first. Exactly which label is stored is under the control of the material shader; using the label of the foremost object regardless of reflections and refractions is merely the default behavior.

- The *basis list* is a list of bases to be used in free-form surface descriptions. Only curves and surfaces use bases. For a list of supported bases, see section 2.7.8.1. The defined bases can be used in all groups that follow, until the end of the object.

- Finally, a list of object groups contains the actual geometric representation. The decision whether to put all geometry into a single object group or to use different groups for different geometric entities is of importance only for free-form surfaces. If two surfaces appear in the same group, they may be connected if the appropriate `connect` statements are used (see below) or if adjacency detection (edge merging) takes place. Surfaces in different groups cannot be connected. Connecting surfaces means that they will be approximated such that there is no crack between them; they will form one continuous combined surface in the range of the connection. The merge *epsilon* that can be specified in the group determines the maximum gap between two surfaces that still leads to the automatic connection of both surfaces. The smaller the epsilon, the closer any two surfaces must be to become merged. The results of automatic edge merging depends on a judicious choice of the merge epsilon. By default, the merge epsilon is 0.0, so no edge merging is computed. Generally, it is recommended to use only a single object group in any object and create multiple objects instead because mental ray will split multigroup objects into multiple single-group objects internally anyway, and explicit objects allow more control.

  At the end of each object group, approximation statements can be given that control the tessellation method. They are valid for both polygonal and free-form surface object groups. In polygonal object groups, the approximation is used only for polygons whose material contains a displacement shader. Free-form surfaces are always controlled by their approximations; see page 110 for details.

The `visible`, `shadow`, `trace`, `caustic`, and `globillum` flags can be overridden by the instance using the standard inheritance mechanism. Instances can specify that a flag in the instanced object is turned on or off, or that it is left unchanged. The object flags are used only if all the instances from the root of the scene DAG down to the object all leave the flag unchanged.

Object groups contain the actual geometry. All geometry needs *vector lists* and *vertex lists*. The *vector list* contains 3D vectors that can describe points in space, normals, texture vertices, basis vectors, motion vectors, and others. Vectors are anonymous, they are triples of floating-point numbers separated by whitespace without inherent meaning. They are numbered beginning with `0`. Numbering restarts at `0` whenever a new object group starts.

mental ray also accepts a compressed binary format for vectors. Instead of three floating-point numbers, a sequence of 12 bytes enclosed in backquotes is accepted. These 12 bytes are the memory image of three floats in IEEE 854 format, using big-endian byte order. This format is intended for increasing translation and parsing speed when ray is connected to a native translator; it should not be used in files modified with text filters. Many filters and editors refuse to accept files containing binary data, or corrupt them.

Vertices build on vectors. In the `.mi` format, there is no syntactical difference between polygon vertices and control points vertices for free-form surfaces; both are collectively referred to as "vertices" in this discussion. All vertices define a point in space and optional vertex normals, motion vectors, derivatives, zero or more textures and basis vectors, and user vectors:

 `v` $index_{int}$
[`n` $index_{int}$]
[`d` $index_{int}$ $index_{int}$ [$index_{int}$ [$index_{int}$ $index_{int}$]]]
[`t` $index_{int}$ [$index_{int}$ $index_{int}$]]
[`m` $index_{int}$]
[`u` $index_{int}$
 ...

Polygon vertices may use all of these. Free-form surface control points may use `v` and `m` only; the others are either computed analytically or are specified in other ways as part of the surface definition.

`v` specifies the point in space,

`n` specifies the vertex normal (ignored when the vertex is used as a curve or surface control point),

`m` specifies the motion vector (the distance the point moves during the shutter open time specified in the `options` statement), and

`t` specifies a texture vertex with an optional X/Y basis vector pair for bump map calculation. There can be up to 64 `t` lines for any given `v` vertex. (The texture and basis vectors are ignored when the vertex is used as a curve or surface control point. Texture and basis information for surfaces is defined using a "texture surface", described below.)

`d` specifies a first and/or second surface derivative. First derivatives describe the UV parametric gradient of a surface; second derivatives describe the curvature. mental ray can compute surface derivatives analytically for free-form surfaces but not for polygons because polygons have no inherent UV coordinate space. Therefore, the d keyword must be used to define explicit surface derivatives for polygons. If d is followed by two indices they are taken to reference the first derivative $d\vec{P}du$ and $d\vec{P}dv$ (with P being the point in space); if three indices follow they are taken to reference the second derivative $d^2\vec{P}du^2$, $d^2\vec{P}dv^2$, and $d^2\vec{P}dudv$; and if five indices follow the first two describe the first derivatives and the next three the second derivatives. Derivatives are not used by mental ray, they are made available to shaders only.

u specifies a user vector. No constraints are imposed on user vectors. mental ray does not operate on them in any way, they are passed through with the vertex and can be picked up by the shader.

Every vertex begins with a v statement and ends with the next v statement or with the start of the geometry description. All occurrences of *index* above reference the vector list; 0 is the first vector in this group. References of different types (for example, v and n) may not reference the same vector. As stated before, all vectors are 3D. If the third coordinate is not used (as is the case for 2D texture vertices, for 2D curve control points, and for 2D surface special points) it should be set to 0.0 by convention. If both the second and third coordinates are unused (as is the case for 1D curve special points), they should both be set to 0.0.

Vertices themselves are numbered independently of vectors. The first vertex in every group is numbered 0. The geometry description is referencing vertices by vertex index, just like vertices are referencing vectors by vector index. This results in a three-stage definition of geometry:

1. List of vectors
2. List of vertices
3. List of geometry

The reason for this three-stage process is that it allows both sharing vectors and sharing vertices. This is best illustrated with an example. Consider two triangles ABC and ABD sharing an edge AB. (This example will use the simplest form of polygon syntax that will be described later in this section.) The simplest definition of this two-triangle object is:

```
object "twotri"
    visible
    group
        0.0  0.0  0.0
        1.0  0.0  0.0
        0.0  1.0  0.0
        1.0  0.0  0.0
        1.0  1.0  0.0
        0.0  1.0  0.0


        v 0
```

```
        v 1
        v 2
        v 3
        v 4
        v 5

        p "material_name" 0 1 2
        p 3 4 5
    end group
end object
```

The first three vectors are used to build the first three vertices, which are used in the first triangle. The remaining three vectors build the next three vertices, which are used for the second triangle. Two vectors are listed twice and can be shared:

```
object "twotri"
    visible
    group
        0.0  0.0  0.0
        1.0  0.0  0.0
        0.0  1.0  0.0
        1.0  1.0  0.0

        v 0
        v 1
        v 2
        v 1
        v 3
        v 2

        p "material_name" 0 1 2
        p 3 4 5
    end group
end object
```

The order of vector references is noncontiguous to ensure that the second triangle is in counterclockwise order. Two vertices are redundant and can also be removed by sharing:

```
object "twotri"
```

```
    visible
    group
        0.0  0.0  0.0
        1.0  0.0  0.0
        0.0  1.0  0.0
        1.0  1.0  0.0


        v 0
        v 1
        v 2
        v 3


        p "material_name" 0 1 2
        p 1 3 2
    end group
end object
```

The need for sharing both vectors and vertices can be shown by specifying vertex normals:

```
object "twotri"
    visible
    group
        0.0  0.0  0.0
        1.0  0.0  0.0
        0.0  1.0  0.0
        1.0  1.0  0.0
        0.0  0.0  1.0


        v 0  n 4
        v 1  n 4
        v 2  n 4
        v 3  n 4


        p "material_name" 0 1 2
        p 1 3 2
    end group
end object
```

In this last example, both vector sharing and vertex sharing takes place. The normal is actually redundant: if no normal is specified, mental ray uses the polygon normal. Defaulting to the polygon normal is slightly more efficient than interpolating vertex normals, if vertex normals are explicitly specified.

Two types of geometry can be contained in the *geometry list*, polygonal geometry and free-from surfaces. In the next sections the syntax of the definitions of polygonal geometry and free-form surfaces is described and illustrated by examples.

An object group permits only one type of geometry, either polygons or surfaces but not both. It is recommended that objects contain only a single object group, so normally objects are either polygonal or surface objects but not both at the same time. Also, vector sharing is supported only for vectors of similar types (point in space, normal, motion, texture, basis vector, derivative, or user vector. A vector may not be referenced by vertices once as a point in space and once as a normal, for example.

2.7.7 Polygonal Geometry

Polygonal geometry consists of polygons. For efficiency reasons, mental ray distinguishes simple convex polygons from general concave polygons or polygons with holes. Both are distinguished by keyword:

c ["*material_name*"] *vertex_ref_list*
cp ["*material_name*"] *vertex_ref_list*
p ["*material_name*"] *vertex_ref_list*
p ["*material_name*"] *vertex_ref_list* hole *vertex_ref_list* ...

If the enclosing object has the `tagged` flag set, mandatory label integers must be given instead of the optional materials:

c *label_number*$_{int}$ *vertex_ref_list*
cp *label_number*$_{int}$ *vertex_ref_list*
p *label_number*$_{int}$ *vertex_ref_list*
p *label_number*$_{int}$ *vertex_ref_list* hole *vertex_ref_list* ...

The `c` keyword selects convex polygons without holes. The results are unpredictable if the polygon is not convex. The `cp` keyword is a synonym for `c` for backwards compatibility; `c` should be used in new translators. The `p` keyword also renders concave polygons correctly, and allows specification of holes, using one or more `hole` keywords, each followed by a *vertex_ref_list*. If all polygons within the same object group are simple convex polygons containing three sides (i.e. triangles), mental ray will pre-process them in a more efficient manner than non-triangular polygons.

A *vertex_ref_list* is a list of non-negative integers *index* that reference vertices in the vertex list of the group described in the previous section. The first vertex in the vertex list is numbered 0.

Any vertex index can be used in both polygon and hole *vertex_ref_lists*. A polygon with *n* vertices is defined by *n* index values in the vertex list following the material name. The order of the polygon vertices is important. A counter-clockwise ordering of the vertices yields a front-facing polygon. The vertex list of a hole may be ordered either way. Any polygon violating this rule, for example because it has been displaced such that its new normal points the wrong way, causes the error message "orientation of triangles inconsistent" and the surface to be dropped.

The material name must have been defined before the object definition that contains the polygon definition, in a statement like

> material "*material_name*"
>
> ...
>
> end material

In both cases, it is recommended to quote the material name to avoid conflicts with reserved words, and to allow arbitrary characters in the name. For a detailed description of material definitions, see section 2.7.4. Once a material name has been specified for a polygon, it becomes the default material. All following polygons may omit the material name. Polygons without explicit material use the same material as the last polygon that does have an explicit material. Not specifying materials improves parsing speed because no names must be looked up in the symbol table.

If no material is specified, polygons remain without material; in this case the material from the closest instance up the scene DAG is used instead. This is called material inheritance. Tagged objects always inherit their material from the instance. It can distinguish polygons by using the `miQ_GEO_LABEL` mode of the *mi_query* function during rendering (not in displacement shaders).

The tessellation of polygons assumes that polygons are "reasonably" planar. This means that every polygon will be tessellated, but the exact subdivision into triangles does not attempt to minimize curvature. If the curvature is low, different tessellations cannot be distinguished, but consider the extreme case where the four corners of a tetrahedron are given as polygon vertices: the resulting polygon will consist of two triangles, but it cannot be predicted which of the four possible triangles will be chosen.

The behavior will be different for convex polygons without holes (c keyword) and polygons which contain holes or are concave (p keyword). Convex polygons without holes are triangulated by picking a vertex on the outer loop and connecting it with every other vertex except its direct neighbors. If polygons are not flagged with the c keyword but do not have any holes an automatic convexity test is performed and if they are indeed convex they are triangulated as described. Convex polygons with holes and concave polygons are triangulated with a different algorithm. In any case a projection plane is chosen such that the extents of the projection of the bounding box of the (outer) loop have maximal size. If the projection of the polygon onto that plane is not one-to-one the results of the triangulation will be erroneous.

If a textured polygon's material contains a displacement map the vertices are shifted along the normals accordingly. If an approximation statement is given triangles are subdivided until the specified criteria are fulfilled; see section 2.7.8.8 for details.

2.7.8 Free-Form Surface Geometry

Free-form surfaces are polynomial patches of any degree up to twenty-one.[5] Supported basis types include Bézier, Taylor, B-spline, cardinal, and basis-matrix form. Any type can be rational or non-rational. Patches can be explicitly or automatically connected to one another, or may be defined to contain explicitly defined points or curves in their approximation. Various approximation types including (regular) parametric, spatial, curvature-dependent, view-dependent, and combinations of these. Surfaces may be bounded by a trimming curve, and may contain holes.

Surface geometry, like polygonal geometry, is defined by a series of sections. An object containing only surface geometry follows this broad outline:

```
object "object_name"
    [ visible   [on|off] ]
    [ shadow    [on|off] ]
    [ trace     [on|off] ]
    [ tagged    [on|off] ]
    [ caustic   [on|off] ]
    [ globillum [on|off] ]
    [ caustic   [mode] ]
    [ globillum [mode] ]
    [ tag label_number_int ]
    [ basis list ]
    group
        [ merge epsilon ]
        vector list
        vertex list
        [ list of curves ]
        surface
        [ list of surface derivative requests ]
        [ list of texture or vector surfaces ]
        ... # more surfaces
        [ list of approximation statements ]
        [ list of connection statements ]
    end group
    ... # more groups
end object
```

[5]The algorithms used impose no inherent limit. The limit may be increased in future versions.

Curves, surfaces, approximations, and connections may be interspersed as long as names are defined before they are used. For example, a curve must come before the surface it is trimming, and an approximation must come after the surface to be approximated. Texture and vector texture surfaces must always directly follow the surface they apply to. The individual sections are:

- The *basis list* must be specified at the beginning of the object definition, just before the group begins. Bases defined in this section are referenced by name in the curve and surface definitions to specify their degrees and types (Bézier, B-spline, etc.).
- The *vector list* in the group is a list of (x, y, z) vectors used to build control points later. This section is the same as the vector section used to build vertices for polygonal geometry.
- The *vertex list* that follows the vector list builds control points out of the vectors. This also works like the vertex list for polygonal geometry, except that no normals and texture vertices can be defined here (i.e., no `n`, `t`, or `d` statements may appear). Normals are defined implicitly by the surface, and textures are defined by *texture surfaces* instead as described below. Surface derivatives are generated if `derivative` keywords are present. Rational curves and surfaces specify additional weights at each vertex reference (see below).
- *Curves* may be defined and used as trimming curves, hole curves, and special curves. This section is optional; if no trimming curve is defined surfaces are untrimmed and end at the boundaries specified by the ranges of the bases used. Trimming a surface means to cut away portions that fall outside an outer boundary curve; holes cut away portions inside the hole curve. Special curves are curves that are always included in the tessellation; they can be used to define features like sharp creases that need to be tessellated consistently. Surfaces may also be connected along trimming curves.
- The surface geometry list consists of `surface` statements, much like polygonal geometry that consists of `p` and `c` statements. A surface is defined by a `surface` statement, optionally followed by surface derivative request statements and one or more `texture surface` or `vector surface` statements.
- *Approximation* statements give additional information about how a surface and its trimming, hole, and special curves are to be approximated with triangles. Various modes such as parametric, regular parametric, curvature-dependent, and view-dependent approximations can be selected, along with the precision. If there are approximation statements in the `options` statement (see Options, Tessellation Quality above), they override any approximation statements in the objects.

For a description of vector lists and vertex lists, refer to page 89.

2.7.8.1 Bases

When surfaces and curves are present within an object group, it is mandatory that at least one basis has been defined within the object. Bases define the degree and type of polynomials (denoted by $N_{i,n}$ below) to be used in the description of curves or surfaces. Curves and surfaces reference bases by name. Every surface needs two bases, one for the U and one for the V parameter direction. Both can have a different degree, but must have the same type (for example, rational Bézier in U and Cardinal in V is not allowed). There are five basis types:

```
basis "basis_name" [rational] taylor degree_int
basis "basis_name" [rational] bezier degree_int
basis "basis_name" [rational] cardinal
basis "basis_name" [rational] bspline degree_int
basis "basis_name" [rational] matrix degree_int stepsize_int basis_matrix
```

A parametric representation may be either non-rational or rational as indicated by the `rational` flag. Rational curves and surfaces specify additional weights at each control point. This flag is optional; it can also be specified in the curves and surfaces that reference the basis.

The *degree* specifies the degree of the polynomials used in the description of curves or surfaces. Recall that the degree of a polynomial is the highest power of the parameter occurring in its definition. When bases of degree 1 are used control points are connected with straight lines. Cardinal bases always have degree 3. The degree and the type combined determine the length of the parameter vector and the number of control points needed for the surface. The meaning of the parameter vector differs for the different basis types. This is described in detail below.

The supported polynomial types for curves and surfaces are `bezier`, `bspline`, `taylor`, `cardinal` and `matrix`.

`taylor` specifies the basis functions:

$$N_{i,n}(t) = t^i$$

`bezier` specifies the basis functions:

$$N_{i,n}(t) = \binom{n}{i} t^i (1-t)^{n-i}$$

`cardinal` specifies third degree curves and surfaces . The Cardinal splines, also known as Catmull-Rom splines, are most easily formulated as a conversion from Bézier form. If we let $B_{i,3}(t)$ be the cubic Bézier basis functions (i.e., the above basis functions $N_{i,n}(t)$ with $n = 3$), then we may write the cardinal basis functions as

$$\begin{aligned}
N_{0,3} &= -\frac{1}{6}B_{1,3}(t) \\
N_{1,3} &= B_{0,3}(t) + B_{1,3}(t) + \frac{1}{6}B_{2,3}(t) \\
N_{2,3} &= \frac{1}{6}B_{1,3}(t) + B_{2,3}(t) + B_{3,3}(t) \\
N_{3,3} &= -\frac{1}{6}B_{2,3}(t)
\end{aligned}$$

`bspline` specifies a non-uniform B-spline representation whose basis functions are given by the following recursive definition:

$$N_{i,0}(t) = \begin{cases} 1 & \text{if } x_i \leq t < x_{i+1} \\ 0 & \text{otherwise} \end{cases}$$

and

$$N_{i,n}(t) = \frac{t - x_i}{x_{i+n} - x_i} N_{i,n-1}(t) + \frac{x_{i+n+1} - t}{x_{i+n+1} - x_{i+1}} N_{i+1,n-1}(t)$$

where, by convention, $0/0 = 0$. $(x_0, \ldots, x_q)$ is known as the knot vector. It must be specified through the parameter lists when using B-spline bases in curves and surfaces (see below).

A `matrix` $(b_{i,j})_{0 \leq i \leq n, 0 \leq j \leq n}$ specifies the basis functions:

$$N_{i,n}(t) = \sum_{j=0}^{n} b_{i,j} t^j$$

When a curve or surface is being evaluated and a transition from one segment or patch to the next occurs, the set of control points (the 'evaluation window') used is incremented by the *stepsize*. The appropriate *stepsize* depends on the representation type expressed through the basis matrix and on the degree.

Consider a curve with k control points $\{v_1, \ldots, v_k\}$. If the curve is of degree n, then $n+1$ control points are needed for each polynomial segment. If the *stepsize* is given as s, then the $(1+i)$th polynomial segment, will use the control points $\{v_{is+1}, \ldots, v_{is+n+1}\}$. For example, for Bézier curves $s = n$, whereas for Cardinal curves $s = 1$. For surfaces, the above description applies independently to each parametric dimension.

The *basis_matrix* specifies the basis functions used to evaluate a parametric representation. For a basis of degree n the matrix must be of size $(n+1) \times (n+1)$. The matrix is laid out in the order $b_{0,0}$, $b_{0,1}$, ... , $b_{0,n}$, ... , $b_{n,n}$. Note that the generalization to the rational case for all representations is admitted in all cases.

As an example, an object containing a nonrational Bézier surface of degree 3 in one parameter direction and degree 1 in the other parameter direction needs two bases defined at the beginning of the object like this:

```
object "mysurface"
    visible
    basis "bez1" bezier 1
    basis "bez3" bezier 3
    group
      ...
```

The surface definition will reference the two bases by their names, `bez1` and `bez3`.

2.7.8.2 Surfaces

A surface specifies a name and a list of control points. For both parametric dimensions it specifies a basis, a global parameter range, and a parameter list. Optionally, it specifies surface derivative requests, texture surfaces, trimming curves, hole curves, special curves and special points. Special curves and points are included as edges and vertices in the approximation (triangulation) of the surface.

surface "*surface_name*" "*material_name*"
"*u_basis_name*" *range u_param_list*
"*v_basis_name*" *range v_param_list*
hom_vertex_ref_list
[*derivative_request*]
[*texture_surface_list*]
[*surface_specials_list*]

If the enclosing object has the `tagged` flag set, a label integer must be given instead of a material name (see page 88). This changes the first line of the preceding syntax block to:

surface "*surface_name*" $label\_number_{int}$

The bases used in the definition of the surface must have been defined in the *basis list* of the object. They are referenced by their *basis_names*. Their *ranges* consist of two floating-point numbers specifying the minimum and maximum parameter values used in the respective direction.

The *parameter_lists* in the basis specifications define the number of patches of the surface and the number of control points. For bases of the types `taylor`, `bezier`, `cardinal` and `matrix` such a *parameter_list* consists of a strictly increasing list of at least two floating-point numbers. For `bspline` bases the *parameter_lists* specify the knot vector. If the B-spline basis to be used is of degree n the knot vector $(x_0, \ldots, x_q)$ must have at least $q + 1 = 2(n + 1)$ elements. Knot values represent a monotone sequence of floating-point numbers but are not necessarily strictly increasing, i.e. $x_i \le x_{i+1}$. Moreover, they must satisfy the following conditions:

(1) $x_0 < x_{n+1}$
(2) $x_{q-n-1} < x_q$
(3) $x_i < x_{i+n}$ *for* $0 < i < q - n - 1$
(4) $x_n \le t_{min} < t_{max} \le x_{q-n}$

where $[t_{min}, t_{max}]$ is the range over which the B-spline is to be evaluated. Equation (1) demands that no more than $n + 1$ parameters at the beginning of the parameter list may have the same value. Equation (2) is the same restriction for the end of the parameter list. Equation (3) says that in the middle of the parameter list, at most n consecutive parameters may have the same value. To generate closed B-spline curves, it is often necessary to write a parameter list where the first n and last n parameters in the list produce initial and final curve segments that should not become part of the curve; in this case equation (4) allows choosing a start and end parameter in the range bounded by the first and last parameter of the parameter list.

The number of control points per direction can be derived from the number of parameters p, the degree of the basis n, and the step size s. Their total number can be calculated by multiplying the numbers taken from the following table for each of the U and V directions.

`type`	min # of parameters	# of control points
`Taylor`	2	$(p-1)\cdot(n+1)$
`Bézier`	2	$(p-1)\cdot n+1$
`cardinal`	2	$p+2$
`basis matrix`	2	$(p-2)\cdot s+n+1$
`B-spline`	$2(n+1)$	$p-n-1$

Note that only certain numbers of control points are possible; for example, if the U basis is a degree-3 Bézier, the number of control points in the U direction can be 4, 7, 10, 13, and so on, but not 3 or 5. For B-spline bases of degree 3 the minimum number of parameters is 8 corresponding to 4 control points.

Each vertex reference in the *hom_vertex_ref_list* is an integer index into the vertex list of the current group in the object (index 0 is the first vertex). When the surface is rational, homogeneous coordinates must be given with the control points, by appending a floating-point weight to every vertex reference integer in the *hom_vertex_ref_list*. There are two methods for specifying weights: either a simple floating-point number that must contain a decimal point to distinguish it from an integer index, or the keyword `w` followed by a weight value that need not contain a decimal point. The `w` keyword method is recommended because it eliminates the requirement that numbers contain decimal points, so translators can use %g format specifiers. Weights are used only if the surface is rational and ignored otherwise. If a weight in a rational surface is missing, it defaults to 1.0.

The surface specials list is used to define trimming curves, hole curves, special curves, and special points (vertex references). A surface may be further modified by approximation and connection statements, as described below.

For example, an object with a simple degree-3 Bézier surface can be written as:

```
object "mysurface"
    visible
    basis "bez3" bezier 3
    group
        0.314772   -3.204608  -7.744229    # vector 0
        0.314772   -2.146943  -6.932366
        0.314772   -1.089277  -6.120503
```

```
            0.314772    -0.031611   -5.308641
            -0.660089   -2.650739   -8.465791    # vector 4
            -0.660089   -1.593073   -7.653928
            -0.660089   -0.535407   -6.842065
            -0.660089   0.522259    -6.030203
            -1.634951   -2.096869   -9.187352    # vector 8
            -1.634951   -1.039203   -8.375489
            -1.634951   0.018462    -7.563627
            -1.634951   1.076128    -6.751764
            -2.609813   -1.543000   -9.908914    # vector 12
            -2.609813   -0.485334   -9.097052
            -2.609813   0.572332    -8.285189
            -2.609813   1.629998    -7.473326

            v 0       v 1       v 2       v 3         # vertices
            v 4       v 5       v 6       v 7
            v 8       v 9       v 10      v 11
            v 12      v 13      v 14      v 15

            surface "surf1" "material"
                    "bez3"  0.0 1.0   0.0 1.0
                    "bez3"  0.0 1.0   0.0 1.0
                    0 1 2 3 4 5 6 7 8 9 10 11 12 13 14 15
        end group
    end object
```

First, 16 vectors are defined, each of which is used to build one vertex (control point). Next, a surface is defined that uses basis `bez3` for both the U and V parameter directions. Since the surface is built from only one 4×4 Bézier patch, the parameter vector after the basis range has only length 2. If there had been two patches in the U direction and three in the V direction, the bases would have been referenced as

```
"bez3"  0.0 1.0 0.0 0.5 1.0
"bez3"  0.0 1.0 0.0 0.33333 0.66667 1.0
```

Alternatively, the parameter vector may be given as

```
"bez3"  0.0 2.0 0.0 1.0 2.0
"bez3"  0.0 3.0 0.0 1.0 2.0 3.0
```

by changing the parameter range of the basis. This has no influence on the geometry of the surface, but generates UV texture coordinates in a different range (here, $[0.0, 2.0] \times [0.0, 3.0]$). However, a different parametrization does affect the texture surface range (see below), and the range of trimming, hole, and special curves (which do not define their own ranges but borrow the range from the surface they apply to).

The optional *surface_specials_list* that completes the surface definition is a sequence of trimming curves, hole curves, special curves, and special points as described in the next section.

2.7.8.3 Surface Derivatives

mental ray can automatically generate surface derivative vectors if requested. First derivatives describe the UV parametric gradient of a surface; second derivatives describe the curvature. They are computed and stored only if requested by *derivative_request* statements in the surface definition:

```
derivative number_int [number_int]
```

There can be one or more `derivative` statements that request first and/or second derivatives. Valid values for *number* are 1 and 2, for first and second derivatives, respectively.

mental ray does not use derivative vectors but makes them available to shaders. First derivatives are presented as two vectors ($d\vec{P}du$ and $d\vec{P}dv$, with P being the point in space); second derivatives are presented as three vectors ($d^2\vec{P}du^2$, $d^2\vec{P}dv^2$, and $d^2\vec{P}dudv$). This is the same format that can be explicitly given for polygonal data using the `d` keyword in vertices. Surfaces always compute the vertex derivatives analytically, explicit vertex derivatives given by `d` keywords are ignored.

2.7.8.4 Texture Surfaces

A plain `surface` statement defines the geometry of the surface. If a texture is to be mapped on the surface, it is necessary to include texture surfaces. A texture surface defines a mapping from raw UV coordinates to texture coordinates as used by shaders. A vector texture is a variation of a texture surface that additionally defines a pair of basis vectors; it is used for bump mapping.

The texture or vector texture directly following a surface defines texture space number `0`, the next defines texture space number 1, and so on, exactly like the first `t` statement after the `v` statement in a vertex used for building polygonal geometry defines texture space number `0`, the next `t` defines texture space number 1, and so on. Basically, texture and vector texture surfaces replace the `t` statements used by polygonal geometry, because attaching textures to control points that usually are not part of the surface is not useful.

Texture spaces is what ends up in the *state* → *tex_list* array where it can be accessed by texture shaders to decide which texture is mapped which way. Texture space `0` is the first entry in that array, which is used by the shader for the first texture listed in the texture list in the material definition. In general, there is one texture space per texture on a material, although shaders making nonstandard use of texture spaces could be written.

The syntax for texture surfaces is a simplified version of geometric surfaces. The *texture_surface_list* in the grammar summary at the beginning of the "Surfaces" section above expands to zero or more copies of the following block:

```
[ volume ] [ vector ] texture
    "u_basis_name" u_param_list
```

"*v_basis_name*" *v_param_list*
vertex_ref_list

Unlike geometric surfaces, no surface name and material name is given. Bases are given like in geometric surfaces. Texture surfaces use the ranges of the geometric surface they are attached to, they are not repeated in the texture surface basis statements. The *vertex_ref_list* follows the same rules as the geometric surface's *vertex_ref_list*. Texture surfaces have no specials such as trimming curves or holes.

The optional `volume` keyword in the texture surface definition disables seam compensation. It should be used for 3D textures where each texture vector should be used verbatim. If the `volume` flag is missing, the tessellator detects textures that span the geometric seam on closed surfaces, and prevents rewinding. Consider a sphere with a 2D texture that is shifted slightly in the U parameter direction: a triangle might have $u_0 = 0.0$ on one side and $u_1 = 0.1$ on the other side. If the texture is shifted towards higher u coordinates by 0.05, u_0 and u_1 will map to texture coordinates $t_0 = 0.95$ and $t_1 = 0.05$, assuming an otherwise normal UV mapping. Even though $u_0 < u_1$, $t_0 >> t_1$, causing a fast "rewind" of the texture. Seam compensation corrects t_1 to 1.05. This is undesirable for 3D textures, which should have the `volume` keyword set. Most problems with strangely shifted textures are caused by inappropriately used or missing `volume` keywords.

The optional `vector` keyword in the texture surface definition is a flag that causes bump basis vectors to be calculated during tessellation. This flag must be used if the texture surface is used for a bump map; all built-in shaders supporting bump maps expect such a pair of bump basis vectors.

For a geometric surface S that maps parameters (u, v) into an object's coordinates (x, y, z) and a texture surface T that maps the same parameters into texture coordinates (s, t), the bump map basis vectors are the derivatives

$$\partial(S \circ T^{-1})/\partial s \partial(S \circ T^{-1})/\partial t$$

of the composite map $S \circ T^{-1}$ from the texture coordinates into object coordinates. They are not normalized and not necessarily orthogonal to each other.

The normal perturbation as suggested by Blinn (see [Watt 92] sec. 6.4, pp. 199–201) is given by

$$\begin{aligned} lclD &= M' - M \\ &= (\partial H/\partial s)A - (\partial H/\partial t)B \end{aligned}$$

with

$$\begin{aligned} lclA &= N \times \partial(S \circ T^{-1})/\partial t \\ B &= N \times \partial(S \circ T^{-1})/\partial s \end{aligned}$$

where

$$N = M/\|M\|$$

is the normalized surface normal with

$$M = \partial(S \circ T^{-1})/\partial s \times \partial(S \circ T^{-1})/\partial t$$

and H a height field defining the bump map, usually the intensity of the picture stored in the texture.

This is an example for the simplest of all texture surfaces, a bilinear mapping:

```
object "mysurface"
    visible
    basis "bez1" bezier 1
    basis "bez3" bezier 3
    group

        # ... 16 vectors used for the surface
        0.0  0.0  0.0          # vector number 16
        0.0  1.0  0.0          # vector number 17
        1.0  0.0  0.0          # vector number 18
        1.0  1.0  0.0          # vector number 19

        # ... 16 vertices used for the surface
        v 16                   # vertex number 16
        v 17                   # vertex number 17
        v 18                   # vertex number 18
        v 19                   # vertex number 19

        surface "surf1" "material"
            "bez3"    0.0 1.0    0.0 1.0
            "bez3"    0.0 1.0    0.0 1.0
            0 1 2 3 4 5 6 7 8 9 10 11 12 13 14 15

        texture
            "bez1"    0.0 1.0
            "bez1"    0.0 1.0
            16 17 18 19
    end group
end object
```

This texture surface defines a bilinear mapping from the UV coordinates computed during surface tessellation to the texture coordinates. To define other than bilinear mappings, the texture surface needs to have more control points than just one at every corner of the surface. Whenever the surface tessellator generates a triangle vertex, it uses the UV coordinate of that vertex to look up the texture surface and interpolate the texture coordinate from the nearest four points of the texture surface. The resulting texture coordinate is stored with the vertex and becomes available in *state* $\rightarrow$ *tex_list* when the material shader is called because a ray has hit the surface.

If more than one texture surface is given, one texture coordinate is computed for each texture surface and stored in sequence in the generated triangle vertices. Each texture surface is said to define a "texture space". They are available in the *state* $\rightarrow$ *tex_list* array in the same order. The number and order of texture surfaces should agree with the number and order of textures given in the texture list in the material definition. (Note that not all material shaders support multiple textures.)

If the material name of a surface is empty (two consecutive double quotes), the surface uses the material from the closest instance (this is called material inheritance).

2.7.8.5 Curves

Curves are two-dimensional parametric curves when they are referenced by surfaces. They are used as trimming curves, hole curves, and special curves. They must be defined before the surface which references them. Curves are three-dimensional parametric curves when referenced by space curves. A curve is defined as:

```
curve "curve_name" "basis_name"
    parameter_list
    hom_vertex_ref_list
    [ special special_point_list ]
```

The *parameter_list* of a curve is a list of monotonically increasing floating-point numbers that define the number of segments of the curve and the number of control points. Curve parameter lists work very much the same way as surface parameter lists except that no range needs to be provided, because they are supplied by the surfaces that reference the curve under consideration as explained in the next section. For details on parameter lists, see the sections on bases and surfaces above.

Each vertex reference in the *hom_vertex_ref_list* is an integer index into the vertex list of the current group in the object (index 0 is the first vertex), optionally followed by the keyword `w` and a weight value. (For backwards compatibility, the `w` keyword may be omitted if the weight is a floating-point value containing a decimal point.) Weights are used only if the curve is rational, they are ignored otherwise. If a weight in a rational curve is missing, it defaults to 1.0. The vertices indexed by the integers in the *hom_vertex_ref_list* should have no normals or textures (no `n` and `t` statements), and the third component of the vector (`v` statement) should be 0.0 because curves are defined in UV space, not 3D space.

The optional *special_point_list* specifies points that are included in the approximation of the curve. After the `special` keyword, a sequence of integers follows that index into the vertex list, just like the integers in the *hom_vertex_ref_list*. The first component of the vector is used as the t parameter; it forces the point on the curve at parameter value t to become part of the curve approximation. Of course t must be in the range of parameters allowed by the surface definition.

2.7.8.6 Trimming, Hole, and Special Curves; Special Points

A surface may reference curves to trim the surface, to cut holes into it, and to specify "special curves" that become part of the tessellation of the surface. Special points in surfaces work like special points in curves, except that they provide a point in the parameter range of the surface, that is, a two-dimensional UV coordinate, rather than a one-dimensional curve parameter. They specify single points on the surface that are to be included in the tessellation. As all curves and points are in UV space, the third component of the vectors provided for them is ignored. None of the above types of curves and points may exceed the range of (0.0, 1.0) at any point.

No two curves may intersect each other, and no curve may self-intersect. This is an important point because trimming curves and holes that are not closing or intersecting themselves or other loops can produce unexpected tessellation results.

Trimming, hole, and special curves and special points are defined at the end of the surface definition. The curves are composed of segments from the list of curves of the surface's group. The *surface_specials_list* given in the previous section is a list of zero or more of the following four items:

```
trim      "curve_name" min max
          ...
hole      "curve_name" min max
          ...
special   "curve_name" min max
          ...
special   vertex_int
          ...
```

The dots indicate that each trim, hole, and special statement may be followed by more than one curve segment or vertex, respectively. All listed segments are concatenated to form a single curve.

The *vertex* integers specify vertices from the vertex section of the current group in the current object. Such a vertex specifies the UV coordinate of the special point that is to be included in the tessellation.

Each of the three types of curves references a curve that has been defined earlier with a `curve` statement. If a single `trim`, `hole`, or `special` statement is followed by more than one curve, the resulting trimming, hole, or special curve is pieced together by concatenating the given curves. The *min* and *max* parameters allow using only part of the curve referenced. *min* and *max* must be in the range of the parameter vector of the curve which in turn must be mapped into the parameter range of the surface. The *min* and *max* parameters of two different curve pieces are independent, they only depend on the curve parameter lists. For example, a trimming curve can be built from two curves, using the first three quarters of the first curve and the last three quarters of the second curve:

```
curve "trim1"
        "bez1" 0.0 1.0 2.0 3.0 4.0
        0 1 2 3 4

curve "trim2"
        "bez1" 0.0 1.0 2.0
        3 5 0

surface "patch1" "mtl"
        "bez3" 0.0 1.0        0.0 1.0
        "bez3" 0.0 1.0        0.0 1.0
        6 7 8 9 10 11 12 13 14 15 16 17 18 19 20 21
        trim "trim1" 0.0 3.0
             "trim2" 0.5 2.0
```

Both trimming curves use the basis `bez1`, which is assumed to be a degree-1 linear curve. Hence, `trim1` connects the UV vertices 0, 1, 2, 3, and 4 with straight lines, and `trim2` connects the vertices 3, 5, and 0. If these two curves are put together by the `trim` statement in the surface definition, all parts of the surface that fall outside the polygon formed by the UV vertices 0, 1, 2, 3, and 5 are trimmed off. The `trim2` curve includes vertex 0 to close the trimming curve. Holes and special curves are constructed exactly the same way. Trimming curves and holes must form closed loops but special curves are not restricted in this way.

Note that trimming and hole curves must be listed in the correct order, outside in. If there is an outer trimming curve, it must be listed first, followed by the holes. If a hole has a hole, the inner hole must be listed after the outer hole. Since curves may never intersect, there is always an unambiguous order - if a curve A encloses curve B, A must be listed before B. Curves that do not enclose one another can be listed in any order.

This example omits the vector and vertex parts of the group in the object. Here is an example that defines a complete object containing a surface with a trimming curve that precisely follows the outer boundary. A trimming curve that follows the outer surface boundary does not actually clip off any part of the surface, but it is still useful if surfaces are to be connected, because connections work on trimming curves.

```
object "mysurface"
    visible
    basis "bez1" bezier 1
    basis "bez3" bezier 3
    group

        # ... 16 vectors used for the surface
        0.0  0.0  0.0    # vector number 16
        1.0  0.0  0.0    # vector number 17
```

```
            1.0  1.0  0.0     # vector number 18
            0.0  1.0  0.0     # vector number 19

            # ... 16 vertices used for the surface
            v 16              # vertex number 16
            v 17              # vertex number 17
            v 18              # vertex number 18
            v 19              # vertex number 19

            curve "trim1"
                "bez1" 0.0  0.25  0.5  0.75  1.0
                16  17  18  19  16

            surface "surf1" "material"
                ...
                trim "trim1"  0.0  1.0
        end group
    end object
```

The trimming curve in the example is linear, using a degree-1 Bézier basis. This means that the parameter vector has five equally-spaced parameters, one for each corner in counter-clockwise order and back to the first corner to close the trimming curve. Trimming and holes always require a closed curve or sequence of curves (they can be pieced together by multiple curves as long as the pieces form a closed loop together). The results are undefined if trimming or hole loops are not closed, or intersect.

If the trimming curve would be a degree-3 Bézier going through four corner points, a parameter vector with $3 \cdot 5 + 1 = 16$ parameters would be required (again, the 5 is the number of corners visited including the return to the first to close the curve).

For details on the parameter vector following the basis name in the definition of the curve, refer to section 2.7.8.5. The bases and parameter vectors for curves and surfaces follow the same rules, except that curves have no explicit range; they always use the implicit range given by the parameter list.

2.7.8.7 Space Curve Geometry

Unlike trimming curves, space curves[2.1]are defined in 3D space. A space curve object may not contain any other type of geometry, such as free-form surfaces or polygons. Space curves are not rendered but serve as input geometry for modeling operations, by passing the space curve object as a parameter to a geometry shader. The curve geometry is defined as a list of space curves, each referencing multiple curve segments.

An object containing space curve geometry follows this outline:

object "*object_name*"
  [tag *label_number*$_{int}$]
  [*basis list*]

```
    group
        [ merge epsilon ]
        vector list
        vertex list
        [ list of curves ]
        space curve
        [ list of curve segment references ]
    end group
    ... # more groups
end object
```

A single space curve definition follows this outline:

```
space curve         "curve_name" min max
                    ...
```

The dots indicate that each space curve statement may be followed by more than one curve segment reference. The *min* and *max* parameters allow using only part of the curve referenced. *min* and *max* must be in the range of the parameter vector of the curve.

Here is an example of a space curve object:

```
object "myspacecurve"
    basis "bezier_1" bezier 1
    group
        0.4 0.4 1.2
        0.6 0.4 1.2
        0.6 0.6 1.2
        0.4 0.6 1.2
        v 0 v 1 v 2 v 3
        curve "curve1" bezier_1
                0. 1. 2. 3. 4.
                0 1 2 3 0
        space curve "sp1"
                "curve1" 0. 4.
    end group
end object
```

2.7.8.8 Approximations

Approximations are defined within an object group and they specify how previously defined polygons, surfaces and curves should be tessellated. Within an object group containing free-form surface geometry the approximation statements are given separately for the surface itself and for curves used by the surface. The `surface` approximation statement sets the approximation technique for the surface itself. If it carries a displacement map this statement refers to the underlying geometric base surface and does not take the displacement into account. One may specify the approximation criteria on the displaced surface with an additional `displace` approximation statement or even leave out the `surface` approximation statement altogether.

If the material of the surface does not contain a displacement shader the `displace` approximation statement is ignored. A `trim` approximation statement applies to all trimming, hole and special curves attached to the given surface or surfaces collectively; it is equivalent to separate `curve` approximations for each individual curve. When the keyword `approximate` is directly followed by an approximation technique it refers to a polygon or a list of polygons. It only has an effect on displacement mapped polygons. If the `options` statement specifies approximation statements for base surfaces and/or displacements, they override the approximation statements in the object. This can be used for quick previews with low tessellation quality, for example.

`approximate`
  technique [min_{int} max_{int}]

`approximate surface`
  technique [min_{int} max_{int}] [`max` max_{int}] "*surface_name*" ...

`approximate displace`
  technique [min_{int} max_{int}] "*surface_name*" ...

`approximate trim`
  technique [min_{int} max_{int}] "*surface_name*" ...

`approximate curve`
  technique [min_{int} max_{int}] "*curve_name*" ...

`approximate space curve`
  technique [min_{int} max_{int}] "*spacecurve_name*" ...

The dots indicate that there may be more than one *surface_name* or *curve_name* following the approximation statement. The given approximation is then used for all named surfaces or curves.

technique stands for one or more of the following:

`view`
`tree`
`grid`
`delaunay`
[`regular`] `parametric` *u_subdiv* [*v_subdiv*]
`any`
`length` *edge*

`distance` *dist*
`angle` *angle*
`spatial` [`view`] *edge*
`curvature` [`view`] *dist angle*
`grading` *angle*

`tree`, `grid`, and `delaunay`[2.1] are mutually exclusive. `parametric` cannot be combined with any of the others except `grid`, which is the default for the parametric case anyway. `regular` can only be used together with `parametric`. `view` has no effect unless one of `length`, `distance`, `spatial`, or `curvature` is also given. Grading can only be used in combination with Delaunay triangulation.

View-dependent approximation is enabled if the `view` statement is present. It controls whether the *edge* argument of the `length` and `spatial` statements, and the `dist` argument of the `distance` and `curvature` statements, are in the space the object is defined in or in raster space.

Tree, grid, and Delaunay approximation algorithms are available for surface approximation. The grid algorithm tessellates on a regular grid of isolines in parameter space; the tree algorithm tessellates in a hierarchy of successive refinements that produces fewer triangles for the same quality criteria; the Delaunay algorithm creates a successive refinement that maximizes triangle equiangularity. criteria. By definition parametric approximations always use the grid algorithm; all others can use either but `tree` is the default. `tree`, `grid`, and `delaunay` have no effect on curve approximations. Delaunay triangulation creates more regular triangles but takes longer to compute.

Parametric approximation subdivides each patch of the surface into $u\_subdiv \cdot degree$ equal-sized pieces in the U parameter direction, and $v\_subdiv \cdot degree$ equal-sized pieces in the V parameter direction. If `regular` the number of pieces the whole surface is subdivided into simply equals the parameter value. *v_subdiv* must be present for `surface` approximations and must be omitted for `curve` and `trim` approximations. Note that the factor is a floating point number, although a patch can only be subdivided an integral number of times. For example, if a factor of 2.0 is given and the surface is of degree three, each patch will be subdivided six times in each parametric direction. If a factor of 0.0 is given, each patch is approximated by two triangles.

Curves are subdivided in $subdiv \cdot degree$ equal pieces by the `parametric` approximation and into *subdiv* equal pieces by the `regular parametric` approximation.

For displacement mapped polygons and displacement mapped surfaces with a `displace` statement `regular parametric` has the same meaning as `parametric` in the approximation. For displacement mapped polygons the *u_subdiv* constant specifies that each edge in the triangulation of the original polygon is subdivided for the displacement 2^{u_subdiv} times. If a `displace` approximation is given for a displacement mapped surface, the initial tessellation of the underlying geometric surface is subdivided in the same way as for polygons. For example, a value of 2 leads to a fourfold subdivision of each edge. Non-integer values for the subdivision constant are admissible. Nothing is done if the expression above is smaller than 2 (i.e. if $u\_subdiv < 1$). The *v_subdiv* constant is ignored for the parametric approximation of displacement maps.

Length/distance/angle (LDA) approximation specifies curvature-dependent approximation according to the criteria specified by the `length`, `distance`, and `angle` statements. These statements can be given in any combination and order, but cannot be combined with parametric approximation in the same `approximate` statement. If they are preceded by the `any` keyword[2.1]the approximation stops as soon as any of the criteria is satisfied.

The `length` statement subdivides the surface or curve such that no edge length of the tessellation exceeds the *edge* parameter. *edge* is given as a distance in the space the object is defined in, or as a fraction of a pixel diagonal in raster space if the `view` keyword is present. Small values such as 1.0 are recommended. For tree and grid approximation the *min* and *max* parameters, if present, specify the minimum and maximum number of recursion levels of the adaptive subdivision. The *min* parameter is a means to enforce a minimal triangulation fineness without any tests. Edges are further subdivided until they satisfy the given criterion is fulfilled or the *max* subdivision level is reached. The defaults are 0 and 5, respectively; 5 is a very high number. Good results can often be achieved with a maximum of 3 subdivisions. For Delaunay approximation, the number *max* following the keyword `max` specifies the maximum number of triangles of the surface tessellation. This number will be exceeded only if required by trimming, hole, and special curves because every curve vertex must become part of the tessellation regardless of the specified maximum.

For displacement mapped polygons and displacement mapped surfaces with a `displace` approximation statement the length criterion in the approximation limits the size of the edges of the displaced triangles and ensures that at least all features of this size are resolved. Subdivision stops as soon as an edge satisfies the criterion or when the maximum subdivision level is reached. The possibility that at an even finer scale new details may show up which would lead again to longer edges of course cannot be ruled out. This caveat about the potential miss of high-frequency detail applies also to the distance and angle criteria.

The `distance` statement specifies the maximum distance *dist* between the tessellation and the actual curve or surface. The value of *dist* is a distance in the space the object is defined in, or a fraction of a pixel diagonal in raster space if the `view` statement is present. As a starting point, a small distance such as 0.1 is recommended. For tree and grid approximation the *min* and *max* parameters, if present, specify the minimum and maximum number of recursion levels of the adaptive subdivision. For Delaunay approximation, the number *max* following the keyword `max` specifies the maximum number of triangles of the surface tessellation.

For displacement mapped polygons and displacement mapped surfaces with a `displace` approximation statement the distance criterion cannot be used in the same way because the displaced surface is not known analytically. Instead, the displacements of the vertices of a triangle in the tessellation are compared. The criterion is fulfilled only if they differ by less than the given threshold. Subdivision is finest in areas where the displacement changes. For example, if a black-and-white picture is used for the displacement map the triangulation will be finest along the borders between black and white areas but the resolution will be lower away from them in the uniformly colored areas. In such a case one could choose a moderately dense parametric `surface` approximation that samples the displacement map at sufficient density to catch small features, and use the curvature-dependent `displace` approximation to resolve the curvature introduced by the displacement map. Even if the base surface is triangulated without adding interior points, as if its trim curve defined a polygon in parameter space, it is still possible to guarantee a certain resolution by increasing the *min* subdivision level. Only the consecutive subdivisions are then performed adaptively.

The `angle` statement specifies the maximum angle *angle* in degrees between normals of adjacent tiles of a displaced polygon or the tessellation of a surface or its displacement or between tangents of adjacent segments of the curve approximation. Large angles such as 45.0 are recommended. For tree and grid approximation the *min* and *max* parameters, if present, specify the minimum and maximum number of recursion levels of the adaptive subdivision. For Delaunay approximation, the number *max* following the keyword `max` specifies the maximum number of triangles of the surface tessellation.

Spatial approximation as specified by a `spatial` statement is a special case of an LDA approximation that specifies only the `length` statement. For backwards compatibility, the `spatial` statement has been retained; it is equivalent to the `length` statement plus an optional `view` statement.

Curvature-dependent approximation as specified by the `curvature` statement is also a special case of LDA approximation, equivalent to a `distance` statement, an `angle` statement, and an optional `view` statement. The `spatial` and `curvature` statements can be combined, but future designs should use `length`, `distance`, and `angle` directly.

Grading applies only to Delaunay triangulation[2.1]controls the density of triangles around the border of the surface. It allows the density of triangles to vary quickly in a smooth transition between a finer curve approximation and a coarser surface approximation. The *angle* constant specifies a lower bound related to the degree of the minimum angle of a triangle. Values from 0.0 to 30.0 can be specified. Small values up to 20.0 are recommended. The default is 0.0. When using high grading values it is recommended to specify a maximum number of triangles because otherwise high grading values might result in a huge number of triangles or endless mesh refinement. The purpose of this option is to prevent a large number of tiny triangles at the trimming or hole curve to abruptly join very large triangles in the interior of the surface.

If no approximation statement is given the parametric technique is used by default with $u\_subdiv = v\_subdiv = 1$ for surfaces, or $u\_subdiv = 1$ in the case of curves and $u\_subdiv = 0$ for polygons.

2.7.8.9 Connections

Connections may be defined within a group to specify the connection between two surfaces along intervals of their respective trimming curves or hole curves. They may be used in place of or in addition to the edge merging performed on the group level. A connection is defined as:

```
connect  "surface_name1"  "curve_name1"  min1  max1
         "surface_name2"  "curve_name2"  min2  max2
```

This statement connects two surfaces $surface\_name_1$ and $surface\_name_2$ by connecting their trimming curves $curve\_name_1$ and $curve\_name_2$. The curves are connected only in the range

$(min_1 \ldots max_1)$ and $(min_2 \ldots max_2)$, respectively. They share the same points, but normals, textures etc. are evaluated on the individual surfaces. Only surfaces that have trimming curves can be connected by an explicit connect statement; for an example for a simple trimming curve that goes around the edge of a surface see the section on curves above. Trimming curves used in connections must satisfy three conditions:

- As always, the trimming curve or sequence of trimming curves must be closed.
- It does not matter whether the trimming curve is oriented clockwise or counterclockwise, but if a sequence of trimming curves is used all pieces must have the same direction.
- The trimming curves along the connected range must run in the same direction in 3D space.

The range values $min_{1,2}$ and $max_{1,2}$ must not exceed the range of the trimming curve segment as referenced by a `trim` statement of the corresponding surface. The minimum value must be less than the maximum value; it is not possible to satisfy the third condition by inverting the range.

Best results are obtained if the curves to be connected are close to each other in world space and have at least approximately the same length. `connect` is not meant to be a replacement for proper modeling. For carefully modeled surfaces it will not be necessary most of the time. Its purpose is to close small cracks between adjacent surfaces that are already not too far from each other. Topologically complex situations with several connections meeting in a point are beyond its scope.

2.7.8.10 Example

Here is an example of two surfaces that meet along one of their edges such that a gap remains. A connection is used to close the gap. The four control points defining the straight trimming curves that are connected are marked as #0, #1, #2, and #3; the control points of the second surface marked `(*)` have been modified slightly to create the gap. This is a complete .mi file that can be rendered directly.

```
verbose on
link "base.so"
$include <base.mi>

options "opt"
    samples      -1 1
    contrast     .1 .1 .1 .1
    trace depth  2 2
end options

camera "cam"
     frame       1
     output      "rgb" "x.rgb"
     focal       50.000000
     aperture    44.724029
```

```
    aspect      1.179245
    resolution 500 424
end camera

instance "cam_inst" "cam" end instance

light "light"
    "mib_light_point" (
        "color"  1 1 1,
        "shadow" on,
        "factor" 1
    )
    origin      140.189178 83.103180 50.617714
end light

instance "light_inst" "light" end instance

material "mtl" opaque
    "mib_illum_phong" (
        "ambience"  .3 .3 .3,
        "ambient"   .5 .5 .5,
        "diffuse"   .7 .7 .7,
        "specular"  1 1 1,
        "exponent"  50,
        "lights"    [ "light_inst" ]
    )
end material

object "obj"
    visible shadow trace


    basis "bez1" bezier 1
    basis "bez3" bezier 3
    group "example"
        0.314772    -3.204608   -7.744229
        0.314772    -2.146943   -6.932366
        0.314772    -1.089277   -6.120503
        0.314772    -0.031611   -5.308641    #0
        -0.660089   -2.650739   -8.465791
        -0.660089   -1.593073   -7.653928
        -0.660089   -0.535407   -6.842065
        -0.660089   0.522259    -6.030203    #1
        -1.634951   -2.096869   -9.187352
        -1.634951   -1.039203   -8.375489
        -1.634951   0.018462    -7.563627
        -1.634951   1.076128    -6.751764    #2
        -2.609813   -1.543000   -9.908914
        -2.609813   -0.485334   -9.097052
        -2.609813   0.572332    -8.285189
        -2.609813   1.629998    -7.473326    #3

        0.000000    0.000000    -5.000000    #0 (*)
```

```
1.224400    0.561979    -6.081950
2.134028    1.155570    -6.855258
3.043655    1.749160    -7.628566
-0.500000   0.700000    -6.000000    #1 (*)
0.249538    1.115849    -6.803511
1.159166    1.709439    -7.576819
2.068794    2.303029    -8.350128
-1.200000   1.000000    -7.000000    #2 (*)
-0.725323   1.669719    -7.525073
0.184305    2.263309    -8.298381
1.093932    2.856899    -9.071690
-2.000000   2.000000    -7.500000    #3 (*)
-1.700185   2.223588    -8.246634
-0.790557   2.817178    -9.019943
0.119071    3.410769    -9.793251

0.0     0.0     0.0
1.0     0.0     0.0
1.0     1.0     0.0
0.0     1.0     0.0

v 0  v 1  v 2  v 3  v 4  v 5  v 6  v 7
v 8  v 9  v 10 v 11 v 12 v 13 v 14 v 15

v 16 v 17 v 18 v 19 v 20 v 21 v 22 v 23
v 24 v 25 v 26 v 27 v 28 v 29 v 30 v 31

v 32 v 33 v 34 v 35

curve "curve1"
     "bez1" 0.0 0.25 0.5 0.75 1.0
     32 33 34 35 32

curve "curve2"
     "bez1" 0.0 0.25 0.5 0.75 1.0
     32 35 34 33 32

surface "patch1" "mtl"
     "bez3" 0.0 1.0          0.0 1.0
     "bez3" 0.0 1.0          0.0 1.0
     0 1 2 3 4 5 6 7 8 9 10 11 12 13 14 15
     trim "curve1" 0.0 1.0

surface "patch2" "mtl"
     "bez3" 0.0 1.0          0.0 1.0
     "bez3" 0.0 1.0          0.0 1.0
     16 17 18 19 20 21 22 23
     24 25 26 27 28 29 30 31
     trim "curve2" 0.0 1.0

approximate surface parametric 1.0 1.0 "patch1"
approximate surface parametric 1.0 1.0 "patch2"
approximate trim    parametric 3.0     "patch1"
```

```
        approximate trim    parametric 3.0      "patch2"

        connect "patch1" "curve1" 0.25 0.5
                "patch2" "curve2" 0.0  0.25
    end group
end object

instance "obj_inst"   "obj"   end instance

instgroup "root"
    "light_inst" "cam_inst" "obj_inst"
end instgroup

render "root" "cam_inst" "opt"
```

Note that the trimming curves curve1 and curve2 have a different orientation, one clockwise and one counterclockwise, because their control point lists are in a different order. This means that where both trimming curves run in parallel, they run in the same direction in 3D space, which is a required condition for trimming curves to be connected. The trimming curves must be closed (another condition) and so run around all four edges of the (square) surfaces. Since only one edge of each surface is connected to the other, the connection ranges select only one quarter (0.5 . . . 0.25 and 0.25 . . . 0.0) of each curve.

The example produces the following image, once rendered without and then with the connect statement:

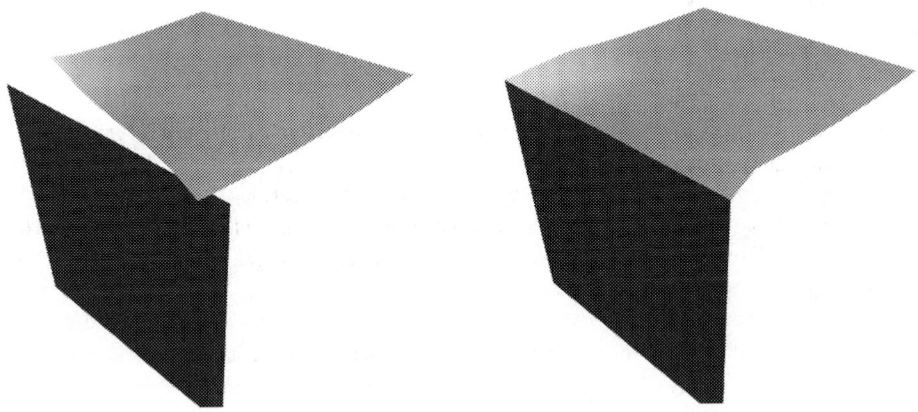

2.7.9 Instances

instance "*name*"
    "*element*" | geometry *function*
    [hide   on | off]

```
    [ visible            on|off ]
    [ shadow             on|off ]
    [ trace              on|off ]
    [ caustic            [ mode ]]
    [ globillum          [ mode ]]
    [ transform          [ matrix ]]
    [ motion transform   [ matrix ]]
    [ motion             off ]
    [ material           "material_name" ]
    [ material           [ "material_name" [ , "material_name" ... ] ] ]
    [ (parameters) ]
end instance
```

Instances place cameras, lights, objects, and instance groups into the scene. Without instances, these entities have no effect; they are not tessellated and are not scheduled for processing. An instance has a *name* that identifies the instance when it is placed into an instance group (see below). Every instance references exactly one element *element*, which must be the name of a camera, a light, an object, or an instance group. If the instanced item is a geometry shader *function*, the scene element created by this special shader is actually used as the instanced item.

The `hide` flag can be set to on to disable the instance and the element it references. This is useful to temporarily suspend an instance to evaluate a subset of the scene, without deleting and later recreating suspended parts. `hide` is `off` by default.

The `visible`, `shadow`, `trace`, `caustic`, and `globillum` modes are inherited down the scene DAG. Flags in instances lower (closer to the objects) override flags in instances higher up. The flags from the instance closest to the object are merged with the corresponding object flags. The resulting values become the effective flags for rendering. If no flags are specified in the relevant instances, only the object flags are used. For the exact definition of these flags refer to the Object section. The caustics *mode* bitmap contains five bits, and the desired behavior is the sum of 1 (to enable caustic casting), 2 (to enable caustic receiving), 4 (to disable caustic casting), and 8 (to disable caustic receiving). Obviously, 1 and 4, and 2 and 8, cannot be mixed, respectively. If *mode* is omitted, the default is 3 (enable casting and receiving). The fifth bit[2.1]contains an 'invisible to photons' flag, that is, if the fifth bit is set photons do not intersect this object. The globillum[2.1]*mode* bitmap is similar.

The `transform` statement is followed by 16 numbers that define a 4×4 matrix in row-major order. The matrix establishes the transformation from the parent coordinate space to the object space of the instanced *element*. If the instance is directly attached to the root instance group (see below), the parent coordinate space is world space. For example, the following matrix translates the instanced element to the coordinate (x, y, z):

```
transform   1 0 0 0
            0 1 0 0
            0 0 1 0
            x y z 1
```

Instance transformations are ignored if the options element explicitly sets the coordinate space to camera space, using the `camera space` statement. This is not recommended. The parent-to-local space transformation direction has the effect that in order to move an instanced object one (local) unit in the (local) +X direction, x must be decremented by 1.

The `motion transform` matrix specifies a transformation from parent space to local space for motion blurred geometry. If not specified, the instance transformation is used for the motion blur transformation. In this case the parent instance determines whether motion blur is active or not. Motion blur is activated by specifying a motion transformation in the scene DAG. This transformation is propagated through the scene DAG in the same way as the instance transformations. The `motion off` statement turns off all motion information inherited up to this point, as if the camera and all instances above did not have motion transforms. This can be used to disable motion transformations for a scene subtree.

If a motion transformation is specified in an object instance, the triangle vertex points of the tessellated geometry are transformed by the matrix product of the accumulated instance matrix and the inverse accumulated motion transformation matrix. The difference vector between the transformed and the untransformed triangle vertex point is used as a motion vector in local object space. If an object has motion vectors attached to the vertices, the motion vector calculated as described above is combined with the object motion vector. A motion transformation can be given for both object and camera instances. If a motion transformation is specified in a camera instance, the effective motion transformation for the triangle vertices is the matrix product of the relative instance and relative camera motion transformation.

The *material_name* is the name of a previously defined material. It is stored along with the instance. Instance materials are inherited down the scene DAG. Materials in instances lower in the scene DAG (closer to the leaves) override materials in instances higher up. The material defined lowest becomes the default material for any polygon or surface in a geometrical object that has no material of its own.

If a bracketed, comma-separated list of *material_names* is given, mental ray will use the n-th material in the list if the polygon or surface label is n. If the label exceeds the length of the list, the first material in the list is used. Polygon and surface labels can be specified in the object definition that have the `tagged` flag set. If this flag is not set, the first material in the list is used. The list may not be empty.

An instance may define parameters. Instance parameters are evaluated during scene preprocessing during preprocessing. Whenever the initial scene traversal finds an instance, it calls the inheritance shader defined in the options element with the parent instance parameters and the parameters of the new instance. The inheritance shader must then compute a new parameter set, which becomes the parent parameters for any future instances found in the *element* subtree below the new instance, if *element* is an instance group (if not, no sub-instances can exist and recursion ends). The inheritance shader is also called if there is no parent instance yet or if the new instance contains no parameters. The final parameter set created by the inheritance shader called for the bottom-level instance (which instances a camera, light, or object) is made available to shaders, in addition to the regular shader parameters.

The instance parameters must be declared just like shader parameters. The `declare` command must name the inheritance function, as specified in the `options` element. All instances share the same declaration. Note that this limits the portability of the scene — it is difficult to merge it with another scene that uses a different parameter inheritance shader.

If `transform`, `motion transform`, and `material` are given without arguments, the respective feature is turned off. This is useful for incremental changes. It is not relevant for the initial definition because these features are off by default when an instance is created.

The *element* may be named in more than one instance. This is called "multiple instancing." If two instances name the same object, the object appears twice in the scene, even though it is stored only once in the scene database. This greatly reduces memory consumption. For example, it is sufficient to create one wheel object for a car, and then instance it four times. All four instances will contain a different transformation matrices to place the wheels in four different locations. (This implies that multiple instancing is not useful in camera space mode because in this mode the transformations are ignored.) It is also possible to apply multiple instancing to object groups to replicate entire sub-scenes.

If the instanced item is a "geometry shader", the *function* is called with shader parameters and the scene element created by the shader is defined in the local coordinate space of the instance. The geometry shader is called just before tessellation takes place. The following example uses a geometry shader *mib_geo_sphere*:

```
instance "sphere"
    geometry "mib_geo_sphere" ()
end instance
```

This example creates a spherical object procedurally. It uses the syntax for anonymous shaders; as usual the named shader syntax using the `shader` keyword and named shader assignments using the "=" sign can also be used. As usual, shader lists may be used; if the shader is correctly written all created objects are put in a group and instanced together. Named shaders created inside or outside procedural object definitions are in global scope and can be shared with other objects.

For a complete example for building scene graphs with instances and instance groups, see below.

2.7.10 Instance Groups

```
instgroup "name"
              "name"
              ...
end instgroup
```

Every scene consists of more than one element. There must be at least one camera and at least one object. In the simplest case, all cameras, lights, and objects can be collected into a single group, forming a "flat scene" because there is no hierarchy. Cameras, lights, and objects are never put into an instance group directly. Instead, an instance must be defined, one for each element, and the instance is then put into the group. (This is why it is called an "instance group.")

Instance groups can be nested. An instance group is placed into a parent instance group exactly like a camera, light, or object: an instance must be defined for the child instance group, and the instance is put into the parent instance group. As with other entities, it is possible to create more than one instance for an instance group; this allows multiple instancing of sub-scenes. There is no limit on the nesting depth of instance groups.

Since the only purpose of instance groups is as a container for instances, the syntax is very simple. After the name of the instance group, one or more names of instances follow. An incremental change to an instance group clears the old instance list (without deleting the instances themselves); to add or remove an instance in an instance group, the incremental change must respecify the entire instance list.

The top-level instance group has no instance. It is called the root instance group. The root instance group stands for the entire scene. It is passed to the `render` command to process the scene. More than one root instance group can exist, but only one can be processed at a time. Camera instances must always be attached to the root instance group, not a lower-level instance group, and it may not be multiply instanced to ensure unambiguity. Multiple cameras can exist in the root instance group, but only one can be passed to the `render` command.

2.8 Contours

In order to get contours, it is necessary to link with the `contour.so` shader library, and a `$include <contour.mi>` statement is also needed. The file `contour.mi` contains declarations of the contour shaders in `contour.so`.

Also, the *contour store shader* has to be specified in the `options` statement. A contour store shader has no parameters and is specified as

```
contour store "contour_store_function" ()
```

2.8.1 Where to Place Contours

A *contour contrast shader* specifies where there should be a contour. Like the contour store shader, the contour contrast function has to be specified in the `options` statement. The parameters of this function specify which difference in depth or surface orientation should cause a contour. For example, to get a contour where the difference in depth is more than 1.0 or the difference in surface normal is more than 60 degrees and between materials, the following contour contrast shader is used

```
contour contrast "contour_contrast_function_levels" (
```

```
        "zdelta"      1.0,
        "ndelta"      60.0,
        "diff_mat"    on,
        "contrast"    on,
        "min_level"   1,
        "max_level"   1
    )
```

(Be aware that if `zdelta` or `ndelta` is set to a very small value, contours will be created also in large regions interior to objects.)

When `diff_mat` is `on`, contours are created between different materials. When `contrast` is `on`, contours are created where the contrast between colors is larger than the `contrast` specified in the options within the `options` statement. The parameters `min_level` and `max_level` tell which levels of reflection and layers of semitransparent materials should have contours on them. When both are set to 1, as here, only the outermost materials get contours and no reflections cause contours.

The hands in the figure shows the influence the parameters of the contour contrast shader has on where contours are created. Top row (left to right): large `zdelta` and `ndelta` give only contours on the outline where the depth difference to the infinitely distant background is large; large `ndelta` and small `zdelta` give contours where there is even a small depth difference; small `ndelta` and `zdelta` gives contours where there is a small change in depth or orientation. Bottom row: Contours on deeper levels of materials seen through a semitransparent material; contours on reflections on a reflective material, for example the reflection of the thumb is visible in the index finger.

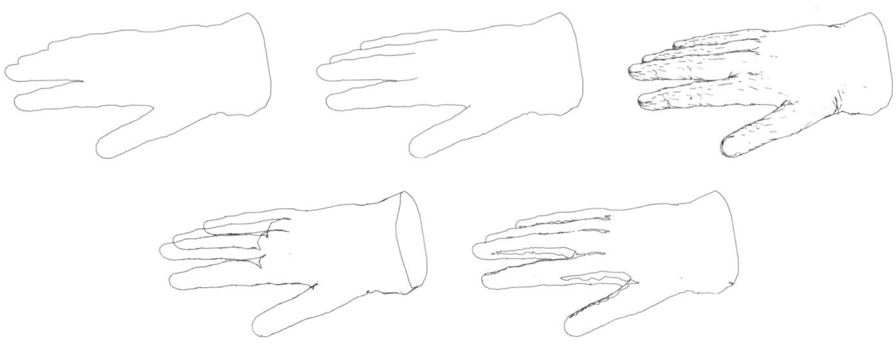

2.8.2 Color and Width of Contours

The contour properties (color, width, etc.) depend on the object the contour is on and its material. For each material that should have a contour, one has to specify a *contour shader*. A material will not get a contour if it does not have a contour shader. The colors consist of four components: red, green, and blue color, and opacity. All four components of the color are normally between 0 and 1.

The width is specified as a percentage of the minimum of image x resolution and y resolution. For example, if the image resolution is 700×500 and a contour width of 1.0 (percent) is specified, the thickness of the line becomes 5 pixels. The color, width, etc. can be parameters, or depend on curvature, distance, color, and illumination.

A material gets a simple contour of constant color and width if it has the `contour_shader_simple` contour shader. For example, the following specifies red contours that are half a percent wide:

```
contour "contour_shader_simple" (
   "color"  1.0 0.0 0.0 1.0,    # solid red
   "width"  0.5                 # in % of image resol
)
```

As another example of a contour shader, contours of color and width that are linearly interpolated between two values, depending on distance to the camera, are specified with the contour shader `contour_shader_depthfade`. Two depths, colors, and widths are specified. If a contour point is more distant than `far_z`, the contour gets color `far_color` and width `far_width`. If a point is nearer than `near_z`, the contour gets color `near_color` and width `near_width`. If the depth is in between, the color and width are linearly interpolated. For example, to get contours that are interpolated between two percent wide red at depth -10 and half a percent wide blue at depth -25, specify

```
contour "contour_shader_depthfade" (
   "near_z"      -10.0,              # from this depth,
   "near_color"   1.0 0.0 0.0 1.0,   # color (red),
   "near_width"   2.0,               # and width (in %)
   "far_z"       -25.0,              # to this depth,
   "far_color"    0.0 0.0 1.0 1.0,   # color (blue),
   "far_width"    0.5                # and width (in %)
)
```

The left figure is a black-and-white illustration of this depthfade contour shader. The right figure is a scene with two materials with different contour type: illumination-dependent contours on the teapot and simple contours on the "floor".

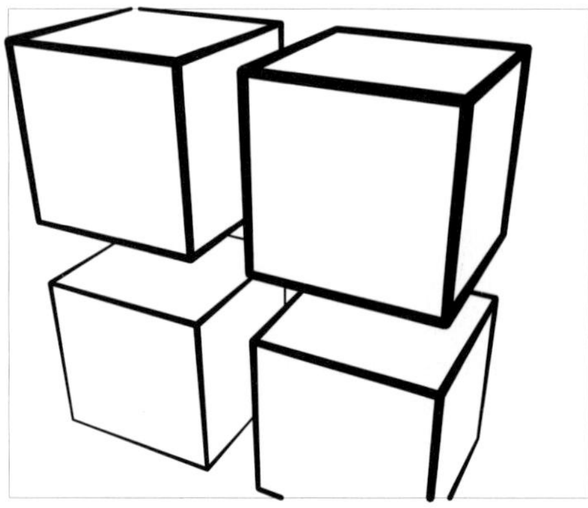

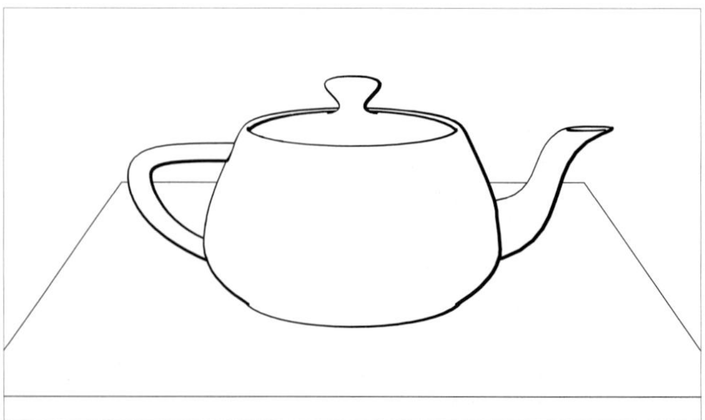

There are many other contour shaders in `contour.so`, and new ones can be written by the user.

2.8.3 Contour Output

After the regular image has been computed, a contour output shader can get the contour line segments and use them to for example render a contour image or write a file with contour information. The user can write contour output shaders using the built-in function *mi_get_contour_line*.

There are three contour output shaders in `contour.so`. They can generate a contour image, a contour image composited over the regular image, and a PostScript file with black contours. The output shader has to be specified in the `camera`.

To get a contour image called `mycontourimage.rgb` in `rgb` format, write

```
output "contour,rgba" "contour_only" ()
output "rgb" "mycontourimage.rgb"
```

To get an image called `mycontourimage2.rgb` (in `rgb` format) containing contours composited over the regular image, write

```
output "contour,rgba" "contour_composite" ()
output "rgb" "mycontourimage2.rgb"
```

The `contour_composite` output shader has two optional Boolean parameters: `glow` and `maxcomp`. The `glow` parameter makes all contours become darker and more transparent near their edges, creating a glow effect. `maxcomp` specifies that when a contour is over another contour, the maximum of the two colors (in each color band) should be used. If `maxcomp` is not specified (or set `off`), normal alpha compositing is used. The `contour_only` output shader also has the `glow` and `maxcomp` parameters, and in addition it has a `background` parameter which determines the background color (default is black).

To get a PostScript file called `mycontourfile.ps` with all contours in black, write

```
output "contour,rgba" "contour_ps" (
   "paper_size"           4,
   "paper_scale"          1.0,
   "paper_transform_b"    0.0,
   "paper_transform_d"    1.0,
   "title"                on,
   "landscape"            on,
   "ink_stroke_dir"       1.0 1.0 0.0,
   "ink_min_frac"         0.1,
```

```
        "file_name"             "mycontourfile.ps"
    )
```

The PostScript file in this example gives A4 paper size with full scale. "paper_size" is an integer, with 0 indicating "letter" size, 1 indicating "executive", 2 indicating "legal", 3–6 indicating "a3", "a4", "a5", "a6", 7–9 indicating "b4", "b5", "b6", and 10 indicating "11x17". The parameter paper_scale scales the PostScript output. Furthermore, the Postscript coordinates are transformed according to the matrix $\begin{pmatrix} 1 & b \\ 0 & d \end{pmatrix}$, where b and d are the parameters "paper_transform_b" and "paper_transform_d". This e.g. enables one to compensate for printers that print out with a slight skew. The Boolean title determines whether a title (consisting of file name and frame number) and a frame around the image are written. The Boolean landscape makes the output be in landscape mode rather than portrait mode. If the parameter ink_stroke_dir is set, each contour segment will have a width that depends on its orientation, giving an ink pen look. For the ink pen look, ink_min_frac specifies the minimum fraction of the original contour thickness (at contour segment orientations perpendicular to the stroke direction). The file_name specifies the name of the file that the contours are written to.

It is also possible to get both the regular image (without contours) and one of the above at the same time. For example, to get the regular image and an image of the contours, write

```
output "rgb" "myimage.rgb"
output "contour,rgba" "contour_only" ()
output "rgb" "mycontourimage.rgb"
```

2.8.4 Faster Contours

If only simple outlines of objects are needed, *contour_shader_simple* can be used with *contour_store_function_simple* and *contour_contrast_function_simple* to get fast contour computations. Furthermore, very simple material shaders should be used (no illumination, shadow, reflection, refraction, or texture computations).

2.9 Scene Example

This example creates two images of a cube, each with a different camera and light:

```
verbose on
link "base.so"
$include <base.mi>

options "opt"
    samples     -1 1
    contrast    .1 .1 .1 .1
```

```
    trace depth  2 2
end options

camera "cam1"
    frame         1
    output        "rgb" "x.rgb"
    focal         100
    aperture      144.724029
    aspect        1.179245
    resolution    500 424
end camera

instance "caminst1" "cam1" end instance

light "light1"
    "mib_light_point" (
        "color"  1 1 1,
        "shadow" on,
        "factor" 1
    )
    origin        141.375732 83.116005 35.619434
end light

instance "lightinst1" "light1" end instance

material "mtl" opaque
    "mib_illum_phong" (
        "ambience"  .3 .3 .3,
        "ambient"   .5 .5 .5,
        "diffuse"   .7 .7 .7,
        "specular"  1 1 1,
        "exponent"  50,
        "lights"    [ "lightinst1" ]
    )
end material

object "obj1"
    visible shadow trace
    group "mesh"
                -7.068787   -4.155799   -22.885710
                -0.179573   -7.973234   -16.724060
                -7.068787    4.344949   -17.619093
                -0.179573    0.527515   -11.457443
                 0.179573   -0.527514   -28.742058
                 7.068787   -4.344948   -22.580408
                 0.179573    7.973235   -23.475441
                 7.068787    4.155800   -17.313791

                v 0   v 1   v 2   v 3   v 4   v 5   v 6   v 7

                c "mtl"  0 1 3 2
                c        1 5 7 3
                c        5 4 6 7
```

```
            c       4 0 2 6
            c       4 5 1 0
            c       2 3 7 6
    end group
end object

instance "inst1" "obj1" end instance

instgroup "world"
    "caminst1" "lightinst1" "inst1"
end instgroup

render "world" "caminst1" "opt"         # render frame 1

incremental camera "cam1"
    frame 2
    aperture 100
end camera

incremental light "light1"
    "mib_light_point" (
        "color"  1 0 1,
    )
end light

render "world" "caminst1" "opt"         # render frame 2
```

Chapter 3

Using and Writing Shaders

All color, displacement, contour, and other computation in mental ray is based on shaders. There are various types of shaders for different situations, such as material shaders to evaluate the material properties of a surface, light shaders to evaluate the light-emitting properties of a light source, lens shaders to specify camera properties other than the default pinhole camera, and so on.

There are external shader libraries that support compatibility with Alias, Autodesk 3D Studio MAX, Dassault CATIA, SOFTIMAGE, SolidWorks, Wavefront, and others. Much of the power of mental ray relies on the possibility to write custom shaders and link them dynamically to mental ray at runtime. Custom shaders are written in C or C++, using the full language and library support available in these languages.

Here are the steps necessary to create a new shader:

- Write a .mi declaration for the shader, providing the shader name, return type, shader parameter names and types, and the version to mental ray.
- Write a C shader parameter data structure that agrees exactly with the .mi parameter declaration. (The mkmishader utility can do this translation.)
- Write the shader function in C or C++, using the correct signature. The shader computes a result from its shader parameters and the state, and by calling shader interface functions provided by mental ray.
- Write a version shader (same name with `_version` appended to the name) that returns a version number that matches the version number in the .mi declaration.
- If required, write initialization and exit shaders (same name as the shader with `_init` and `_exit` appended, respectively).
- Compile and link the shader, and create a shared library (DSO or DLL). This step can be omitted but DSO/DLLs are easiest to use and much faster to link than objects or sources. Libraries must be installed on all machines on the net that are used as clients or network rendering servers.

- Use a `$include` statement in the scene .mi file to load the .mi declaration and a `link` (or `code` or `$code`) statement to load the shader DSO/DLL (or source code).

Note that if the shader is expected to work on Windows NT, all four function definitions (the shader, the version function, and the init and exit shaders) must be preceded with `DLLEXPORT`. This is a pseudo type specifier that makes the functions visible to users of the generated shader library. On Unix systems `DLLEXPORT` evaluates to an empty word.

The shader is then ready to be used in the scene. These steps are described in detail below.

3.1 Dynamic Linking of Shaders

Shaders are written as C or C++ subroutines, stored in files with the extension "`.c`". To use these shaders in a scene, they must be dynamically linked into mental ray at runtime. mental ray accepts shaders in three forms:

- Directly as source code. The .mi file offers the `code` statement and the standalone renderer has a `-code` option. Both accept a source file with a `.c` extension.
- In object format. Source files can be compiled to object code using Unix commands such as "`cc -O -c source.c`" (assuming that the shader source is in a file named `source.c`). The command may vary on some platforms, consult the manual (see "`man cc`)". On Windows NT systems, shared libraries are called DLLs. This is the most common form on systems that do not support DSOs; it is faster than source because mental ray does not have to compile the shader. The compilation leaves a `source.o` file with the extension `.o` in the current directory. This file can be passed to mental ray using the `link` statement in the .mi file, or with the `-link` option of the standalone renderer.
- In DSO format. DSO stands for Dynamic Shared Object. DSOs are supported on most platforms, such as SGI systems running IRIX 5.2 or higher. The operating system version can be found by running the Unix command "`uname -r`". DSOs have the extension `.so` on SGI systems and other extensions on other systems, but it is highly recommended to use `.so` on all systems. This makes it possible to use the same name on all systems regardless of type. mental ray automatically substitutes `.dll` for `.so` on Windows NT platforms.

To create a DSO, first compile the shader source to object format using `cc` as described above, then run the Unix command "`ld -shared source.o`", again assuming that the object file is called `source.o`. This `ld` command applies to SGI IRIX; refer to "`man ld`" on other platforms. Using DSOs is the fastest way to load shaders, there is very little overhead. DSOs, like object files, are loaded using `link` statements or `-link` options.

The commands to create a DSO depend on the operating system type. To create a DSO named *example.so* from a source file *example.c*, use the following commands. Insert the `-g` command line option after `-c` to insert debugging information, or insert `-O` to compile an optimized version. On most systems `-g` and `-O` cannot be combined. Refer to the compiler documentation for details.

Linux x86

```
gcc -c -O2 -fPIC shader.c
ld -export-dynamic -shared -o shader.so shader.o
```

Linux Alpha

```
gcc -c -O2 -fPIC -mieee shader.c
ld -export-dynamic -shared -o shader.so shader.o
```

SGI IRIX

```
cc opt shared o example.so example.c
```

HP/UX

```
cc -c -Aa +z example.c
ld -b -o example.so example.o
```

IBM AIX

```
cc -c example.c
ld -o example.so example.o -bE:example.exp extra.so
     -bI:keep.exp -bM:SRE -T512 -H512 -lc
```

`example.exp` is a user supplied export file for the shader and must contain the names of the exported symbols, one at a line. `keep.exp` is the list of symbols exported by mental ray, either for use by shaders or for internal linking purposes. It is supplied with mental ray and can be referenced using an absolute path name. `extra.so` must be supplied to allow linking with shader libraries that are preloaded during runtime (such as `physics.so`) if functions from that library are used directly.

Convex SPP-UX 5.x

```
cc -c -D_REENTRANT -DPARALLEL -Aa +z example.c
ld -b -o example.so example.o /usr/lib/libc.1 -lm
```

Sun Solaris 2

```
cc -c -D_REENTRANT example.c
ld -G -o example.so example.o -ldl
```

(Using Sun CC; gcc can also be used.)

Digital Unix V4.0

```
cc -c -newc -O2 -ieee_with_no_inexact -D_REENTRANT example.c

ld -expect_unresolved '*' -shared -o example.so example.o
```

Windows NT

```
cl /c /O2 /MD /nologo example.c
link /nologo /DLL /nodefaultlib:LIBC.LIB
     /OUT:example.dll example.obj shader.lib
```

(Using Visual C++ 6.x or up; earlier versions are too buggy.) `shader.lib` is a stub library that is provided with mental ray. It is necessary because Windows NT cannot automatically share symbols between modules sharing a process. Note that the Visual C++ optimizer may introduce bugs into your code, causing (possibly intermittent) malfunctions that are very hard to find. Always test without optimization (without `/O2`)! Or use Intel's Proton/Electron compilers.

Compiling and creating DSOs requires that a C development environment is installed on the system. If the `cc` and `ld` commands are not found, make sure that a development environment exists. On most platforms, it is a separate product that must be purchased separately. Dynamically loading a DSO does not require compilers or development options.

SGI offers a range of processors, with later processors having more instruction set features than earlier ones. While newer processors and newer operating system versions can execute older programs (as long as they all use the ELF object format), programs and shaders should be compiled for newer instruction sets to improve performance. Four instruction sets have been defined by MIPS, called mips1 through mips4. mips3 is about 30% faster than mips2 on the same system. mips4 should be used if a very large virtual address space (4 terabytes) is required to keep large numbers of large textures. Choose the *opt* options string according to the following table:

IRIX	instruction set	CPU	word size	*opt*
5.x	mips2	R4000 and up	32 bits	
6.x	mips2	R4000 and up	32 bits	`-32`
6.x	mips3	R4400 and up	32 bits	`-n32`
6.x	mips4	R8000 and up	64 bits	`-64`

In any case, the options *must* agree with the version of mental ray. See the abi(5) manual page for more details. Use the Unix `file` command on mental ray and the shader library and make sure that they both report the same number of bits and the same MIPS version. If there is a mismatch, the run-time linker will print a message like:

```
/my/shader.so: 1234:ray: rld: Fatal Error:
    cannot successfully map soname '/my/shader.so'
    under any of the filenames /my/shader.so
```

The run-time linker always tries to match executables and libraries, which allows multiple ABIs to reside on the same system without conflicts. If the filename of the DSO given as an absolute pathname mental ray only tries to load that particular file. If it is given as a relative path, mental ray searches the DSO in a list of paths that can be supplied via the command line parameter (`-ld_path`) or the environment variable (`MI_LIBRARY_PATH`). There is also a default search path (`/usr/local/mi/lib;.`). A search list is a colon-separated (Unix) or semicolon-separated (Unix or Windows NT) list of paths to be searched. (Windows NT uses colons for drive letters.)

Note that source code (`.c` extension) is normally portable, unless nonportable system features (such as *fsqrt* on SGIs) are used. This means that the shader will run on all other vendors' systems unchanged. If the compilation fails and the shaders therefore are undefined, mental ray will — when calls of the undefined shaders are attempted — return `miFALSE`, which will generally leave the pixel sample black.

Neither object files (`.o` extension) nor DSOs (`.so` extension) are portable. They must be compiled separately for each platform and, usually, for each major operating system release. For example, a Hewlett-Packard object file will not run on an SGI system, and an SGI IRIX 4.x object file cannot be used on an IRIX 6.x system, and vice versa. Also note that pointers are 32-bit values on some systems and 64-bit values on others, and that most but not all (IBM) processors require that 64-bit values such as `doubles` are stored at memory addresses evenly divisible by 8.

On SGI systems, a shader can be debugged after it has been called for the first time, which attaches it to the program and makes its symbols available to the debugger. For this to work, the `-g` option must be given to the `cc` and `ld` commands in all stages — compilation, linking, and shared-library building. Also, only DSO shaders are debuggable, not shaders loaded in object (`.o`) or source (`.c`) form.

On non-SGI systems, debugging shaders is, unfortunately, difficult. The reason is that most debuggers cannot deal with parts of a program that have been dynamically linked. In general, the debugger will refuse to set breakpoints in dynamically linked shaders, and will step over calls to these shaders as if they were a single operating system call. Some vendors are working on fixing these problems, but at this time the only option on non-SGI systems is using *mi_info* or *mi_debug* statements in the shader sources. Avoid *printf* because it is lost on server hosts and because it can cause problems at runtime.

Windows NT shader libraries must use at least one shader interface call (any true C function beginning with *mi_*), or an error message "`DLL_SetModuleHandle not found`" will occur.

When a shared library is loaded that contains a function *module_init*, that function is called just after the library was loaded, before the first shader in it is called. Conversely, if it contains a function *module_exit*, that function is called just before the library is unloaded, after the last call to a shader in this library. Note that in the case of irrecoverable errors at any time after the library was loaded *module_exit* is not guaranteed to be called. Neither *module_init* nor *module_exit* may rely on any shader interface services that assume that a rendering operation is in progress. Message functions such as *mi_info* are available. **Note**: this feature is not supported on IBM systems and should not be used for portable shaders.

3.2 Coordinate Systems

Internal space is the coordinate system mental ray uses to present intersection points and other points and vectors to shaders. All points and vectors in the state except bump basis vectors (which are in object space) are presented in internal space, namely, `org`, `dir`, `point`, `normal`, `normal_geom`, `motion` and `derivs`. The actual meaning of internal space is left undefined, it varies between different versions of mental ray and depends on the `space` statement in the `options` block in the .mi file. **A shader must not assume that internal space is identical to world space**, even though this is true in most scenes.

World space is the coordinate system in which modeling and animation takes place.

Object space is a coordinate system relative to the object's origin. The modeler that created the scene defines the object's origin. Most translators use the center of the bounding box of the object as the object origin.

Camera space is a coordinate system in which the camera is at the coordinate origin (0, 0, 0) with an *up* vector of (0, 1, 0) and looking down the negative Z axis.

In addition to these 3D coordinate spaces, *raster space* is a two-dimensional pixel location on the screen bounded by (0, 0) in the lower left corner of the image, and the rendered image resolution. The center of the pixel in the lower left corner of raster space has the coordinates (0.5, 0.5).

Screen space is defined such that $(-1, -1/a)$ is in the lower left corner of the screen and $(1, 1/a)$ is in the the upper right, where a is the aspect ratio of the screen (the relation between its width and height).

Most shaders never need to transform between spaces. Texture shaders frequently need to operate in object space; for example, in order to apply bump basis vectors to *state→normal*, the normal must be transformed to object space before the bump basis vectors are applied, and back to internal space before the result is passed to any mental ray function such as *mi_trace_reflection*. mental ray offers 18 functions to convert points, vectors and normals between coordinate spaces:

function	*operation*
mi_point_to_world(s,p_r,p)	internal point to world space
mi_point_to_camera(s,p_r,p)	internal point to camera space
mi_point_to_object(s,p_r,p)	internal point to object space
mi_point_from_world(s,p_r,p)	world point to internal space
mi_point_from_camera(s,p_r,p)	camera point to internal space
mi_point_from_object(s,p_r,p)	object point to internal space
mi_vector_to_world(s,v_r,v)	internal vector to world space
mi_vector_to_camera(s,v_r,v)	internal vector to camera space
mi_vector_to_object(s,v_r,v)	internal vector to object space
mi_vector_from_world(s,v_r,v)	world vector to internal space
mi_vector_from_camera(s,v_r,v)	camera vector to internal space
mi_vector_from_object(s,v_r,v)	object vector to internal space
mi_normal_to_world(s,v_r,v)	internal normal to world space
mi_normal_to_camera(s,v_r,v)	internal normal to camera space
mi_normal_to_object(s,v_r,v)	internal normal to object space
mi_normal_from_world(s,v_r,v)	world normal to internal space
mi_normal_from_camera(s,v_r,v)	camera normal to internal space
mi_normal_from_object(s,v_r,v)	object normal to internal space

Point and vector transformations are similar, except that the vector versions ignore the translation part of the matrix. Normal transformations are similar to vector transformations, except that the transpose of the inverse transformation matrix is used. In this way it is ensured that if a vector and a normal are orthogonal in one coordinate system they remain orthogonal after they have been transformed to a different coordinate system. This holds for arbitrary, not necessarily orthogonal transformations.

The length of vectors is preserved only if the transformation matrix does not scale. The *mi_point_transform* and *mi_vector_transform* functions are also available to transform points and vectors between arbitrary coordinate systems given by a transformation matrix. *mi_vector_transform_T* transforms with the transpose of the matrix and can be used for the transformation of normals.

3.3 Shader Type Overview

There are many types of shaders, all of which can be substituted by user-written shaders:

- **material shaders** describe the visible material of an object. They are the only mandatory part of any material description. Material shaders are called whenever a visible ray (eye ray, reflected ray, refracted ray, or transparency ray) hits an object. Material shaders have a central function in mental ray.
- **volume shaders** are called to account for atmospheric effects encountered by a ray. The state (see below) distinguishes two types of volume shaders: the standard *volume* shader that is called in most cases, and the *refraction volume* shader that is taken from the object material at the current intersection point, and becomes the standard *volume* shader if a refraction or transparency ray is cast. Many material shaders substitute a new standard *volume* shader based on inside/outside calculations. Volume shaders, unlike other shaders, accept an input color (such as the one calculated by the material shader at the last intersection point) that they are expected to modify.
- **light shaders** implement the characteristics of a light source. For example, a spot light shader would use the illumination direction to attenuate the amount of light emitted. A light shader is called whenever a material shader uses a built-in function to evaluate a light. Light shaders normally cast shadow rays if shadows are enabled to detect obscuring objects between the light source and the illuminated point.
- **shadow shaders** are called instead of material shaders when a shadow ray intersects with an object. Shadow rays are cast by light sources to determine visibility of an illuminated object. Shadow shaders are basically light-weight material shaders that calculate the transmitted color of an object without casting secondary or shadow rays. Frequently, material shaders are written such that they can also be used as shadow shaders.
- **environment shaders** are called instead of a material shader when a visible ray leaves the scene entirely without intersecting an object. Typical environment shaders evaluate a texture mapped on a virtual infinite sphere enclosing the scene (virtual because it is not part of the scene geometry).
- **photon shaders** are used to propagate photons through the model in order to simulate caustics and global illumination[2.1]. Photon shaders are used in a preprocessing step in which photons are emitted from the light sources into the model (just as a real light source emits photons into the world). Each photon is traced through the scene using a technique called photon tracing which is similar to ray tracing. As with ray tracing a photon is reflected of a specular mirror surface in the mirror direction. The most important difference is the fact that the photon shader modifies the photon energy *before* reflecting the photon unlike ray tracing which traces a ray and then modifies the result accordingly (for example multiplies it with the specular reflection coefficients). Photon shaders also store information about the incoming photon in a global photon map which contains all photons stored in the model. This photon map is then used by the material shaders during the rendering step (ray tracing step) to simulate caustics and global illumination[2.1]. Frequently, material shaders are written such that they can also be used as photon shaders (and also shadow shaders).

- **photon emitter shaders** are used to control the emission of photons from a light source. Combined with the light shaders it is possible to simulate complex light sources with complex emission characteristics. Photon emitters are only used if caustics or global illumination[2.1] are enabled, to construct a photon map before the actual rendering takes place.

- **texture shaders** come in three flavors: color, scalar, and vector. Each calculates and returns the respective type. Typical texture shaders return a color from a texture image after some appropriate coordinate transformation, or compute a color at a location in 3D space using some sort of noise function. Their main purpose is to relieve other shaders, such as material or environment shaders, from performing color and other computations. For example, if a marble surface were needed, it should be written as a texture shader and not a material shader because a texture shader does not have to calculate illumination by light sources, reflections, and so on. It is much easier to write a texture shader than a material shader. mental ray never calls a texture shader directly, it is always called from one of the other types of shaders.

- **displacement shaders** are called during tessellation of polygonal or free-form surface geometry, a procedure that creates triangles to be rendered. Displacement shaders are called to shift the created vertices along their normals by a scalar distance returned by the shader. mental ray supports approximation controls that allow adjusting the tessellation to better resolve curvature introduced by displacement shaders.

- **geometry shaders** are run before rendering begins. They create geometry procedurally by using a function call library that closely follows the .mi2 scene description language. Unlike displacement shaders, which are called once per vertex, geometry shaders are responsible for creating an entire object or object hierarchy (each of which, when tessellated later, can cause displacement shader calls).

- **contour shaders** come in four different flavors: contour store functions, contour contrast shaders, contour shaders, and contour output shaders. For details see chapter 2.8.

- **lens shaders** are called when a primary ray is cast by the camera. They may modify the eye ray's origin and direction to implement cameras other than the standard pinhole camera, and may modify the result of the primary ray to implement effects such as lens flares.

- **output shaders** are different from all other shaders and receive different parameters. They are called when the entire scene has been completely rendered and the output image resides in memory. Output shaders operate on the output image to implement special filtering or compositing operations. Output shaders are not associated with any particular ray because they are called after the last ray is completed.

The following diagram illustrates the path of a ray cast by the camera. It first intersects with a sphere at point A. The sphere's material shader first casts a reflection ray that hits a box, then a refraction ray that intersects the sphere at its other side T, and finally it casts a transparency ray that also intersects the sphere, at D. (This example is contrived, it is very unusual for a material shader to cast both a refraction and a transparency ray.) The same material shader is called at points A, T, and D. In this example, the reflection trace depth may have prevented further reflection rays to be cast at T and D.

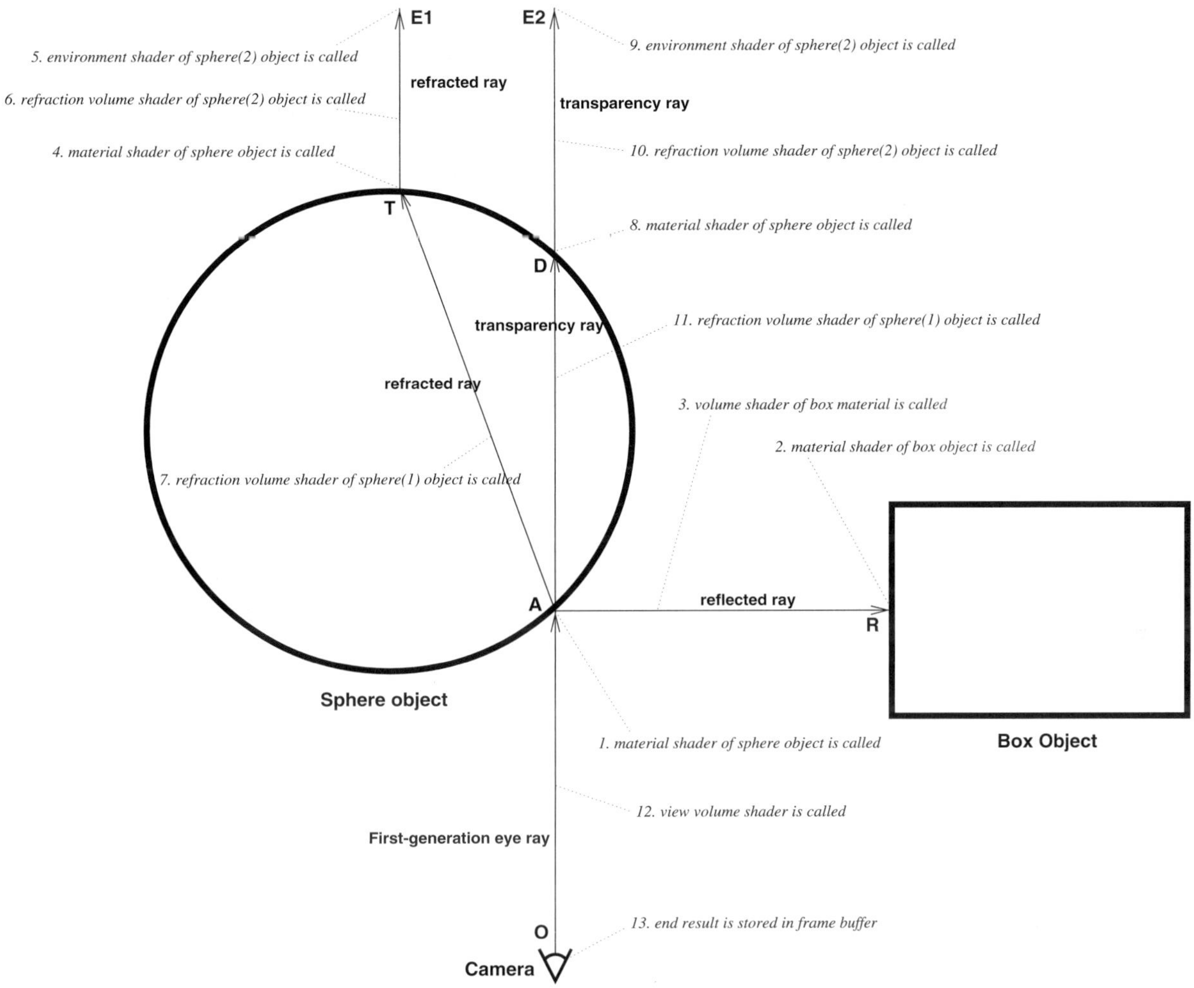

The annotations set in *italics* are numbered; the events described happen in the sequence given by the numbers.

Since material shaders may do inside/outside calculations based on the surface normal or the parent state chain (see below), the volume shaders are marked (1) and (2), depending on whether the volume shader left by A or by T/D in the *refraction volume* field of the state. The default refraction volume shader is the one found in the material definition, or the standard volume shader if the material defines no volume shader. For details on choosing volume shaders, see the section on writing material and volume shaders. Note that the volume shaders in this diagram are called immediately after the material shader returns.

The next two diagrams depict the situation when the material shader at the intersection point M requests a light ray from the light source at L, by calling a function such as *mi_sample_light*. This results in the light shader of L to be called. No intersection testing is done at this point. Intersection testing takes place when shadows are enabled and the light shader casts *shadow rays* by calling *mi_trace_shadow*. This function is called only once but may result in more than one shadow shader call. There are four different modes for shadow casting, listed in the order of increased computational cost:

- **shadow off**
  No shadows are computed, and no shadow shaders are called. Call to *mi_trace_shadow* return immediately without modifying the result color.
- **shadow on**
  For each obscuring object (A and B), a shadow ray is generated with the origin L and the intersection point A or B, and the shadow shaders of objects A and B are called to modify the light emitted by the light source based on the transparency attributes of the obscuring object. No shadow ray is generated for the segment from B to M because no other obscuring object whose shadow shader could be called exists. Although shadow rays always go from the light source towards the illuminated point in this mode, the order in which the shadow shaders are called is undefined. If an object without shadow shader is found, or if a shadow shader returns `miFALSE`, it is assumed that no light reaches the illuminated point and the search for more obscuring objects is stopped (although the light shader has the option of ignoring this result and supplying some light anyway). See the first diagram below. The volume shader of the illuminated object M is applied to the entire distance between M and L.
- **shadow sort**
  Same as the previous method, but shadow shaders are called in distance order, object closest to the light source first. In the first diagram, steps 4 and 5 may be reversed.
- **shadow segments**
  This mode is more sophisticated than the others. Shadow rays become similar to visible rays; they travel in segments from the illuminated point to the first obscuring object, then from there to the next obscuring object, and so on until the light source is reached. This means that shadow rays travel in the opposite direction, and one shadow ray's end point becomes the next shadow ray's origin. Volume shaders are called for each of these segments, and every shadow shader must perform inside/outside calculations to store the correct volume shader in *state* $\rightarrow$ *volume* much like material shaders to. This mode is preferred if volume effects should cast shadows.

Note that the shadow segment mode requires complex shadow shaders to behave differently. Every shadow shader must be able to work with all these modes, so shadow shaders that deal with volumes or depend on the ray direction must test *state* $\rightarrow$ *options* $\rightarrow$ *shadow* to determine the mode. In case an incorrectly implemented shadow shader fails to call *mi_trace_shadow_seg* to evaluate other shadows, mental ray will call *mi_trace_shadow_seg* and then call the shadow shader again, thus simulating the effect.

The first diagram shows the ray casting order and the ray directions for the **shadow on** and **shadow sort** modes:

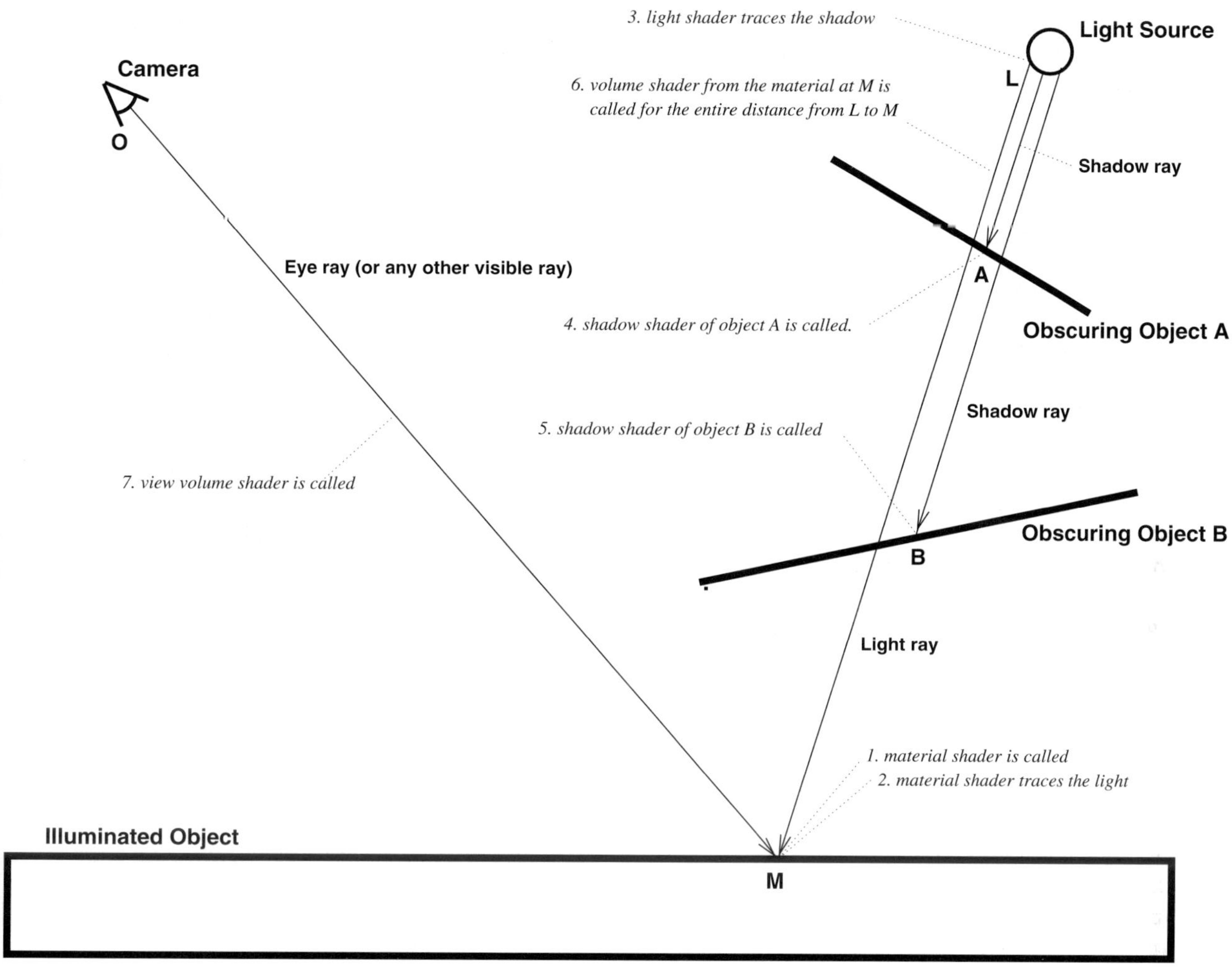

The next diagram shows the same situation in **shadow segments** mode:

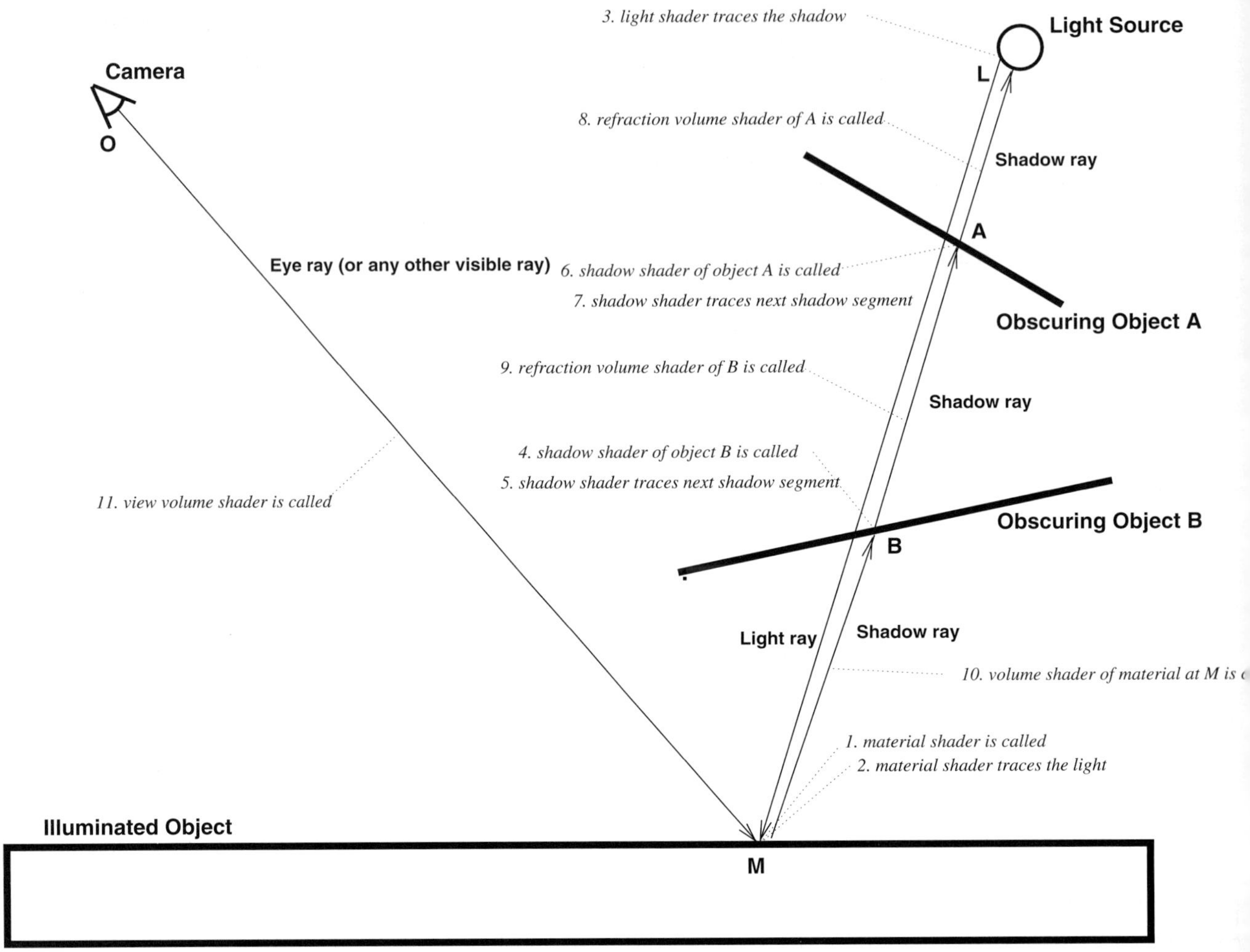

The following diagram illustrates the path of a photon shot from the light source in the caustics or global illumination[2.1] preprocessing phase. First a photon is traced from the light source. It hits object A, and the photon material shader of object A is called. The photon material shader stores energy at the intersection point and determines how much energy is reflected and how much is refracted, and the directions of reflection and transmission. It then traces a new photon from A, in the reflection direction, or in the transmission direction, or both. The reflected photon hits object B, and the photon material shader of object B is called. The photon material shader of object B stores energy at the intersection point and shoots a new photon.

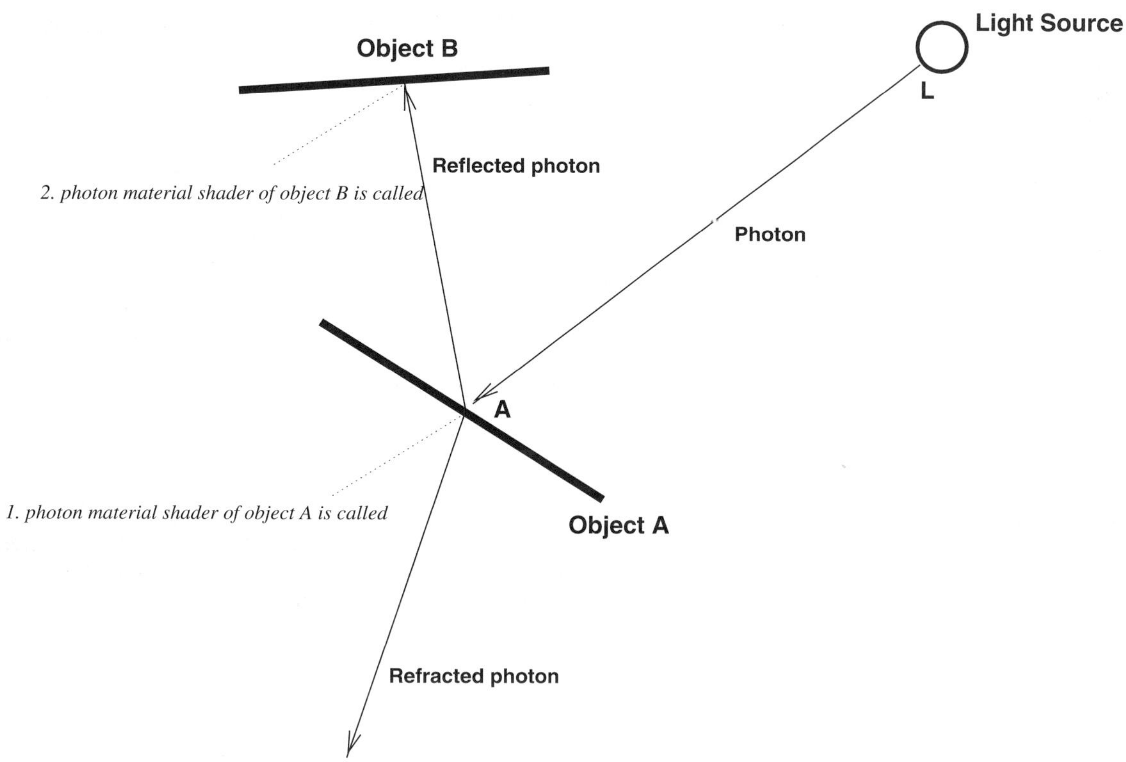

The remainder of this chapter describes how to write all types of shaders. First, the concepts of ray tracing state parameter passing common to all shaders are presented, followed by a detailed discussion of each type of shader.

3.4 State Variables

Every shader needs to access information about the current state of mental ray, and information about the intersection that led to the shader call. This information is stored in a single structure known as the *state*. Not all information in the state is of interest or defined for all shaders; for example, lens shaders are called before an intersection is done and hence have no information such as the intersection point or the normal there. It is recommended to call the state parameter that shaders receive as a formal parameter *state* because some macros provided in the `mi_shader.h` include file that require access to the state rely on this name (namely, the typed *mi_eval_** variants). The state, and everything else needed to write shaders, is defined in `mi_shader.h`, which must be included by all shader source files.

Before a shader is called, mental ray prepares a new state structure that provides global information to the shader. This state may be the same data structure that was used in the previous call (this is the case for shaders that modify another shader's result, like lens, shadow, and volume shaders); or it may be a new state structure that is a copy of the calling shader's state with some state variables changed (this is done if a secondary ray is cast with one of the tracing functions provided by mental ray). For example, if a material shader that is using state A casts a reflected ray, which hits another object and causes that object's material shader to be called with state B, state B will be a copy of state A except for the ray and intersection information, which will be different in states A and B. State A is said to be the *parent* of state B. The state contains a parent pointer that allows sub-shader to access the state of parent shaders. If a volume shader is called after the material shader, the volume shader modifies the color calculated by the material shader, and gets the same state as the material shader, instead of a fresh copy.

The state also contains a *child* pointer that, together with the parent pointer, forms a double-linked list of states. After a shader casts a ray, the state used by the ray remains available after the trace call returns. This means that the shader has full access to the intersection information, label value, and all other state variables used by the child shader. For example, the shader for a completely transparent object may decide to copy *state* → *child* → *label* to *state* → *label* after *mi_trace_transparency* returns. Only the most recent discarded child state is retained; *state* → *child* → *child* is undefined.

This means that it is possible to pass information from one shader to another in the call tree for a primary ray, by one of two methods: either the parent (the caller) changes its own state that will be inherited by the child, or the child follows the parent pointer. The state contains a *user pointer* that a parent can store the address of a local data structure in, for passing it to sub-shaders. Since every sub-shader inherits this pointer, it may access information provided by its parent. A typical application of this are inside/outside calculations performed by material shaders to find out whether the ray is inside a closed object to base the interpretation of parameters such as the index of refraction on.

Note that the state can be used to pass information from one shader to sub-shaders that are lower in the call tree. Care must be taken not to destroy information in the state because some shaders (shadow, volume, and the first eye shader) re-use the state from the previous call. In particular, the state cannot be used to pass information from one primary (camera) ray to the next. Static variables can be used in the shader for this purpose, but care must be taken to avoid multiple access on multiprocessor shared-memory machines. On such a machine, all processors share the same set of static variables, and every change by one processor becomes immediately visible to all other processors, which may be executing the same shader at the same time. Locking facilities are available in mental ray to protect critical sections that may execute only once at any time.

Here is a complete list of state variables usable by shaders. Variables not listed here are for internal use only and should not be accessed or modified by shaders. Some variables are available only in some types of shaders; see the "State Variables by Shader Type" section below. The first table lists all state variables that remain unchanged for the duration of the frame:

3.4.1 Frame

type	*name*	*content*
int	version	shader interface version
miTag	camera_inst	tag of camera instance
miCamera *	camera	camera information
miRc_options *	options	general rendering options

The camera data structure pointed to by *camera* has the following fields. None of these may be written to by a shader.

type	*name*	*content*
miBoolean	orthographic	orthographic rendering
float	focal	focal length of the camera
float	aperture	aperture of the camera
float	aspect	aspect ratio $\frac{y}{x}$
miRange	clip	Z clipping distances
int	x_resolution	image width in pixels
int	y_resolution	image height in pixels
int	window.xl	left image margin
int	window.yl	bottom image margin
int	window.xh	right image margin
int	window.yh	top image margin
miTag	volume	camera volume (atmosphere)
miTag	environment	camera environment shader
miTag	lens	lens shader or lens shader list
miTag	output	output shader or output shader list
int	frame	frame number
float	frame_time	frame time in seconds
float	x_offset[2.1]	x offset of image in pixels
float	y_offset[2.1]	y offset of image in pixels

The option data structure pointed to by *option* has the following format. The option structure may not be written to by shaders.

type	*name*	*content*
miBoolean	trace	ray tracing turned on?
miBoolean	scanline	scanline mode turned on?
miBoolean	motion	motion blur turned on?
char	shadow	no, normal, segmented, sorted
char	filter	nonlocal sampling filter
char	acceleration	ray tracing algorithm
char	face	front, back, or both faces
char	field	odd or even fields, or off
int	reflection_depth	max reflection trace depth
int	refraction_depth	max refraction trace depth
int	trace_depth	max combined trace depth
int	photon_reflection_depth	max photon reflection trace depth
int	photon_refraction_depth	max photon refraction trace depth
int	photon_trace_depth	max combined photon trace depth
miBoolean	samplelock	noise animation locking on/off
miBoolean	caustic	caustics on/off
miBoolean	globillum$^{2.1}$	global illumination on/off
miBoolean	finalgather$^{2.1}$	final gather on/off
miPointer	image [ ]	frame buffers for output shaders

version The version number of the interface and the state structure. Useful to check if the version is compatible with the shader. Version 1 stands for mental ray 1.8, version 2 stands for 1.9 and 2.0.

camera_inst The camera instance is a data structure in the mental ray database that contains transformation information about the camera. Like all other tags in the state, a pointer to that data structure can be obtained by calling *mi_db_access* with the tag as the only argument. This function returns a void pointer to the accessed data structure. After the pointer is no longer used, the pointer must be "returned" by calling *mi_db_unpin* with it. Failure to do so will abort rendering.

The following parameters are in the *state→camera* structure:

orthographic This flag is `miTRUE` if the renderer is in orthographic mode, and `miFALSE` if it is in perspective mode.

focal The focal length of the camera (the distance from the origin in camera space to the viewing plane that the image pixels are mapped on).

aperture The aperture of the camera (the width of the viewing plane in camera space).

aspect The aspect ratio (the ratio of the width and height of the viewing plane in camera space).

clip — This data structure has two members, *min* and *max*, that specify the hither and yon clipping planes in camera space. Objects will be clipped if their Z coordinate in camera space is less than -*max* or greater than -*min*.

x_resolution — The x resolution of the image in pixels.

y_resolution — The y resolution of the image in pixels.

window — The window specifies the lower left and the upper right pixel of the sub-region of the image to be rendered. If *xl* and *yl* are `0` and *xh* and *yh* match or exceed the resolution minus one, the entire image is rendered. The window is clipped to the resolution. Pixels outside the window are set to black.

volume — The global volume (atmosphere) shader from the camera that is used for attenuating rays outside of objects, such as the primary ray from the camera to the first object intersection. Material shaders inherit this volume shader because the `volume` state variable defaults to the camera volume, but shaders may override the volume. See below.

environment — The environment (reflection map) shader of the camera. It is used to assign a color to primary eye rays that leave the scene without ever intersecting an object. Material shaders that do not define their own environment shaders for evaluation of local reflection maps inherit the camera environment shader. Reflection maps give the illusion of true raytraced reflections by looking up a texture based on the reflection direction.

lens — The list of lenses applied to the standard pinhole camera. Each lens shader in this list is called when a primary ray leaves the camera.

output — The list of output shaders and file outputs attached to the camera. File outputs are encoded in special `miFunction` data structures that contain a file name and various miscellaneous data instead of a shader reference.

frame — The current frame number. In field mode, this is the field number, two successive frames rendered by mental ray are combined into a single output frame by an output shader. In field mode, the odd frame is the first frame and the even frame is the second.

frame_time — The current frame number, expressed as a time in seconds. The relation between *frame* and *frame_time* depends on the frame rate. Both numbers are taken verbatim from the input scene, mental ray does not change or verify either number. If the frame time is omitted in the .mi file, it is set to `0.0`.

x_offset — [2.1]The X offset of the rendered image. The default value is `0.0` which means that the image will be centered on the camera's axis.

y_offset — [2.1]The Y offset of the rendered image. The default value is `0.0` which means that the image will be centered on the camera's axis.

The following parameters are in the *state→options* structure:

trace — If this flag is `miTRUE`, secondary ray tracing (reflection and refraction) is enabled. If it is `miFALSE`, only eye and transparency rays are evaluated, refraction rays degenerate to transparency rays, lens shaders cannot modify the ray origin and direction, and no shadows are computed regardless of the `shadow` flag.

scanline — If this flag is `miTRUE`, the scanline algorithm is enabled for primary rays. If `scanline` is `miFALSE`, primary rays are cast using pure ray tracing, which may slow down the rendering process.

motion — If this flag is `miTRUE`, motion blurring is enabled; if it is `miFALSE`, motion blurring is disabled even if motion vectors are present.

shadow — This ASCII character controls shadow casting. If it is `0`, shadows are disabled (shadow off); if it is `1`, normal shadows are computed in undefined order with volume shaders applied to the light ray (shadow on); if it is `'l'`, shadow shaders are called in sorted order from the light source towards the illumination point (shadow sort); if it is `'s'`, shadows are computed by tracing the segments between the illumination point, the occluding objects and the light source and applying volume shaders to these segments (shadow segment).

filter — Nonlocal filtering weighs samples according to their distance from the pixel center. Possible values are `'b'` for box, `'t'` for triangle, and `'g'` for gauss.

acceleration — The ray tracing algorithm. This is either `'c'` (an algorithm based on ray classification), or `'b'` (a BSP algorithm), or `'g'` (a hierarchical uniform grid algorithm). The latter two are often, but by no means always, faster. Note that by default, primary rays are computed using a scanline algorithm if possible.

face — This variable specifies whether front-facing, back-facing, or all triangles are taken into account. All others are ignored, resulting in speed improvements. This is also called *back face culling*. The possible values are `'f'` (front), `'b'` (back), and `'a'` (all).

field — Field rendering, if turned on, renders only the even or odd scanlines of an image. Two successive renders are then combined to a full frame, resulting in smoother animations. `0` turns off field rendering, `'e'` renders only even scanlines (top is odd), and 'o' renders only odd scanlines.

reflection_depth

The maximal allowed number of recursive reflections. A reflection ray will only by cast when this limit is not exceeded. If set to 0, no secondary reflection rays will be cast. See `reflection_level` below.

refraction_depth

The maximal allowed number of recursive refractions. A refraction ray will only be cast if this number is not exceeded. If set to 0, no secondary refraction or transparency rays will be cast. See `refraction_level` below.

trace_depth

The maximal summed trace depth. mental ray will allow this many segments of the ray tree when it is followed through the scene, with any combination of reflections and refractions permitted by the previous two values until the total trace depth is reached. A ray will only be cast if this number is not exceeded.

photon_reflection_depth

The maximal allowed number of recursive photon reflections. Similar to `reflection_depth`. Default is 5.

photon_refraction_depth

The maximal allowed number of photon refractions. Similar to `refraction_depth`. Default is 5.

photon_trace_depth

The maximal summed photon trace depth. The maximum number of photon bounces is limited by this number. Default is 5.

caustic

Specifies whether caustics are being simulated or not.

globillum

[2.1]Specifies whether global illumination is being simulated or not.

finalgather

[2.1]Specifies whether illumination is computed with final gathering. Final gathering can be combined with global illumination and caustics.

samplelock

Whether to let the sampling of area light sources, motion blur, and depht-of-field be static or depend on the frame number. The default is on, meaning static sampling.

image[ ]

An array of pointers to frame buffers. It is available only in output shaders. The type is `miPointer` to ensure network transparency, requiring access with `image[i].p`; the real type is `miImg_image *`. The array is indexed with the predefined indices `miRC_IMAGE_RGBA`, `miRC_IMAGE_Z`, `miRC_IMAGE_N`, `miRC_IMAGE_M`, and `miRC_IMAGE_TAG`, each corresponding to one of the standard frame buffers that are enabled with appropriate output statements. If a frame buffer was not enabled, the corresponding pointer is 0.

All frame buffers have the same resolution as specified in the camera.

The frame buffer pointers can be passed to the buffer access functions, *mi_img_get_color*, *mi_img_put_color*, etc. For each type of frame buffer, there are functions to retrieve and store a pixel value that accept the frame buffer pointer as their first argument. Motion vector data can be accessed with the normal-vector access functions; the data format is identical.

3.4.2 Image Samples

The state variables in the next table describe an eye (primary) ray. There is one eye ray for every sample that contributes to a pixel in the output image. If a material shader that evaluates a material hit by a primary ray casts secondary reflection, refraction, transparency, light, or shadow rays, all shaders called as a consequence will inherit these variables unmodified:

type	*name*	*content*
`miScalar`	`raster_x`	X coordinate of image pixel
`miScalar`	`raster_y`	Y coordinate of image pixel
`miFunction *`	`shader`	current shader
`miLock`	`global_lock`	lock shared by all shaders
`short`	`thread`	current thread

raster_x — The X coordinate of the point in raster space to be rendered. Raster space is the pixel grid of the rendered image file, with 0/0 at the lower left corner.

raster_y — The Y coordinate of the point in raster space to be rendered. In output shaders executing in parallel mode[2.1]because *state* → *dist* is nonzero, it contains the number of the first scanline of the scanline block to write.

shader — This pointer points to a data structure describing the current shader. The fields usable by shaders are `lock`, which is a lock shared by all calls to this shader, `miTag next_function` for chained shaders such as lens shaders, and `char parameters[]` which contains the shader parameters. The latter is redundant for the current shader because the parameter pointer is also passed as the third shader argument, but it can be used to find the parameters of parent shaders. This should be used with care because the C data structure of parent shader parameter lists is not generally known.

global_lock — This lock is shared by all shaders, regardless of their name. It can be used to lock critical sections common to all shaders. For example, it could be used to protect a nonreentrant user-defined random-number generator, or initialization of a more specific set of locks. It is pre-initialized by mental ray; do not initialize or delete it.

thread The current thread number. This is a faster way of finding the thread number than calling *mi_par_localvpu*.

3.4.3 Rays

Whenever a ray is cast the following state variables are set to describe the ray:

type	*name*	*content*
miState *	parent	state of parent shader
miState *	child	state of child shader
miRay_type	type	type of ray: reflect, light...
miCBoolean	scanline	from scanline algorithm
void *	cache	RC intersection cache
miVector	org	start point of the ray
miVector	dir	direction of the ray
float	time	shutter interval time
miTag	volume	volume shader of primitive
miTag	environment	environment shader
int	reflection_level	current reflection ray depth
int	refraction_level	current refraction ray depth

parent Points to the state of the parent ray. In the first lens shader, it is NULL. In subsequent lens shaders, it points to the previous lens shader. In the material shader that is called when the primary ray hits an object, it points to the last lens shader's state, or is NULL if no lens shader has been applied. For material shaders called when a secondary reflection or refraction ray hits an object, it points to the parent material shader that cast the ray. In light shaders and environment shaders, it points to the state of the shader which requested the light or environment lookup. For shadow shaders, it points to the state of the light shader that started the shadow trace. In volume shaders, its value is the same as for a material or light shader of the same ray.

child Points to the state of the most recent child ray. After a function that created a separate state returns, this state is still accessible to the caller of the function through this pointer. For example, *mi_trace_refraction* constructs a state when hitting geometry before calling the material shader attached to that geometry with this state. After it returns, the new state can be accessed by the caller of *mi_trace_refraction* to access *state* → *user*, *state* → *label*, and all other local information.

type Specifies the reason for this ray. This is an enumerator:

miRAY_EYE	primary rays from the camera

`miRAY_TRANSPARENT`	transparency rays cast by a material shader
`miRAY_REFRACT`	refraction rays cast by a material shader
`miRAY_REFLECT`	reflection rays cast by a material shader
`miRAY_SHADOW`	light rays cast from a light source
`miRAY_LIGHT`	rays cast by a material shader when a light source is evaluated (which may result in the light source casting shadow rays back)
`miRAY_ENVIRONMENT`	rays that sample an environment (reflection) map
`miRAY_DISPLACE`	is set for displacement shaders
`miRAY_NONE`	is a catch-all for other types of rays.
`miPHOTON_LIGHT`	is a photon emitted from a light source.
`miPHOTON_REFLECT_SPECULAR`	is a photon reflected specularly from a surface.
`miPHOTON_REFLECT_GLOSSY`	is a photon reflected glossily from a surface.
`miPHOTON_REFLECT_DIFFUSE`	is a photon reflected diffusely from a surface.
`miPHOTON_TRANSMIT_SPECULAR`	is a photon transmitted specularly through a surface.
`miPHOTON_TRANSMIT_GLOSSY`	is a photon transmitted glossily through a surface.
`miPHOTON_TRANSMIT_DIFFUSE`	is a photon transmitted diffusely through a surface.

`miPHOTON_TRANSPARENT` is a photon transmitted directly (ie., without refraction) through a surface.

The ray type (`state->type`) can be queried using the following macros:

`miRAY_PRIMARY(raytype)` is true if the raytype is a primary or a transparency ray.

`miRAY_SECONDARY(raytype)` is true if the raytype corresponds to a ray generated at an intersection point.

`miRAY_PHOTON(raytype)` is true if the raytype is one of the `miPHOTON_*` rays. This macro can be used to separate the photon tracing part of a shader from the regular ray tracing part.

scanline This flag is set if the current intersection was found by means of the scanline algorithm.

cache This variable is used by the renderer internally to improve speed. Its existence determines which shaders may call which tracing functions. By setting this pointer to 0, the shader can ease these restrictions and call tracing functions that are not normally legal for this type of shader. For details, see the section *Shaders and Trace Functions* below.

org The origin (start point) of the ray in internal space. In the primary material shader, it is set by the last lens shader, or is (0, 0, 0) if there is no lens shader and the default non-orthogonal pinhole camera is used. In all other material shaders, it is the previous intersection point. In light and shadow shaders, it is the origin of the light source. If the light source does not have an origin, it is undefined.

dir The direction of the ray in internal space. This is basically the normalized difference between `point` and `org`, pointing towards the current intersection point (except in the case of directional light sources that have no origin; in this case the light direction is used). Light and non-segmented shadow rays point from the light source to the intersection.

time The time of the ray in the shutter interval. If motion blurring is turned off, the time is always 0. Otherwise, it is systematically sampled in the range from 0 to the shutter time.

volume

The volume shader to be applied to the ray. The volume shader is called immediately after the material shader returns, without any change to the state. The volume shader changes the result color of the material shader to take the distance the ray to the material has traveled into account. For primary rays this is the `volume` of the camera, for reflection and light rays the `volume` of the parent, and for refraction and transparency rays the `refraction_volume` of the parent. Note that the `mi_trace_refract` and `mi_trace_transparent` functions copy `refraction_volume` to `volume` to ensure that sub-shaders use the volume shader that applies to the interior of the object. Volume shaders are also applied to light rays.

environment

The active environment shader. For primary rays this is the environment of the camera. For reflection and refraction rays the active shader is taken from the material, if it specifies an environment shader. If it does not, the environment shader defaults to the environment shader in the camera, if present. The purpose of the environment shader is to provide a color if a ray leaves the scene entirely.

reflection_level

The reflection level of the ray. It may range from 0 for primary rays to `reflection_depth` minus one. The `trace_depth` imposes another limit: The sum of `reflection_level` and `refraction_level` must be one less than `trace_depth`. A shader may decrement or reset the reflection level to circumvent the restrictions imposed by the trace depth state variables.

refraction_level

The refraction level of the ray. This is equivalent to the reflection level but applies to refraction and transparency (which is a variation of refraction that does not take the index of refraction into account) rays. A shader may decrement or reset the reflection level to circumvent the restrictions imposed by the trace depth state variables.

3.4.4 Intersection

The variables in the next table are closely related to the previous. They describe the intersection of the ray with an object, and give information about that object and how it was hit.

type	*name*	*content*
miTag	refraction_volume	volume shader for refraction
miUint	label	object label for label file
miTag	instance	instance of object
miTag	light_instance	instance of light
miScalar [4]	bary	barycentric coordinates
miVector	point	intersection (ray end) point
miVector	normal	interpolated normal at point
miVector	normal_geom	geometry normal at point
miCBoolean	inv_normal	true if normals were inverted
miScalar	dot_nd	dot prod of normal and dir
double	dist	length of the ray
void *	pri	identifies hit box
int	pri_idx	identifies hit primitive in box
double	shadow_tol	safe zone to prevent self-shadows
miScalar	ior	index of refraction of medium
miScalar	ior_in	index of r. of previous medium

refraction_volume The volume at the other side of the object. This is set to the volume shader of the material. It will be applied to refraction rays. This is implemented by copying `refraction_volume` to `volume` (which is the shader that gets called when the material shader returns) in the `mi_trace_refract` and `mi_trace_transparent` functions. The material shader may decide that the ray is leaving and not entering the object, and look in the state's parents for an outside volume shader.

label The label of the hit object. Every object may contain a label that is made available by this variable. When the primary material shader returns, the `label` is copied from the state to the "tag" frame buffer, if one was created by an appropriate `output` statement in the `camera`. The primary material shader is free to change this variable to any value to put different values into the tag frame buffer.

instance The instance of the object containing the primitive hit by the ray.

light_instance If the ray is a light ray or the corresponding shadow ray: the light instance. If the ray hit a visible area light source, `light_instance` is set to that light instance.

bary The three barycentric coordinates of the intersection in the hit primitive. The fourth value is reserved for implicit patches and is not currently used. Barycentric coordinates are weights that specify the contribution by each vertex or control point. The sum of all barycentric coordinates is 1.

point The intersection point (end point of the ray) in internal space.

normal

The (interpolated) surface normal at the intersection point if vertex normals are present, or the uninterpolated geometric normal of the primitive otherwise, in internal space. It points to the side of the primitive from which it is hit by the ray, and is normalized to within the precision of a `float`. Care should be taken when calculating the length of the normal; the result of this calculation might be very slightly greater than 1 because a `float` has only a little over six significant digits. This can cause math functions like `acos` to return `NaN` (Not a Number, an illegal result), which usually results in white pixels in the output if the `NaN` finds its way into a result color.

normal_geom

The uninterpolated normal of the hit primitive in internal space. It points to that side of the primitive from which it is hit by the ray. It is normalized.

inv_normal

If a ray hits geometry from behind (that is, if the dot product of the ray direction and the normal is positive), mental ray inverts both *normal* and *normal_geom* and sets *inv_normal* to `miTRUE`.

dot_nd

The negative dot product of the normal and the direction (after the normals have been inverted in the case of backfacing geometry). In the case of light rays, it is the negative dot product of the light ray direction and the normal at the point which is to be illuminated.

dist

The length of the ray, which is the distance from `org` to `point` if there is an origin, in internal space. A value lower or equal to `0.0` indicates that no intersection was found, and that the length is infinite. In output shaders, it is `0` for sequential shaders or the number of scanlines to write, beginning at *raster_y*, for parallel output shaders[2.1].

material

The material of the primitive hit by the ray. (If a visible area light source has been hit, `material` is set to the inherited instance material, if available.) The data can be accessed using *mi_db_access* followed by *mi_db_unpin*. This is generally not necessary because all relevant information is also available in the state.

pri

This number uniquely identifies the current box. All primitives are grouped in boxes. When casting light rays, mental ray may check whether the primitive's normal is pointing away from the light and ignore the light in this case; for this reason some shaders, such as ray-marching volume shaders, assign `0` to *pri* before sampling a light. Shaders other than volume shaders should restore *pri* before returning. When a visible area light source is hit, *pri* is set to NULL. Some *mi_query* modes do not work if *pri* has been modified.

pri_idx

Together with *pri*, this number uniquely identifies the primitive in the current box. This value is used by mental ray internally.

shadow_tol — If a shadow ray is found to intersect the primitive in shadow, at a distance of less than this tolerance, the intersection is ignored. This prevents self-shadowing in the case of numerical inaccuracies.

ior — This field is intended for use by material shaders that need to keep track of the index of refraction for inside/outside determination. It is not used by mental ray. The *mi_mtl_refraction_index* shader interface function stores the index of refraction of the medium the ray travels through in this state variable.

ior_in — Like *ior*, this field helps the shader with inside/outside calculations. It contains the "previous" index of refraction, in the medium the ray was traveling through before the intersection. Like *ior*, *ior_in* is neither set nor used by mental ray, it exists to allow the material shader to inherit the previous index of refraction to subsequent shaders.

3.4.5 Textures, Motion, Derivatives

The following table is an extension to the previous. These variables give information about the intersection point for texture mapping. They are defined when the ray has hit a textured object:

type	*name*	*content*
`miVector *`	`tex_list`	list of texture coordinates
`miVector *`	`bump_x_list`	list of X bump basis vectors
`miVector *`	`bump_y_list`	list of Y bump basis vectors
`miVector`	`tex`	texture coord (tex shaders)
`miVector`	`motion`	interpolated motion vector
`miVector *`	`derivs[5]`	list of surface derivatives

tex_list — A pointer to an array containing the texture coordinates of the intersection point in all texture spaces. When material shaders that support multiple textures on a surface call a texture lookup function, they must specify which texture coordinate to use, usually by choosing one of the texture vertices in *tex_list* and copying it to *tex*.

bump_x_list — A pointer to an array containing the x bump basis vectors in all texture spaces. The vectors are in object space.

bump_y_list — A pointer to an array containing the y bump basis vectors in all texture spaces. The vectors are in object space.

tex — The texture coordinates where the texture should be evaluated. This variable is available only in texture shaders; it is set by the caller (for example, a texture lookup from a material shader).

motion The motion vector of the intersection point. If the object has no motion vectors (m statements in the vertices in the scene description file), the motion vector is a null vector.

derivs[ ] A pointer to an array containing the surface derivative vectors. If the object is a free-form surface object, the surface derivative vectors derivs[0] ... derivs[4] contain $\partial\vec{x}/\partial u$, $\partial\vec{x}/\partial v$, $\partial^2\vec{x}/\partial u^2$, $\partial^2\vec{x}/\partial v^2$, $\partial^2\vec{x}/\partial u\partial v$, respectively. Here $\vec{x}$ denotes the intersection point. For polygonal objects the surface derivatives are taken from the .mi file. If the object has no first derivative vectors, the first two vectors are null vectors. If the object has no second derivative vectors, the last three vectors are null vectors. Since surface derivatives are calculated approximately, the vectors $\partial\vec{x}/\partial u$, $\partial\vec{x}/\partial v$ and the normal vector at the intersection point are not necessarily orthogonal to each other.

3.4.6 User Fields

Finally, the user field allows a shader to store a pointer to an arbitrary data structure in the shader. Subsequent shaders called as a result of operations done by this shader (such as casting a reflection ray or evaluating a light or a texture) inherit the pointer and can read and write this shader's local data. Sub-shaders can also find other parent's user data by following state parent pointers, see above. With this method, extra parameters can be provided to and extra return values received from sub-shaders.

However, once the shader that has set the user pointer returns, the user pointer is lost. Its purpose is to pass information to sub-shaders down the call graph, not to pass information from one invocation of a shader to the next (for example, to the next primary ray). This implies that it is not a good idea to use *mi_mem_allocate* to obtain the pointer because by definition this could result in millions of allocations, which is inefficient. Long-term shader user data should be stored in *state* → *shader* → *user.p* instead, typically allocated in the init shader and released in the exit shader.

The user variables are initialized to 0.

type	*name*	*content*
void *	user	user data pointer
int	user_size	user data size (optional)

The shader pointer can be used to access the shader parameters, as *state*→*parameters*. This is redundant for the current shader because this pointer is also passed as the third shader argument, but it can be used to find a parent shader's parameters.

3.4.7 State Variables by Shader Type

The following table describes which state variables are available in which types of shaders:

G geometry shader
D displacement shader
P photon shader and photon volume shader
E photon emitter shader
Le lens shader
M material shader and texture shader
T texture shader
V volume shader
Lg light shader
S shadow shader
Cs contour store shader
C contour contrast shader and contour shader
O output shader

In the following table,

r means that the shader may read this variable but should not modify it because it may have unknown effects on parent or child shaders.

R means that the shader may read this variable but may never modify it because shader interface functions or other parts of mental ray depend on unchanged values.

rw means that the shader may read or write this variable; if it writes it is good practice to restore the original contents before returning to avoid surprises in parent or volume shaders. *pri*, in particular, **must** be restored. Most shaders do not need to modify most of these.

x means that the shader is free to read and write, and need not restore any values. These are "scratchpad" variables for shader communication, and not used by mental ray.

– means that the shader may neither read nor write this field. Its contents are undefined.

In the case of the *options* and *camera* variables, the shader may write neither the pointer nor any field of the options and camera structures. Note that during rendering (between the *rendering* and *rendering finished* messages), the camera and the options may differ from the scene file specifications because phenomenon requirements and conflict detection may make adjustments. For example, a lens shader might have requested ray tracing to be turned off even though it was turned on in the scene file. In this case, shaders called during rendering would see a *trace* flag that is off, and other shaders such as geometry or displacement shaders do not.

variable	G	D	P	E	Le	M	V	Lg	S	Cs	C	O
version	R	R	R	R	R	R	R	R	R	R	R	R
camera_inst	R	R	R	R	R	R	R	R	R	R	R	R
camera	R	R	R	R	R	R	R	R	R	R	R	R
options	R	R	R	R	R	R	R	R	R	R	R	R
global_lock[1]	–	rw	rw	rw	rw	rw	rw	rw	rw	rw	rw	–
raster_x	–	–	–	–	R	R	R	R	R	R	–	–
raster_y	–	–	–	–	R	R	R	R	R	R	–	R
parent	–	–	R	R	R	R	R	R	R	R	–	–
type	R	R	R	R	R	R	R	R	R	R	–	R
scanline	–	–	–	–	r	r	r	r	r	r	–	–
inv_normal	–	–	r	–	r	r	r	r	–	r	–	–

variable	G	D	P	E	Le	M	V	Lg	S	Cs	C	O
reflection_level	–	–	rw	rw	rw	rw	rw	rw	rw	rw	–	–
refraction_level	–	–	rw	rw	rw	rw	rw	rw	rw	rw	–	–
org	–	–	rw	rw	rw	rw	rw	rw	rw	rw	–	–
dir	–	–	rw	rw	rw	rw	rw	rw	–	rw	–	–
dist	–	–	rw	rw	rw	rw	rw	rw	rw	rw	–	R
time	–	–	R	R	R	R	R	R	R	R	–	–
ior	x	x	x	x	x	x	x	x	x	x	x	x
ior_in	x	x	x	x	x	x	x	x	x	x	x	x
material	–	r	r	r	–	r	r	r	r	r	–	–
volume	–	–	rw	rw	rw	rw	rw	rw	rw	rw	–	–
environment	–	–	–	–	rw	rw	rw	–	–	rw	–	–
refraction_volume	–	–	rw	rw	–	rw	rw	–	–	rw	–	–
label	–	r	r	r	rw	rw	rw	rw	rw	rw	–	–
instance	R	R	R	–	R	R	R	R	R	R	–	–
light_instance	–	–	–	R	–	–	R[2]	R	R	–	–	–
pri[3]	–	–	r	–	rw	rw	rw	rw	rw	rw	–	–
pri_idx	–	–	r	–	r	r	r	r	r	r	–	–

variable	G	D	P	E	Le	M	V	Lg	S	Cs	C	O
bary[4]	–	–	r	–	r	r	r	r	r	r	–	–
point	–	r	r	–	rw	rw	rw	rw	rw	rw	–	–
normal	–	r	r	–	rw	rw	rw	rw	rw	rw	–	–
normal_geom	–	–	r	–	rw	rw	rw	rw	rw	rw	–	–
dot_nd	–	–	r	–	rw	rw	rw	rw	–	rw	–	–
shadow_tol	–	–	r	–	r	r	r	r	r	r	r	–
tex_list	–	rw	rw	–	rw	rw	rw	rw	rw	rw	–	–
bump_x_list	–	–	rw	–	rw	rw	rw	rw	rw	rw	–	–
bump_y_list	–	–	rw	–	rw	rw	rw	rw	rw	rw	–	–
motion	–	–	rw	rw	rw	rw	rw	rw	rw	rw	–	–
derivs[4]	–	–	rw	–	rw	rw	rw	rw	rw	rw	–	–
tex	x	x	x	x	x	x	x	x	x	x	x	x
shader	R	R	R	R	R	R	R	R	R	R	R	R
child	–	–	R	R	R	R	R	R	R	R	–	–
thread	R	R	R	R	R	R	R	R	R	R	R	R
user	x	x	x	x	x	x	x	x	x	x	x	x
user_size	x	x	x	x	x	x	x	x	x	x	x	x

1 *global_lock* is accessed with *mi_lock* and *mi_unlock* only.
2 If *state* → *type* is `miRAY_SHADOW`
3 Set to 0 to cast rays from empty space. Do not set to other values.
4 If the object contains surface derivatives

See page 271 for a similar table listing available shader interface functions.

3.5 Shader Parameter Declarations

In addition to the state variables that are provided by mental ray and are shared by all shaders, every shader has *shader parameters*. In the .mi scene file, shader references look much like a function call: the shader name is given along with a list of parameters. Every shader call may have a different list of parameters. mental ray does not restrict or predefine the number and types of shader parameters, any kind of information may be passed to the shader. Typical examples for shader parameters are ambient, diffuse, and specular colors for material shaders, attenuation parameters for light shaders, and so on. An empty parameter list in a shader call (as opposed to a shader declaration) has a special meaning; see the note at the end of this chapter.

In this manual, the term "parameters" refers to shader parameters in the .mi scene file; the term "arguments" is used for arguments to C functions.

Shaders need both state variables and shader parameters. Generally, variables that are computed by mental ray, or whose interpretation is otherwise known to mental ray, and that are useful to different types or instances of shaders are found in state variables. Variables that are specific to a shader, and that may change for each instance of the shader, are found in shader parameters. mental ray does not access or compute shader parameters in any way, it merely passes them from the .mi file to the shader when it is invoked.

To interpret these parameters in the .mi file, mental ray needs a declaration of parameter names and types that is equivalent to the C struct that the shader later uses to access the parameters. The declaration in the .mi file must be exactly equivalent to the C struct, or the shader will misinterpret the parameter data structure constructed by mental ray. (Using the mkmishader utility ensures that both declarations agree, see section 3.23.) This means that three parts are needed to write a shader: the .mi declaration, the C parameter struct, and the C source of the shader. The .mi declaration is normally stored in a separate file that is included into the .mi scene file using a `$include` statement.

The syntax of .mi shader declarations is fully described in section 2.1. Here, only a brief overview is given. Shaders must be declared with shader name, return type, and the types and names of all parameters. Options such as the shader version may be specified also:

```
declare shader
    [ type ] "shader_name" (
        type "parameter_name",
        type "parameter_name",
        ...
        type "parameter_name"
    )
    [ version version_int ]
    [ options ]
end declare
```

For example, a simple material shader containing ambient, diffuse, and specular colors, transparency, an optional array of bump map textures, and an array of lights could be declared in the .mi file as:

```
declare shader
    color "my_material" (
        color         "ambient",
        color         "diffuse",
        color         "specular",
        scalar        "shiny",
        scalar        "reflect",
        scalar        "transparency",
        scalar        "ior",
        vector texture "bump",
        array light   "lights"
    )
    version 1
end declare
```

If there is only one array, there is a small efficiency advantage in listing it last. It is recommended that the largest array (arrays of large structs are larger than arrays of primitives) is given as the last parameter. The material shader declared in this example can be used in a `material` statement like this:

```
material "mat1"
    "my_material" (
        "specular" 1.0 1.0 1.0,
        "ambient"  0.3 0.3 0.0,
        "diffuse"  0.7 0.7 0.0,
        "shiny"    50.0,
        "bump"     "tex1",
        "lights"   [ "light1", "light2", "light3" ],
        "reflect"  0.5
    )
end material
```

Note that the parameters can be defined in any order that does not have to agree with the order in the declaration, and that parameters can be omitted. Omitted parameters default to 0. This example assumes that the texture `tex1` and the three lights have been defined prior to this material definition. Again, be sure to use the names of the textures and lights, not the names of the texture and light shaders. All names in the above two examples were written as strings enclosed in double quotes to disambiguate names from reserved keywords, and to allow special characters in the names that would otherwise be illegal.

When choosing names, avoid double colons and periods, which have a special meaning when accessing structured shader return values and interface parameters in phenomenon subshaders.

When the shader `my_material` is called, its third argument will be a pointer to a data structure built by mental ray from the declaration and the actual parameters in the .mi file. In order for the C source of the shader to access the parameters, it needs an equivalent declaration in C syntax that must agree exactly with the .mi declaration. The type names can be translated according to the following table:

.mi syntax	*C syntax*
boolean	miBoolean
integer	miInteger
scalar	miScalar
vector	miVector
transform	miMatrix
color	miColor
shader	miTag *of a miFunction*
color texture	miTag *of a miFunction or miImg_image*
scalar texture	miTag *of a miFunction or miImg_image*
vector texture	miTag *of a miFunction or miImg_image*
light	miTag *of a miInstance for a light*
material	miTag *of a miMaterial*
geometry	miTag *of a miObject, miGroup, or miInstance*
struct	struct
array	int, int, *type*[1]

It is strongly recommended to use the same parameter names in the C declaration as in the .mi declaration. Also, structures in either declaration should be reflected in the other, even if not enclosed in arrays, to ensure that mental ray inserts the same padding as the C compiler.

Arrays are more complicated than the types in this table because the size of the array is not known at declaration time. The C declaration of an array consists of a start index prefixed with `i_`, the size of the array prefixed with `n_`, and the array itself, declared as an array with one element. mental ray will allocate the structure as large as required by the actual array size at call time. To access array element i in the range $0 \ldots n\_array - 1$, the C expression $array[i + i\_array]$ must be used. This expression allows mental ray to store the shader parameters in virtual shared memory regardless of the base address of the shader parameter structure, which is different on every machine on the network.

For the above example .mi declaration, the equivalent C structure declaration using mental ray types looks like this:

```
struct my_material {
    miColor  ambient;
    miColor  diffuse;
    miColor  specular;
    miScalar shiny;
    miScalar reflect;
    miScalar transparency;
    miScalar ior;
    miTag    bump;
    int      i_lights;
    int      n_lights;
    miTag    lights[1];
};
```

Note that here the order of structure members must match the order in the .mi declaration exactly. For example, suppose a shader has a .mi declaration containing an array of integers:

```
declare shader
    color "myshader" ( array integer "list" )
    version 1
end declare
```

The C declaration for the shader's parameters is:

```
struct myshader {
     int       i_list;
     int       n_list;
     miInteger list[1];
};
```

A shader that needs to operate on this array, for example printing all the array elements to stdout, would use a loop like this:

```
int *list   =  mi_eval_integer(paras->list);
int i_list = *mi_eval_integer(&paras->i_list);
int n_list = *mi_eval_integer(&paras->n_list);
int i;
for (i=0; i < n_list; i++)
     mi_info("%d", list[i_list + i]);
```

assuming that paras is the third shader argument and has type `struct myshader *`. The use of the `i_list` parameter may seem strange to C programmers, who may wish to hide it in a macro like

```
#define EL(array,nel) array[i_##array + nel]
```

This macro requires an ANSI C preprocessor; K&R preprocessors do not support the ## notation and should use /**/ instead. This macro is not predefined in shader.h. The reason for this peculiar way of accessing arrays is improved performance. The array `list[1]` has space for only one element, because the actual number of array elements depends on the shader instance in the .mi file, which may list an arbitrary number of elements. Since mental ray is based on a virtual shared database that moves pieces of data such as shader parameters transparently from one machine to another, no such piece of data may contain a pointer. Pointers would not be valid in another machine's virtual address space. Adjusting the pointer on the other machine is impractical because it would significantly reduce performance for some scenes, and would require knowledge of the structure layout for finding the pointers that may not be available in versions of mental ray not based on a .mi front-end parser. Therefore, the array is appended to the parameter structure, so the entire block can be moved to another machine in a single network transfer. It is safe to access the first element of the array, because space for it is always allocated by declarations such as `list[1]`, but the second is a problem because in a C declaration like

```
struct myshader {
     int        i_list;
     int        n_list;
     miInteger list[1];
     miScalar  factor;
     miBoolean bool;
};
```

the second element, `list[1]`, occupies the same address as `factor`, and the third overlays `bool`. The situation becomes more complex for arrays of structures. The solution is to put the value of the first element after the last "regular" shader parameter, `bool` in this example, followed by the other element values. This means that the first few C array elements that overlay other parameters must be skipped. The `i_` variable tells the shader exactly how many. In the example, `i_list` would be 3. Assuming the following shader instance, used as part of a material, texture, or some other definition requiring a shader call:

```
"myshader" (
     "factor" 1.4142136,
     "list"   [ 42, 123, 486921, 777 ],
     "bool"   on
)
```

mental ray would arrange the values in memory like this:

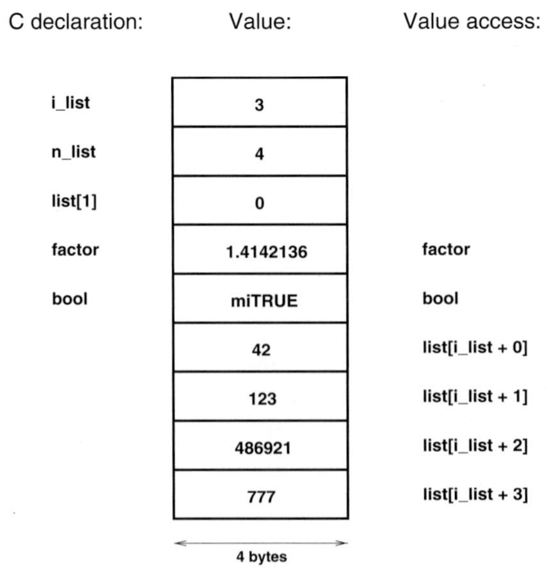

On multithreaded machines, it is possible that any given shader runs in multiple threads simultaneously. When this happens, they share all static variables defined in the sources, all shader parameters, and the user pointer. The only things that are separate in separate threads are "auto" variables on the stack, and the state variables. Also, mental ray makes sure that an init shader runs once, in a single thread, before the actual shader runs in one or more threads. This makes init shaders the natural place to set up the shader user pointer, perhaps to store preprocessed shader parameters. See section 3.21.13 for more information on multithreaded shader design.

Shaders should never write to shader parameters because they might be accessed by other threads or hosts or by future frames, and because shader and interface assignments might exist that would be destroyed.

3.6 Parameter Assignments and mi_eval

The chapter on the .mi scene description language explains assignment of shaders and phenomenon interface parameters to shader parameters. Assignments replace the constant value of a parameter with a link to a shader that gets called automatically when the shader asks for the value of the parameter, or a link to the phenomenon interface which is looked up, respectively.

Shader assignments simplify the development of small, simple shaders called *base shaders* that can be combined into larger shaders or phenomena. For example, assignments make it possible to apply a texture to any shader parameter simply by replacing the constant value of a parameter with an assignment to a texture shader. It is no longer necessary for shader writers to anticipate which parameters should be texturable, and adding additional shader parameters of type `color texture` to the parameter list, just in case.

For example, consider this shader assignment example from page 50:

```
declare shader
   color "phong" (color "ambient",
                  color "diffuse",
                  color "specular")
   version 1
end declare

declare shader
   struct {color "a", color "b"}
         "texture" (color texture "picture")
   version 1
end declare

color texture "fluffy" "/tmp/image.rgb"

shader "map" "texture" (
   "picture"   "fluffy")

shader "mtlsh" "phong" (
```

```
"ambient"    0.3 0.3 0.3,
"diffuse"    = "map.a",
"specular"   = "map.b")
```

The author of the *phong* shader can focus on the purpose of the shader (Phong illumination) without having to consider texturing at all. The texture is applied later as a shader assignment to the parameters of *phong*. This example further illustrates that shaders may have structured return values, in this case in the shader *texture* which returns both *a* and *b*, which can be picked up individually using the dot-member notation.

Frequently, shaders do not access all their parameters. Consider a multiplexing material shader that calls one of two material shaders depending on whether the incident ray hit the front face or the back face of the material. It would be very inefficient to evaluate both material shaders and then choose one of the two returned colors. For this reason, mental ray does not pre-evaluate all assignments before calling a shader. Instead, the shader itself must ask for the value of one of its parameters explicitly. This is done with the *mi_eval* function. The signature of *mi_eval* is

```
void      *mi_eval           (miState    *state,
                              void       *param)
miBoolean *mi_eval_boolean   (miBoolean  *param)
miInteger *mi_eval_integer   (miInteger  *param)
miScalar  *mi_eval_scalar    (miScalar   *param)
miVector  *mi_eval_vector    (miVector   *param)
miScalar  *mi_eval_transform (miScalar   *param)
miColor   *mi_eval_color     (miColor    *param)
miTag     *mi_eval_tag       (miTag      *param)
```

The typed variants of *mi_eval* are implemented as macros that perform all necessary typecasting, as a convenience for shader writers. There are three cases handled by *mi_eval*:

- If there is no assignment to the parameter whose address is passed, *mi_eval* simply returns that parameter. Being a macro, it can do so without measurable loss of performance.
- If the parameter is assigned to a shader, the shader will be called automatically and a pointer to the returned value is returned. If the shader was called before in the same context (such as the current phenomenon execution), the shader is not called again and a pointer to the cached previous result is returned.
- If the parameter is assigned to the interface of the phenomenon the shader is defined in, *mi_eval* returns a pointer to the value stored in the interface.

In any case, the end result is that *mi_eval* returns a pointer to the parameter value, no matter where it comes from. If the shader accessed its parameters directly, without using *mi_eval*, it would get garbage (such as `0` or `NaN`) if the parameter is assigned. For arrays, *mi_eval* must be applied to the array itself, as well as the `i_`*array* and `n_`*array* integers. Once the address of the array has passed through *mi_eval*, the array pointer is subscripted normally without applying *mi_eval* to each element. This is a convention; only entire arrays should be assigned to other shaders or to the phenomenon interface if present, but not individual array members.

For example, the *phong* shader in the example above would be implemented as:

```
struct phong {
   miColor       ambient;
   miColor       diffuse;
   miColor       specular;
};

int phong_version(void) {return(1);}

miBoolean phong(
   miColor       *result,     /* returned illum color */
   miState       *state,      /* ray tracer state */
   struct phong  *paras)      /* phong parameters */
{
   miColor       *diffuse;    /* final diffuse param */
   miColor       *specular;   /* final specular param */
   miScalar      shiny;       /* phong exponent */
   int           n, i;        /* light counter */
   miTag         *lights;     /* global light list */
   miInteger     samples;     /* # of samples taken */
   miColor       color;       /* color from light */
   miColor       sum;         /* summed sample colors */
   miVector      dir;         /* direction to light */
   miScalar      dot_nl;      /* normal <dot> dir*/
   miScalar      spec_f;      /* specular factor */

   *result  = *mi_eval_color (&paras->ambient);
   diffuse  =  mi_eval_color (&paras->diffuse);
   specular =  mi_eval_color (&paras->specular);
   shiny    = *mi_eval_scalar(&paras->shiny);

   mi_query(miQ_NUM_GLOBAL_LIGHTS, state, 0, &n);
   mi_query(miQ_GLOBAL_LIGHTS,     state, 0, &lights);

   for (i=0; i < n; i++) {
       sum.r = sum.g = sum.b = 0;
       samples = 0;
       while (mi_sample_light(&color, &dir, &dot_nl,
                              state, lights[i],
                              &samples)) {

           spec_f = mi_phong_specular(shiny, state,
                                              &dir);
           sum.r += color.r * (dot_nl * diffuse->r +
                               spec_f * specular->r);
           sum.g += color.r * (dot_nl * diffuse->g +
                               spec_f * specular->g);
           sum.b += color.r * (dot_nl * diffuse->b +
```

```
                                    spec_f * specular->b);
            }
            if (samples) {
                result->r += sum.r / samples;
                result->g += sum.g / samples;
                result->b += sum.b / samples;
            }
        }
        result->a = 1;
        return(miTRUE);
    }
```

Note that *mi_eval_color* is called early to obtain pointers to parameters once. If there is a large number of lights, this saves a large number of *mi_eval_color* calls later. Although *mi_eval* et al. employ caching and fast lookups, this makes the shader faster than it were if the code were written like this:

```
dot_nl * mi_eval_color(&paras->diffuse)->r
```

in the inner loop.

3.7 Shader Versioning

The parameter set of a shader must always be correctly described by its declaration in the .mi scene file. It is a common source of errors to have a mismatch between the .mi and the .c shader parameters. This can lead to incorrect rendering results but can also cause shader crashes, for example if the shader mistakes a floating-point number for an array length.

For this reason it is highly recommended to attach version numbers to both the .mi declaration and the shader itself. Version numbers are positive integers, and should begin with 1 (0 is the default if the version number is missing). For example, the .mi declaration of a shader *myshader* might be defined as:

```
declare shader
    color "myshader" (parameters)
    version 42
end declare
```

There are two ways to ensure that the version number is correct. The recommended method is writing a pseudo-shader that provides the version number:

```
DLLEXPORT int myshader_version(void) {return(42);}
```

```
DLLEXPORT miBoolean myshader(
   miColor         *result,
   miState         *state,
   struct myshader *paras)
{
   ...
}
```

Before mental ray calls a shader for the first time, just before looking for its initialization shader (whose name would be `myshader_init`), mental ray checks whether a function exists whose name is the shader name followed by `_version`. If it does, it is called and the version number is compared with the version number in the .mi declaration. If there is a mismatch, an error message is printed. If the version shader does not exist, a warning message is printed.

The second method for shader version comparison is an explicit comparison in the shader using *mi_query*:

```
#define MYSHADER_VERSION 42

DLLEXPORT miBoolean myshader(
   miColor         *result,
   miState         *state,
   struct myshader *paras)
{
   int             version;

   mi_query(miQ_DECL_VERSION, state, 0, &version);
   if (version != MYSHADER_VERSION)
       mi_error("myshader: wrong declaration");
   ...
}
```

It is actually preferable to do this in the initialization shader to reduce the overhead of checking the version number every time the shader is called.

It is *very important* to always increment the version number every time the shader parameters change. Problems introduced by mismatches are hard to find, especially if the shader versions on client and server hosts do not agree.

The following sections discuss the various types of shaders, and how to write custom shaders of those types. Basic concepts are introduced step by step, including supporting functions and state variables supplied by mental ray. All support functions are summarized at the end of this chapter.

3.8 Material Shaders

Material shaders are the primary type of shaders. All materials defined in the scene must at least define a material shader. Materials may also define other types of shaders, such as shadow, volume, and environment shaders, which are optional and of secondary importance.

When mental ray casts a visible ray, such as those cast by the camera (called *primary rays*) or those that are cast for reflections and refractions (collectively called *secondary rays*), mental ray determines the next object in the scene that is hit by that ray. This process is called *intersection testing*. For example, when a primary ray cast from the camera through the viewing plane's pixel (100, 100) intersects with a yellow sphere, pixel (100, 100) in the output image will be painted yellow. (The actual process is slightly complicated by supersampling and filtering, which can cause more than one primary ray to contribute to a pixel.)

The core of mental ray has no concept of "yellow." This color is computed by the material shader attached to the sphere that was hit by the ray. mental ray records general information about the sphere object, such as point of intersection, normal vector, transformation matrix etc. in a data structure called the *state*, and calls the material shader attached to the object. More precisely, the material shader, along with its parameters (called *shader parameters*), is part of the material, which is attached to or inherited by the polygon or surface that forms the part of the object that was hit by the ray. Objects are usually built from multiple polygons and/or surfaces, each of which may have a different material.

The material shader uses the values provided by mental ray in the state and the variables provided by the .mi file in the shader parameters to calculate the color of the object, and returns that color. In the above example, the material shader would return the color yellow. mental ray stores this color in its internal sample list, which later gets filtered to compute frame buffer pixels, and then casts the next primary ray. Note that if the material shader has a bug that causes it to return infinity or NaN (Not a Number) in the `result` color, the infinity or NaN is stored as 1.0 in color frame buffers. This results in white pixels in the rendered image. This is true for subshaders such as texture shaders also.

With an appropriate `output` statement (see page 74), mental ray computes depth, label, normal-vector, and motion vector frame buffers in addition to the standard color frame buffer, and any user frame buffer defined with `frame buffer` statements in the options block. The color returned by the first-generation material shader is stored in the color frame buffer (unless a lens shader exists; lens shaders also have the option of modifying colors). The material shader can control what gets stored in the depth, label, normal-vector, and motion-vector frame buffers by storing appropriate values into $state \rightarrow point.z$, $state \rightarrow label$, $state \rightarrow normal$, and $state \rightarrow motion$, respectively. It can also store data in the user frame buffers with an appropriate call to *mi_fb_put*. Depth is the negative Z coordinate.

Material shaders normally do quite complicated computations to arrive at the final color of a point on the object:

- The shader parameters usually include constant ambient, diffuse, and specular colors and other parameters such as transparency, and possibly optional textures that need to be evaluated to compute the actual values at the intersection point. If textures are present, texture shaders are called by using one of the lookup functions provided by mental ray. Alternatively, shader assignment may be used for texturing. Texture shaders are discussed in the next section.

- The illumination computation sums up the contribution from various light sources listed in the shader parameters. To obtain the amount of light arriving from a light source, a light shader is called by calling a light trace or sample function provided by mental ray. Light shaders are discussed in a separate section below. After the illumination computation is finished, the ambient, diffuse, and specular colors have been combined into a single material color (assuming a more conventional material shader).
- If the material is reflective, transparent, or using refraction, as indicated by appropriate shader parameters, the shader must cast secondary rays and apply the result to the material color calculated in the previous step. (Transparency is a variation of refractive transparency where the ray continues in the same direction, while refraction rays may alter the direction based on an index of refraction.) Secondary rays, like primary rays, cause mental ray to do intersection testing and call another material shader if the intersection test hit an object. For this reason, material shaders must be reentrant. In particular, a secondary refraction or transparency ray will hit the back side of the same object if `face both` is set in the camera and the object is a closed volume.

Note that the shader parameters of a material shader are under no obligation to define and use classical parameters like ambient, diffuse, and specular color and reflection and refraction parameters. Here is a full-featured example for the C source of the shader declared in the previous section:

```
#include <stdio.h>
#include <mi/shader.h>

int my_material_version(void) {return(1);}

miBoolean my_material(
   miColor              *result,
   miState              *state,
   struct my_material *paras)
{
   miColor              *diffuse, *specular;
   miVector             bump, dir;
   miColor              color;
   int                  num, i_lights, n_lights;
   miTag                *lights;
   miScalar             factor;

   /*
    * bump map
    */
   state->tex = state->tex_list[0];
   mi_call_shader((miColor *)&bump, miSHADER_TEXTURE,
                  state, *mi_eval_tag(&paras->bump));
```

```
if (bump.x != 0 || bump.y != 0) {
    mi_vector_to_object(state, &state->normal,
                        &state->normal);
    state->normal.x+=bump.x * state->bump_x_list->x
                    +bump.y * state->bump_y_list->x;
    state->normal.y+=bump.x * state->bump_x_list->y
                    +bump.y * state->bump_y_list->y;
    state->normal.z+=bump.x * state->bump_x_list->z
                    +bump.y * state->bump_y_list->z;
    mi_vector_from_object(state, &state->normal,
                          &state->normal);
    mi_vector_normalize(&state->normal);
    state->dot_nd = mi_vector_dot(&state->normal,
                                  &state->dir);
}

/*
 * illumination
 */
*result  = *mi_eval_color  (&paras->ambient);
diffuse  =  mi_eval_color  (&paras->diffuse);
specular =  mi_eval_color  (&paras->specular);
i_lights = *mi_eval_integer(&paras->i_lights);
n_lights = *mi_eval_integer(&paras->n_lights);
lights   =  mi_eval_tag    ( paras->lights);

for (num=0; num < n_lights; num++) {
    miColor    color, sum;
    miInteger  samples = 0;
    miScalar   dot_nl;

    sum.r = sum.g = sum.b = 0;
    while (mi_sample_light(&color, &dir, &dot_nl,
                           state,
                           lights[i_lights + num],
                           &samples)) {

         sum.r += dot_nl * diffuse->r * color.r;
         sum.g += dot_nl * diffuse->g * color.g;
         sum.b += dot_nl * diffuse->b * color.b;

         factor = mi_phong_specular(
                    *mi_eval_scalar(&paras->shiny),
                    state, &dir);
         sum.r += factor * specular->r * color.r;
         sum.g += factor * specular->g * color.g;
         sum.b += factor * specular->b * color.b;
    }
    if (samples) {
         result->r += sum.r / samples;
         result->g += sum.g / samples;
         result->b += sum.b / samples;
```

```
        }
    }
    result->a = 1;

    /*
     * reflections
     */
    factor = *mi_eval_scalar(&paras->reflect);
    if (factor > 0) {
        miScalar f = 1 - factor;
        result->r *= f;
        result->g *= f;
        result->b *= f;

        mi_reflection_dir(&dir, state);
        if (mi_trace_reflection (&color,state,&dir) ||
            mi_trace_environment(&color,state,&dir)) {

             result->r += factor * color.r;
             result->g += factor * color.g;
             result->b += factor * color.b;
        }
    }

    /*
     * refractions
     */
    factor = *mi_eval_scalar(&paras->transparency);
    if (factor > 0) {
        miScalar ior = *mi_eval_scalar(&state->ior);
        miScalar f = 1 - factor;
        result->r *= f;
        result->g *= f;
        result->b *= f;
        result->a  = f;

        if (mi_refraction_dir(&dir, state, 1.0, ior)
         && mi_trace_refraction (&color, state, &dir) ||
            mi_trace_environment(&color, state, &dir)) {

             result->r += factor * color.r;
             result->g += factor * color.g;
             result->b += factor * color.b;
             result->a += factor * color.a;
        }
    }
    return(miTRUE);
}
```

Four steps are required for computing the material color in this shader. First, the normal is perturbed by looking up a vector in the vector texture, and using the bump basis vectors to determine the orientation of the perturbation (the lookup always returns an XY vector). The second step loops over all light sources in the light array parameter, adding the contribution of each light according to the Phong equation. In the case of area lights, the light is sampled more than once, until the light sampling function is satisfied.

Finally, reflection and refraction rays are cast if the appropriate parameters are nonzero. In both cases, first the direction vector `dir` is computed using a built-in function, and a ray is cast in that direction. If either trace function returns `miFALSE`, indicating that no object was hit, the material's environment map that forms a sphere around the entire scene is evaluated. When all computations are finished, the calculated color, including the alpha component, is returned in the `result` parameter. The shader returns `miTRUE` indicating that the computation succeeded.

The *mi_eval* functions permit shader assignments, which let shaders base their computations on parameters that are driven by other shaders. For example, the diffuse component of the above example is a good candidate for attachment to a texture shader. This works only if *mi_eval* is used properly.

3.9 Texture Shaders

Texture shaders evaluate a texture and typically return a color, scalar, or vector (but like any shader, return values can be freely chosen and may even be structures of multiple values). Textures can either be procedural, for example evaluating a 3D texture based on noise functions or calling other shaders, or they can do an image lookup. The .mi format provides different `texture` statements for these two types, one with a function call and one with a texture file name. Refer to section 2.7.3 for details.

Texture shaders are not first-class shaders. This means that mental ray never calls one by itself and provides no special support for them. Texture shaders are called exclusively by other shaders. There are four ways of calling a texture shader from a material shader or other shaders: either by simply calling the shader by name like any other C function, or by requesting the value of a shader parameter using *mi_eval* (the recommended method, see below), or by using a built-in convenience function like *mi_lookup_color_texture*, or with a statement like

```
mi_call_shader_x(result, miSHADER_TEXTURE, state, tag, args);
```

The *tag* argument references the texture function. The texture function is a data structure in the scene database that contains a reference to the C function itself, plus a pointer to a user argument block *arg* that is passed to the texture shader when it is called. User arguments are rarely used, and *mi_call_shader_x* is the only way to pass them to a shader. Although the texture shader could also be called directly with a statement such as

```
soft_color(result, state, &soft_color_paras);
```

the caller would have to write the required arguments into the user argument structure *soft_color_paras* itself; it would not have access to shader parameters specified in the .mi file.

The recommended way of calling subshaders is implicitly with *mi_eval*, which does not require the calling shader to be aware that a subshader provides the value. This makes shaders very flexible by allowing them to be combined in arbitrary ways from the scene file, without changing and recompiling shader sources. However, there are cases when not the value of a shader but a shader itself is passed as a parameter, and *mi_call_shader_x* provides a good way of calling such shaders.

Unlike material shaders, texture shaders usually return a simple color or scalar or other return value. There are no lighting calculations or secondary rays. This greatly simplifies the task of changing a textured surface. For example, a simple texture shader that does a simple, non-antialiased lookup in a texture image could be written as:

```
#include <stdio.h>
#include <mi/shader.h>

int mytexture_version(void) {return(1);}

miBoolean mytexture(
   register miColor     *result,
   register miState     *state,
   struct image_lookup *paras)
{
   miImg_image          *image;
   int                  xs, ys;
   miTag                texture;

   texture = *mi_eval_tag(&paras->texture);
   image = mi_db_access(texture);
   mi_query(miQ_IMAGE_WIDTH,  state, texture, &xs);
   mi_query(miQ_IMAGE_HEIGHT, state, texture, &ys);
   mi_img_get_color(image, result, state->tex.x * xs,
                                   state->tex.y * ys);
   mi_db_unpin(texture);
   return(miTRUE);
}
```

This shader assumes that the texture coordinate can be taken from *state→tex*, where the caller (usually a material shader) has stored it, probably by selecting a texture coordinate from *state→tex_list*. The caller can use *mi_query* to determine the number of valid textures in *state→tex_list*. A more complicated shader that better anti-aliases image textures with a simple box filter might look like this:

```
#include <stdio.h>
#include <mi/shader.h>

int mytexture2_version(void) {return(1);}

miBoolean mytexture2(
   register miColor     *result,
```

```
    register miState    *state,
    struct image_lookup *paras)
{
    miTag               texture;
    miImg_image         *image;
    int                 xs, ys;
    miColor             col00, col01, col10, col11;
    register int        x, y;
    register miScalar   u, v, nu, nv;

    texture = *mi_eval_tag(&paras->texture);
    image = mi_db_access(texture);
    mi_query(miQ_IMAGE_WIDTH,  state, texture, &xs);
    mi_query(miQ_IMAGE_HEIGHT, state, texture, &ys);
    x = u = state->tex.x * (xs - 1);
    y = v = state->tex.y * (ys - 1);
    u -= x;
    v -= y;
    nu = 1 - u;
    nv = 1 - v;

    mi_img_get_color(image, &col00, x,   y);
    mi_img_get_color(image, &col01, x+1, y);
    mi_img_get_color(image, &col10, x,   y+1);
    mi_img_get_color(image, &col11, x+1, y+1);

    result->r = nv * (nu * col00.r + u * col01.r) +
                 v * (nu * col10.r + u * col11.r);
    result->g = nv * (nu * col00.g + u * col01.g) +
                 v * (nu * col10.g + u * col11.g);
    result->b = nv * (nu * col00.b + u * col01.b) +
                 v * (nu * col10.b + u * col11.b);
    result->a = nv * (nu * col00.a + u * col01.a) +
                 v * (nu * col10.a + u * col11.a);

    mi_db_unpin(texture);
    return(miTRUE);
}
```

The implementation of the body of this shader is similar to the built-in *mi_lookup_color_texture* function if called with *paras→texture*, except that this function also recognizes if the texture is a shader (and calls *mi_call_shader* in this case), and unlike the example above it supports filtered multi-level pyramid texture filtering. Also, both examples above will fail if any texture coordinate is less than `0` or equal to or greater than 1.

This shader can further be extended by applying texture transformations to *state→tex* before it is used for the lookup, for example for rotated, scaled, repeating, or cropped textures. The shader may also decide that a scaled-down texture was missed, and return `miFALSE`. The material shader must then skip this texture if *mi_call_shader* returns `miFALSE`.

Both of the above shaders have shader parameters that consist of a single texture. Textures always have type miTag. Image file textures are read in by the translator and provided as a tag of type miSCENE_IMAGE.

A texture shader using higher quality elliptical filtering might look like this:

```
#include <stdio.h>
#include <mi/shader.h>

int mytexture3_version(void) {return(1);}

miBoolean mytexture3(
   register miColor      *result,
   register miState      *state,
   struct image_lookup   *paras)
{
   miTag                 texture;
   miVector              p[3], t[3];
   miMatrix              ST;

   texture = *mi_eval_tag(&paras->texture);

   mi_texture_filter_project(p, t, state,
                             0.5, paras->space);

   my_remap_parameter(&t[0], &t[0], state, paras);
   my_remap_parameter(&t[1], &t[1], state, paras);
   my_remap_parameter(&t[2], &t[2], state, paras);

   mi_texture_filter_transform(ST, p, t);

   return(mi_lookup_filter_color_texture(result, state,
                         texture,
                         &paras->filter_options, ST));
}
```

This example assumes that *paras* contains the definition of the elliptical filter options and the texture space index. The implementation of the function *my_remap_parameter* is not given here, it would transform the texture coordinates according to some parameters in *paras*, for example perform texture replication, rotation or valid range checking. Note that the checking for miFALSE return values of *mi_texture_filter_project* and *mi_texture_filter_transform* is missing in this example.

3.10 Volume Shaders

Volume shaders may be attached to the camera or to a material. They modify the color returned from an intersection point to account for the distance the ray traveled through a volume. The most common application for volume shaders is atmospheric fog effects; for example, a simple volume shader may simulate fog by fading the input color to white depending on the ray distance.

By definition, the distance *dist* given in the state is 0.0 and the intersection *point* is undefined if the ray has infinite length.

Volume shaders are normally called in three situations. When a material shader returns, the volume shader that the material shader left in the *state→volume* variable is called, without copying the state, as if it had been called as the last operation of the material shader. Copying the state is not necessary because the volume shader does not return to the material shader, so it is not necessary to preserve any variables in the state.

Unless the `shadow segment` mode is in effect, volume shaders are also called when a light shader has returned; in this case the volume shader *state→volume* is called once for the entire distance from the light source to the illuminated point (i.e., to the point that caused the material shader that sampled the light to be called). In `shadow segment` mode, volume shaders are not called for light rays but for every shadow ray segment from the illuminated point towards the light source. Some volume shaders may decide that they should not apply to light rays; this can be done by returning immediately if the *state→type* variable is `miRAY_LIGHT`.

Finally, volume shaders are called after an environment shader was called. Note that if a volume shader is called after the material, light, or other shader, the return value of that other shader is discarded and the return value of the volume shader is used. The reason is that a volume shader can substitute a non-black color even if the original shader has given up. Volume shaders return `miFALSE` if no light can pass through the given volume, and `miTRUE` if there is a non-black result color.

Material shaders have two separate state variables dealing with volumes, *volume* and *refraction_volume*. If the material shader casts a refraction or transparency ray, the tracing function will copy the refraction volume shader, if there is one, to the volume shader after copying the state. This means that the next intersection point finds the refraction volume in *state→volume*, which effectively means that once the ray has entered an object, that object's interior volume shader is used. However, the material shader is responsible to detect when a refraction ray exits an object, and overwrite *state→refraction_volume* with an appropriate outside volume shader, such as *state→camera→volume*, or a volume shader found by following the *state→parent* links.

Since volume shaders modify a color calculated by a previous material shader, environment shader, or light shader, they differ from these shaders in that they receive an input color in the *result* argument that they are expected to modify. A very simple fog volume shader could be written as:

```
#include <stdio.h>
#include <mi/shader.h>

int myfog_version(void) {return(1);}

miBoolean myfog(
   register miColor      *result,
   register miState      *state,
   register struct myfog *paras)
{
   register miScalar     fade;
```

```
    register miColor       *fogcolor;
    register miScalar      max;

    if (state->type == miRAY_LIGHT)
         return(miTRUE);

    max      = *mi_eval_scalar(&state->maxdist);
    fogcolor =  mi_eval_scalar(&state->fogcolor);
    fade     = state->dist > max ? 1.0
                                 : state->dist / max;

    result->r = fade      * fogcolor->r
              + (1-fade) * result->r;
    result->g = fade      * fogcolor->g
              + (1-fade) * result->g;
    result->b = fade      * fogcolor->b
              + (1-fade) * result->b;
    result->a = fade      * fogcolor->a
              + (1-fade) * result->a;

    return(miTRUE);
}
```

This shader linearly fades the input color to *state→fogcolor* (probably white) within *state→maxdist* internal space units. Objects more distant are completely lost in fog. The length of the ray to be modified can be found in *state→dist*, its start point in *state→org*, and its end point in *state→point*. This example shader does not apply to light rays, light sources can penetrate fog of any depth because of the `miRAY_LIGHT` check. In this case, the shader returns `miTRUE` anyway because the shader did not fail; it merely decided not to apply fog. Note that the shader parameters are evaluated with *mi_eval* after the *if* statement to ensure that no unnecessary work is done by obtaining parameter values that are not going to be used.

If this shader is attached to the camera, the atmosphere surrounding the scene will contain fog. Every *state→volume* will inherit this camera volume shader, until a refraction or transparency ray is cast. The ray will copy the material's volume shader, *state→refraction_volume*, if there is one, to *state→volume*, and the ray is now assumed to be in the object. If the material has no volume shader to be copied, the old volume shader will remain in place and will be inherited by subsequent rays.

Some volume shaders employ ray marching techniques to sample lights from empty space, to achieve effects such as visible light beams. Before such a shader calls *mi_sample_light*, it should store 0 in *state→pri* to inform mental ray that there is no primitive to illuminate, and to not attempt certain optimizations such as backface elimination. Shaders other than volume shaders may do this too, but must restore *pri* before returning. Some *mi_query* modes do not work if *pri* has been modified.

3.11 Environment Shaders

Environment shaders provide a color for rays that leave the scene entirely, and for rays that would exceed the trace depth limit. Environment shaders are called automatically by mental ray if a ray leaves the scene, or when a ray exceeds the trace depth. It can also be done explicitly by shaders using the *mi_trace_environment* function:

```
mi_reflection_dir(&dir, state);
if (/* do ray tracing? */)
    mi_trace_reflection (&color, state, &dir);
else
    mi_trace_environment(&color, state, &dir);
 /* use the returned color */
```

Environment shaders, like any other shader, may return `miFALSE` to inform the caller that the environment lookup failed. If mental ray falls back on calling the environment shader, it returns the value returned by the environment shader, not necessarily `miFALSE`.

In both the explicit case and the automatic case (when a ray cast by a function call such as *mi_trace_reflection* leaves the scene without intersecting with any object) mental ray calls the environment shader found in *state→environment*. In primary rays, this variable is initialized with the global environment shader in the camera (also found in *state→camera→environment*). Subsequent material shaders get the environment defined in the material if present, or the camera environment otherwise. Material shaders never inherit the environment from the parent shader, they always use the environment in the material or the camera. All other types of shaders inherit the environment from the parent shader.

Here is an example environment shader that uses a texture that covers an infinite sphere around the scene:

```
#include <stdio.h>
#include <mi/shader.h>

int myenv_version(void) {return(1);}

miBoolean myenv(
   register miColor      *result,
   register miState      *state,
   register struct myenv *paras)
{
   register miScalar     theta;
   miVector              coord;

   theta = fabs(state->dir.z)*HUGE < fabs(state->dir.x)
          ? state->dir.x > 0
                 ? 1.5*M_PI
                 : 0.5*M_PI
          : state->dir.z > 0
```

```
                    ? 1.0*M_PI + atan(state->dir.x /
                                      state->dir.z)
                    : 2.0*M_PI + atan(state->dir.x /
                                      state->dir.z);
    if (theta > 2 * M_PI)
        theta -= 2 * M_PI;

    coord.x = 1 - theta / (2 * M_PI);
    coord.y = 0.5 * (state->dir.y + 1.0);
    coord.z = 0;

    state->tex = coord;
    return(mi_call_shader(result, miSHADER_TEXTURE,
                          state, *mi_eval_tag(
                                  &paras->texture)));
}
```

This shader gets a single parameter in its shader parameter structure, a `miTag` for a texture shader. The texture is evaluated by storing the texture coordinate in *state→tex* and calling the texture shader with *mi_call_shader*. For a description of texture shaders and how to call them, see the Texture section above.

3.12 Light Shaders

Light shaders are called from other shaders by sampling a light using the *mi_sample_light* or *mi_trace_light* functions, which perform some calculations and then call the given light shader, or directly if a ray hits a source. *mi_sample_light* may also request that it is called more than once if an area light source is to be sampled. For an example for using *mi_sample_light*, see the section on material shaders above. *mi_trace_light* performs less exact shading for area lights, and is provided for backwards compatibility only.

The light shader computes the amount of light contributed by the light source to a previous intersection point, stored in *state→point*. The calculation may be based on the direction *state→dir* to that point, and the distance *state→dist* from the light source to that ray. There may also be shader parameters that specify directional and distance attenuation. Directional lights have no location; *state→dist* is undefined in this case.

Light shaders are also responsible for shadow casting. Shadows are computed by finding all objects that are in the path of the light from the light source to the illuminated intersection point. This is done in the light shader by casting "shadow rays" after the standard light color computation including attenuation is finished. Shadow rays are cast from the light source back towards the illuminated point (or vice versa if shadow segment mode is enabled), in the same direction of the light ray. Every time an occluding object is found, that object's shadow shader is called, if it has one, which reduces the amount of light based on the object's transparency and color. If an occluding object is found that has no shadow shader, it is assumed to be opaque, so no light from the light source can reach the illuminated point. For details on shadow shaders, see the next section.

Here is an example for a simple point light that supports no attenuation, but casts shadows:

```
#include <stdio.h>
#include <mi/shader.h>

int mypoint_version(void) {return(1);}

miBoolean mypoint(
    register miColor        *result,
    register miState        *state,
    register struct mypoint *paras)
{
    *result = *mi_eval_color(&paras->color);
    return(mi_trace_shadow(result, state));
}
```

The shader parameters are assumed to contain the light color. The shadows are calculated simply by giving the shadow shaders of all occluding objects the chance to reduce the light from the light source by calling *mi_trace_shadow*. The shader returns `miTRUE` if some light reaches the illuminated point.

There is a useful trick that can improve performance significantly: the light shader should trace shadow rays only if the contribution from the light is greater than some threshold, for example because distance or angle attenuation has left so little of the light color (less than 1/256, for example) that it does not matter whether this contribution is counted or not. If this is the case, the shader might skip shadow calculation (significantly increasing speed in a complex scene) and return (miBoolean)2 to indicate that if this is a small area light source, there is no point in continuing to sample it because all the other samples are not going to make a contribution either. Returning 2 does not work well for large area light sources because some parts of the light may be closer than others and may exceed the threshold for returning early. Consider the following alternate shader body:

```
{
   *result = *mi_eval_color(&paras->color);
   apply_distance_attenuation(result);
   apply_angle_attenuation(result);
   if (result->r < .005 && result->g < .005
                       && result->b < .005)
       return((miBoolean)2);
   else
       return(mi_trace_shadow(result, state));
}
```

The point light can be turned into a spot light by adding directional attenuation parameters for the inner and outer cones and a spot direction parameter to the shader parameters, and change the shader to reduce the light intensity if the illuminated point falls between the inner and outer cones, and turns the light off if it does not fall into the outer cone at all:

```
#include <stdio.h>
#include <mi/shader.h>

int myspot_version(void) {return(1);}

miBoolean myspot(
   miColor             *result,
   miState             *state,
   struct soft_light *paras)
{
   miScalar            d, t;
   miScalar            inner, outer;

   d = mi_vector_dot(&state->dir,
                    mi_eval_vector(&paras->direction));
   if (d <= 0)
        return(miFALSE);

   mi_query(miQ_LIGHT_SPREAD, state, 0, &outer);
   if (d < outer)
        return(miFALSE);
```

```
        *result = *mi_eval_color (&paras->color);
        inner   = *mi_eval_scalar(&paras->inner);
        if (d < inner) {
             t = (outer - d) / (outer - inner);
             result->r *= t;
             result->g *= t;
             result->b *= t;
        }
        return(result->r < .005 && result->g < .005
                                && result->b < .005
            ? (miBoolean)2
            : mi_trace_shadow(result, state));
    }
```

Again, `miFALSE` is returned if no illumination takes place, and `miTRUE` otherwise. Note that none of these light shaders takes the normal at the illuminated point into account; the light shader is merely responsible for calculating the amount of light that reaches that point. The material shader (or other shader) that sampled the light must use the *dot_nd* value returned by *mi_sample_light*, and its own shader parameters such as the diffuse color, to calculate the actual fraction of light reflected by the material.

If the light shader is also to be used for a visible area light source, it needs to check whether *state*$\rightarrow$*type* is different from `miRAY_LIGHT`. If so, a ray has intersected the the area light source directly. In this case, no shadow rays have to be checked, and the light color can directly be assigned to *result*.

3.13 Shadow Shaders

As described in the previous section, light shaders may trace shadow rays between the light source and the point to be illuminated. When this ray hits an occluding object, that object's shadow shader is called, if present. (If the object has no shadow shader, the object is assumed to block all light.) Shadow shaders accept an input color that is dimmed according to the transparency and color of the occluding object. If the resulting color is black, that is, if the object is fully opaque, the shadow shader should return `miFALSE`.

If there is more than one occluding object between the light source and the illuminated point, the order in which the shadow shaders of the occluding objects are called is undefined, unless shadow sorting is turned on. Shadow shaders that rely on being called in the correct order, the one closest to the light source first, should define `shadow sort` in their shader declaration to ensure that shadow sorting is enabled if the shader is used.

Shadow shaders should check for shadow segment mode. If shadow segments are turned on, shadow shaders must behave rather differently, similar to computing transparency in material shaders. The shadow ray points from the previous intersection (or the illumination point for the initial segment) to the current intersection point. It should set up *state* $\rightarrow$ *refraction_volume* for the next shadow segment, obtain the illumination by calling *mi_trace_shadow_seg*, and then apply the usual modifications.

Shadow shaders should distinguish two cases:

- *state* → *options* → *shadow* is 1 or '1'
  All shadow ray origins are at the light source, and their intersection point is on the intersection object whose shadow shader was called. The *mi_trace_shadow* call by the light shader calls all shadow shaders.
- *state* → *options* → *shadow* is 's'
  Shadow rays travel in the opposite direction and form a chain from the illuminated point towards the light source. Each shadow ray's origin is the previous ray's end point. The shadow shader must perform inside/outside calculations and leave the correct volume shader in *state* → *volume*. The *mi_trace_shadow* call by the light shader only calls the first shadow shader closest to the illuminated point; that shadow shader must call *mi_trace_shadow_seg* after choosing the volume.

If a new material shader is written, it is often necessary to also write a matching shadow shader. The shadow shader performs a subset of the calculations done in the material shader: it may evaluate textures and transparencies, but it will not sample lights and it will not cast secondary rays (other than shadow rays in shadow segment mode). The shader writer can either write a separate shadow shader, or let the material shader double as shadow shader by building the scene such that the material shader appears twice in the material definition. Most shaders take the latter approach. It relies on the material shader to omit all calculations that are necessary only in the material shader when called as a shadow shader. The shader can find out whether it is called as a material shader or as a shadow shader by checking if *state*→*type* is `miRAY_SHADOW`: if yes, this is a shadow shader. This sharing of shaders pays off only when the texture computations are very complicated, or if the same complex inside/outside calculation is done for material shaders and for shadow shaders in shadow segment mode.

The following shadow shader is a separate shader that attenuates the light that passes through the object based on two shader parameters, the diffuse color and the transparency. Material shaders usually also have ambient and specular colors, but the best approach is to pass the diffuse color to shadow shaders because it describes the "true color" of the object best. Note that the scene can be arranged such that although the shadow shader is separate from the material shader, it still gets a copy of the material shader's shader parameters so the shadow shader can access the "true" material parameters. In a .mi file, this is done by declaring the shadow shader with no parameters and naming none in the `shadow` statement in the material definition (just give `()`). This sharing of parameters even if the shader itself is not shared avoids having to duplicate a large set of parameters.

```
#include <stdio.h>
#include <mi/shader.h>

int myshadow_version(void) {return(1);}

miBoolean myshadow(
   miColor        *result,
   miState        *state,
```

```
        struct myshadow *paras)
{
        miScalar          opacity;
        miScalar          f, omf;

        if (state->options->shadow == 's') {
            set up state->refraction_volume;
            if (!mi_trace_shadow_seg(result, state))
                result->r =
                result->g =
                result->b = 0;
        }
        opacity = 1 - *mi_eval_scalar(&paras->transp);
        if (opacity < 0.5) {
            f = 2 * opacity;
            result->r *= f * diffuse.r;
            result->g *= f * diffuse.g;
            result->b *= f * diffuse.b;
        } else {
            f = 2 * (opacity - 0.5);
            omf = 1 - f;
            result->r *= f + omf * diffuse.r;
            result->g *= f + omf * diffuse.g;
            result->b *= f + omf * diffuse.b;
        }
        return(result->r != 0 ||
               result->g != 0 ||
               result->b != 0);
}
```

In non-segmented shadow mode, the *org* variable in the state always contains the position of the light source responsible for casting the shadow rays. The `point` state variable contains the point on the shadow-casting object. The *dist* state variable is the distance to the light source (except for directional lights, which have no origin). In shadow segment mode, shadow rays travel in the opposite direction; *org* is the previous intersection (or the illumination point for the initial segment), and *dir* points towards the light source.

3.14 Photon Shaders

Photon shaders are used in the photon tracing phase to compute the photon maps that are used to simulate caustics and global illumination[2.1]. Like shadow shaders, they are specified in materials, and can share the material shader's parameters, or its implementation. Photon shaders need to use the *mi_photon_reflection_** and *mi_photon_transmission_** functions to reflect or transmit photons. They can also, if desired, use the built-in functions to generate new photon directions: *mi_reflection_dir_** and *mi_transmission_dir_**.

The following is a simple photon shader example that handles the interaction between a photon and a simple transmitting material. Notice how the incoming energy is modified *before* the new photon is transmitted; this is according with the fact that photons move in the *opposite* direction of the rays in the raytracing phase.

```
#include "shader.h"

struct ptparm {
   miScalar trans; /* fraction of light transmitted */
   miScalar ior;   /* index of refraction */
};

int ptrans_photon_version(void) {return(1);}

miBoolean ptrans_photon(
   miColor        *result,
   miState        *state,
   struct ptparm  *paras)
{
   miVector       dir;
   miColor        new_energy;
   miScalar       trans;

   mi_refraction_dir(&dir, state, 1.0,
                     *mi_eval_scalar(&paras->ior));

   trans = *mi_eval_scalar(&paras->trans);
   new_energy.r = result->r * trans;
   new_energy.g = result->g * trans;
   new_energy.b = result->b * trans;

   mi_photon_transmission_specular(&new_energy,
                                   state, &dir);
   return(miTRUE);
}
```

This photon shader only handles transmission and it only generates one photon. It is recommended to produce only one photon in a photon shader. If the photon shader supports several types of reflection or transmission, it should use *mi_choose_scatter_type* to select only one of these per photon interaction such that only one photon is propagated. If several photons are generated in a photon shader, the number of photons in the photon map might grow very quickly without obtaining the necessary quality.

Incoming photons should be stored on materials with a diffuse surface. This is done in the photon shader by calling *mi_store_photon*.

To benefit from the photon maps (consisting of the photons stored by the photon shaders), the material shaders should include the illumination from the photon maps using mi_compute_irradiance. This is illustrated in the following example of a simple diffuse surface simulated using a material shader and its corresponding photon shader.

pdif_photon is a simple example of a photon shader that stores a photon; *pdif* is material shader that displays the photon map. Since the *pdif_photon* shader only computes caustics, it does not reflect the photon off the diffuse surface. The *pdif* material shader does not compute direct illumination from the light sources and only takes the caustic into account.

```
#include "shader.h"

struct pdparm {
   miColor diffuse;
};

int pdif_photon_version(void) {return(1);}

miBoolean pdif_photon(
   miColor          *result,
   miState          *state,
   struct pdparm    *paras)
{
   mi_store_photon(result, state);
   return(miTRUE);
}

int pdif_version(void) {return(1);}

miBoolean pdif(
   miColor          *result,
   miState          *state,
   struct pdparm    *paras)
{
   miColor          irrad, *diffuse;

   mi_compute_irradiance(&irrad, state);
   diffuse = mi_eval_color(&paras->diffuse);

   result->r = irrad.r * diffuse->r;
   result->g = irrad.g * diffuse->g;
   result->b = irrad.b * diffuse->b;
   result->a = 1.0;
   return(miTRUE);
}
```

In a scene consisting of a glass lens that creates a caustic on a ground plane, four shaders need to be attached:

- The material of the glass object references a refractive material shader (not described here).
- The material of the glass object references *ptrans_photon* as photon shader.
- The material of the ground plane object references *pdif* as material shader.
- The material of the ground plane object references *pdif_photon* as photon shader.

Here is a more complete example of a photon shader. It simulates both diffuse, glossy, and specular reflection, and can be used for both caustics (both caustic generation and receiving) and global illumination.

```
miBoolean dgs_material_photon(
    miColor              *energy,
    miState              *state,
    struct dgs_material  *paras)
{
    struct               dgs_material m;
    miColor              color;
    miVector             dir;
    miScalar             ior_in, ior_out;
    miRay_type           type;
    miBoolean            ok;

    /*
     * Make a local copy of the parameters (light
     * sources are not used here)
     */

    m.diffuse  = *mi_eval_color (&paras->diffuse);
    m.glossy   = *mi_eval_color (&paras->glossy);
    m.specular = *mi_eval_color (&paras->specular);
    m.shiny    = *mi_eval_scalar(&paras->shiny);
    m.shiny_u  = *mi_eval_scalar(&paras->shiny_u);
    m.shiny_v  = *mi_eval_scalar(&paras->shiny_v);
    m.transp   = *mi_eval_scalar(&paras->transp);
    m.ior      = *mi_eval_scalar(&paras->ior);

    /*
     * Insert photon in map if this is a diffuse
     * surface.
     */

    if (m.diffuse.r > miEPS ||
        m.diffuse.g > miEPS ||
        m.diffuse.b > miEPS)
            mi_store_photon(energy, state);

    /*
     * Choose scatter type for new photon
     */

    type = mi_choose_scatter_type(state, m.transp,
                                  &m.diffuse,
                                  &m.glossy,
                                  &m.specular);
    /*
     * Shoot new photon: Compute new photon color
     * (compensating for Russian roulette) and shoot
     * new photon in a direction determined by the
```

```
     * scattering type
     */

    switch (type) {
                   /* no reflection. or transmission */
      case miPHOTON_ABSORB:
        return(miTRUE);

                   /* specular reflection (mirror) */
      case miPHOTON_REFLECT_SPECULAR:
        color.r = energy->r * m.specular.r;
        color.g = energy->g * m.specular.g;
        color.b = energy->b * m.specular.b;
        mi_reflection_dir_specular(&dir, state);
        return mi_photon_reflection_specular(&color,
                                         state, &dir);

                   /* glossy reflection (Ward model) */
      case miPHOTON_REFLECT_GLOSSY:
        color.r = energy->r * m.glossy.r;
        color.g = energy->g * m.glossy.g;
        color.b = energy->b * m.glossy.b;
        if (m.shiny)
                   /* isotropic glossy reflection */
            mi_reflection_dir_glossy(&dir, state,
                                          m.shiny);
        else {     /* anisotropic glossy reflection */
            miVector u, v;
            miASSERT(m.shiny_u > 0 && m.shiny_v > 0);
            anis_orientation(&u, &v, state);
            mi_reflection_dir_anisglossy(&dir, state,
                       &u, &v, m.shiny_u, m.shiny_v);
        }
        return(mi_photon_reflection_glossy(&color,
                                        state, &dir));

                   /* diffuse (Lamberts cosine law) */
      case miPHOTON_REFLECT_DIFFUSE:
        color.r = energy->r * m.diffuse.r;
        color.g = energy->g * m.diffuse.g;
        color.b = energy->b * m.diffuse.b;
        mi_reflection_dir_diffuse(&dir, state);
        return mi_photon_reflection_diffuse(&color,
                                         state, &dir);

                   /* specular transmission */
      case miPHOTON_TRANSMIT_SPECULAR:
        color.r = energy->r * m.specular.r;
        color.g = energy->g * m.specular.g;
        color.b = energy->b * m.specular.b;
        refraction_index(state, &m, &ior_in, &ior_out);
        miASSERT(ior_in >= 1 && ior_out >= 1);
```

```
            return(ior_out == ior_in
                ? mi_photon_transparent(&color,state)
                : mi_transmission_dir_specular(&dir,
                                  state, ior_in, ior_out)
                ? mi_photon_transmission_specular(
                                  &color, state, &dir)
                : miFALSE);
            }

                      /* glossy transmiss. (Ward model) */
          case miPHOTON_TRANSMIT_GLOSSY:
            color.r = energy->r * m.glossy.r;
            color.g = energy->g * m.glossy.g;
            color.b = energy->b * m.glossy.b;
            refraction_index(state, &m, &ior_in, &ior_out);
            miASSERT(ior_in >= 1 && ior_out >= 1);

            if (m.shiny)
                      /* isotropic glossy transmission */
                ok = mi_transmission_dir_glossy(&dir,
                          state, ior_in, ior_out, m.shiny);
            else {    /* anisotropic glossy transmission */
                miVector u, v;
                miASSERT(m.shiny_u > 0 && m.shiny_v > 0);
                anis_orientation(&u, &v, state);
                ok = mi_transmission_dir_anisglossy(&dir,
                               state, ior_in, ior_out, &u,
                               &v, m.shiny_u, m.shiny_v);
            }
            if (ok)
            return(ok ? mi_photon_transmission_glossy(
                               &color, state, &dir)
                      : miFALSE);

                      /* diffuse transm. (translucency) */
          case miPHOTON_TRANSMIT_DIFFUSE:
            color.r = energy->r * m.diffuse.r;
            color.g = energy->g * m.diffuse.g;
            color.b = energy->b * m.diffuse.b;
            mi_transmission_dir_diffuse(&dir, state);
            return(mi_photon_transmission_diffuse(&color,
                                        state, &dir));

          default:      /* Unknown scatter type */
            mi_error("unknown scatter type in dgs photon shader");
            return(miFALSE);
        }
    }
```

The first thing that happens in *dgs_material_photon* is that the reflection parameters are evaluated with *mi_eval_**. Then the photon is stored if the surface is diffuse and the photon is not directly from the light source. Second, the function *mi_choose_scatter_type* is called. Based on the transparency and reflection coefficients, it decides whether the photon should be absorbed, reflected diffusely, glossily, or specularly, or refracted diffusely, glossily, or specularly. If absorption is not chosen, *mi_choose_scatter_type* changes the reflection coefficients of the chosen reflection or refraction type to compensate for the fact that the photon "survived". This is a method known as "Russian Roulette".

If the photon is absorbed, *dgs_material_photon* simply returns at this point. If the photon should be reflected or refracted, the energy of the new photon is computed, a new direction is computed (using the built-in functions to compute reflection and refraction directions), and the photon is emitted in that direction.

Instead of using Russian Roulette to determine whether the photon should be absorbed or not, one could also emit a new photon for each type of reflection and refraction that has a non-zero reflection coefficient. Each emitted photon should have an energy that is the energy of the incoming photon multiplied by the reflection coefficient for that reflection (or refraction) type. However, this means that each photon emitted from the light source can cause *many* photons to be stored, some with very insignificant energy. The advantage of using Russian Roulette is that all the stored photons have comparable energies — no storage is wasted saving photons with low energy.

Obviously scene creation is simplified if the material shaders are written such that they also function as photon shaders, and also as shadow shaders, because the same shader can be attached to the respective materials three times, as material shader, photon shader, and shadow shader. If no parameters are specified for the photon and shadow shader references, mental ray will pass the material shader arguments to them, so they need not be duplicated twice. A shader can find the context in which it is called by examining $state \rightarrow type$.

3.15 Photon Emitter Shaders

Photon emitter shaders are used in the photon tracing phase to control the emission of photons from the light sources. There exists a number of built-in photon emitters that handle the following types of light sources:

- Point lights: emit photons with equal flux in all directions around the point light.
- Spot lights: emit photons with equal flux within the cone specified by the spotlight parameters.
- Directional lights: emit photons with equal *radiance* (based on the energy). Since a directional light source is strictly non-physical, the energy concepts are different from the other light sources.
- Disc area lights: emit photons from different points on the disc in directions based on a cosine distribution.
- Rectangle area lights: emit photons from different points on the rectangle in directions based on a cosine distribution.

- Sphere area lights: emit photons with equal flux from the surface of the sphere based on a cosine distribution at each surface point.
- Cylinder area lights: emit photons with equal flux from the surface of the cylinder based on a cosine distribution. No photons are emitted from the two disc-shaped "ends" of the cylinder.

Unless there are good reasons, these light sources should be used since they are well optimized. This is particularly true for the point light and sphere light which use a projection map to limit the emission of photons to the directions in which caustic generating objects are found. The appropriate built-in photon emitters are automatically applied if no photon emitter is specified in the light source definition.

If more complex light sources are needed, it can be necessary to write a specialized shader. For example, this could be necessary for a spot light that should support intensity fading near the edges of the cone. Note that the light emitter shader is not called if the light has zero energy; such lights are ignored by mental ray during photon tracing.

An example of a simple point light that emits photons uniformly in all directions around the current point is given in the following shader[1]. The shader receives information about the light source from *state* $\rightarrow$ *light_instance*.

```
#include <stdio.h>
#include <math.h>
#include "shader.h"

int point_emitter_version() {return(1);}

void point_emitter_init(
   miState          *state,
   void             *p,
   miBoolean        *inst_init_req)
{
   miTag            light_tag;
   miMatrix         *T;

   if (!p)
       *inst_init_req = miTRUE;
   else {
       miVector org, *torg;
       torg = mi_mem_allocate(sizeof(miVector));

       mi_query(miQ_INST_ITEM, state,
                state->light_instance, &light_tag);
       mi_query(miQ_INST_LOCAL_TO_GLOBAL, state,
                state->light_instance, &T);
       mi_query(miQ_LIGHT_ORIGIN, state,
                light_tag, &org);
```

[1]This is just a simple example shader — the builtin point light emitter is much more efficient.

```
            mi_point_transform(torg, &org, *T);
            state->shader->user.p = torg;
        }
    }

    void point_emitter_exit(
        miState         *state,
        void            *p)
    {
        if (state->shader->user.p && p) {
            mi_mem_release(state->shader->user.p);
            state->shader->user.p = NULL;
        }
    }

    miBoolean point_emitter(
        miColor         *energy,
        miState         *state,
        void            *p)
    {
        state->org = *(miVector *)state->shader->user.p;
        do
            mi_scattering_dir_diffuse(&state->dir, state);

        while ((state->dir.x * state->dir.x +
                state->dir.y * state->dir.y +
                state->dir.z * state->dir.z) > 1.0);

        mi_vector_normalize(&state->dir);
        mi_photon_light(energy, state);
        return(miTRUE);
    }
```

This shader does not take any parameters. Instead it extracts all information about the light source with *mi_query*. This shader can be attached to a light definition using the `photon` statement. Note the choice of direction using *mi_scattering_dir_diffuse* and rejection sampling: instead of limiting the computed directions to points in a circle, rectangular directions are computed and rejected if they fall outside the circle. This is more efficient than computing polar coordinates, adjusting for uniform density, and converting to rectangular coordinates. The *org* and *dir* or any other ray state variables are undefined when the shader is called, the shader must come up with its own directions.

If a photon emitter shader returns `miFALSE`, photon emission from the current light source is aborted at that point and no more photons are cast from this light source. It is recommended that photon emitter shaders return `miTRUE` only if they called *mi_photon_light* because otherwise mental ray will keep calling the shader for a long time without ever storing a photon.

3.16 Lens Shaders

Lens shaders are called for primary rays from the camera. The camera is normally a simple pinhole camera. A lens shader modifies the origin and direction of a primary ray from the camera. More than one lens shader may be attached to the camera; each modifies the origin and direction calculated by the previous one. By convention, all rays up to and including the one leaving the last lens are called "primary rays". The origin and direction input parameters can be found in the state, in the *origin* and *dir* variables. The outgoing ray is cast with *mi_trace_eye*, whose return color may be modified before the shader itself returns. Lens shaders are called recursively; a call to *mi_trace_eye* will call the next lens shader if there is another one.

Here is a sample lens shader that implements a fish-eye lens:

```
#include <stdio.h>
#include <mi/shader.h>

int fisheye_version(void) {return(1);}

miBoolean fisheye(
   miColor  *result,
   miState  *state,
   void     *paras)
{
   miVector camdir, dir;
   miScalar x, y, r, t;

   mi_vector_to_camera(state, &camdir, &state->dir);
   t = state->camera->focal / -camdir.z /
                            (state->camera->aperture/2);
   x = t * camdir.x;
   y = t * camdir.y * state->camera->aspect;
   r = x * x + y * y;
   if (r < 1) {
        dir.x = camdir.x * r;
        dir.y = camdir.y * r;
        dir.z = -sqrt(1 - dir.x*dir.x - dir.y*dir.y);
        return(mi_trace_eye(result, state,
                            &state->org, &dir));
   } else {
        result->r = result->g =
        result->b = result->a = 0;
        return(miFALSE);
   }
}
```

This shader does not take the image aspect ratio into account, and is not physically correct. It merely bends rays away from the camera axis depending on their angle to the camera axis. Rays that fall outside the circle that touches the image edges are set to black (note that alpha is also set to 0). The rays are bent according to the square of the angle, which approaches the physically correct deflection for small values of π. This example shader has no shader parameters, which is why the type of the *paras* parameter is `void *`.

Be sure to derive the ray origin from *state* $\rightarrow$ *org*, not *state* $\rightarrow$ *point*, which is undefined in lens shaders and can cause incorrect and empty or extremely noisy pictures.

3.17 Output Shaders

Output shaders are functions that are run after rendering has finished. They modify the resulting image or images. Typical uses are output filters and compositing operations. Output shaders can directly access all rendered frame buffers and make modifications to these frame buffers, but they do not return a result like other shaders do. They still get a result pointer as their first argument, for symmetry with the other types of shaders, but this pointer should not be used.

Until version 2.0.20 of mental ray, output shaders had a different prototype (there was no result pointer argument) and a different state called `miOutstate`, which contained frame buffers but very few other state variables, so output shaders could not use any shader interface function that required an argument of type `miState`. For backwards compatibility, these shaders are still supported, but not recommended and not described in this book. mental ray distinguishes old-style output shaders by a null or missing version number in the declaration. Old-style output shaders did not support shader initialization and cleanup and the *mi_eval* family of functions; new ones do.

It is important to specify a non-null shader version number in the declaration of output shaders! If none is specified, mental ray issues a warning and calls the output shader with an `miOutstate`, which will probably crash it.

All output shaders must be declared like any other type of shader, and the same types of arguments can be declared. This includes textures and lights. Nonprocedural textures can be looked up using functions like *mi_lookup_color_texture* and *mi_query*. Lights can also be looked up with *mi_query*. Since rendering has completed, it is not possible to look up procedural textures or to use tracing functions such as *mi_sample_light*.

Here is a simple output shader that depth-fades the rendered image towards total transparency:

```
#include <stdio.h>
#include <mi/shader.h>

struct out_depthfade {
   miScalar   near;    /* no fade closer than this */
   miScalar   far;     /* farther objects disappear */
};

int out_depthfade_version(void) {return(1);}

miBoolean out_depthfade(
   void                 *result,
```

```
    register miState        *state,
    struct out_depthfade    *paras)
{
    register int            x, y;
    miColor                 color;
    miScalar                depth, fade;
    miScalar                near, far;
    miImg_image             *fb_color, *fb_depth;

    near     = *mi_eval_scalar(&paras->near);
    far      = *mi_eval_scalar(&paras->far);
    fb_color = state->options->image[miRC_IMAGE_RGBA].p;
    fb_depth = state->options->image[miRC_IMAGE_Z].p;

    for (y=0; y < state->camera->y_resolution; y++)
        if (mi_par_aborted())
            break;
        for (x=0; x<state->camera->x_resolution; x++) {
            mi_img_get_color(fb_color, &color, x, y);
            mi_img_get_depth(fb_depth, &depth, x, y);

            if (depth >= far || depth == 0.0)
                color.r=color.g=color.b=color.a = 0;
            else if (depth > near) {
                fade = (far - depth) / (far - near);
                color.r *= fade;
                color.g *= fade;
                color.b *= fade;
                color.a *= fade;
            }
            mi_img_put_color(fb_color, &color, x, y);
        }
    return(miTRUE);
}
```

Note the call to *mi_par_aborted*, which stops the shader if the user has instructed mental ray to stop whatever it is doing. This call was inserted in the line loop because it should be called periodically, but not too often to avoid slowing it down.

This shader is stored in a file `out_depthfade.c` and installed in the .mi file with a `code` statement and a declaration:

```
code "out_depthfade.c"
declare shader
    "out_depthfade" (scalar "near", scalar "far")
    version 1
end declare
```

It is actually more efficient to precompile the shader, store it in a DSO file, anmd use the `link` statement instead of `code`. See the beginning of this chapter (page 129) for details. The declaration should appear before the first reference to the shader in a `camera` statement. Note the non-null version statement. The shader is referenced in an `output` statement in the camera:

```
camera "cam"
    output "rgba,z" "out_depthfade"
                        ("near" 10.0, "far" 100.0)
    output "rgb" "filename.rgb"
    samples 0 1
    ...
end camera
```

Note that the output shader statement appears before the output file statement. The output shader must get a chance to change the output image before it is written to the file `filename.rgb`. It is possible to insert another file output statement before the output shader statement; in this case two files would be written, one with and one without depth fading.

Note also that the output shader has a type string `"rgba,z"`. This string tells mental ray to render both an RGBA and a Z (depth) frame buffer. The RGBA buffer would have been rendered anyway because the file output statement requires it, but the depth buffer would not have been rendered without the `z` in the type string. In this case, all depth values returned by *mi_img_get_depth* would be 0.0.

By default, depth buffers are not interpolated; instead the min depth within the pixel is used. If the depths should be interpolated, use the output type `"rgba,+z"`. Refer to the Functionality chapter for more information on frame buffer interpolation.

This shader does not anti-alias very well because there is only one depth value per pixel. The shader makes pixels for which a depth of 0.0 is returned totally transparent to fade edges of objects correctly that have no other object behind them. By definition, *mi_img_get_depth* returns 0.0 for a position x, y if no object was hit at that pixel.

3.17.1 Parallel Output Shaders

Output shaders can be parallelized. If the declaration includes the `parallel` flag[2.1], mental ray will call the output shader multiple times with small portions of the frame buffer. The calls are distributed over all local threads. This can improve the performance significantly if the local machine has more than one CPU, but requires special attention to multithreading issues in the shader.

mental ray splits the frame buffer into blocks of scanlines. Each call to the output shader is expected to operate on one such block. It can still *read* the entire frame buffer, but it is expected to *write* only the assigned scanlines. The call order is unpredictable. The shader writer must make sure that reading does not read lines that have already been written, or are currently being written, by another thread.

Basically, if the output shader reads lines outside its assigned block, it must use an init shader to make a copy of the frame buffer, and an exit shader to delete the copy when it has finished.

Typically, the copy of the frame buffer is attached to *state* → *shader* → *user.p* in the instance init shader. Special care must be taken to delete allocated pointers in case multiple output statements reference the same named shader, to avoid a memory leak.

The scanline block to operate on is defined by mental ray in the state variables *raster_y*, which defines the first scanline to write, and *dist*, which contains the number of scanlines. If *dist* is 0, this shader is not called in parallel mode; this must be checked to make the shader compatible with older mental ray versions that do not support parallel output shaders.

Here is the previous example shader again, with support for parallelism:

```
miBoolean out_depthfade(
   void                     *result,
   register miState         *state,
   struct out_depthfade     *paras)
{
   register int             x, y, ye;
   miColor                  color;
   miScalar                 depth, fade;
   miScalar                 near, far;
   miImg_image              *fb_color, *fb_depth;

   near     = *mi_eval_scalar(&paras->near);
   far      = *mi_eval_scalar(&paras->far);
   fb_color = state->options->image[miRC_IMAGE_RGBA].p;
   fb_depth = state->options->image[miRC_IMAGE_Z].p;

   if (state->dist > 0) {
        y  = state->raster_y;      /* parallel mode */
        ye = state->dist + y;
   } else {
        y  = 0;                    /* sequential mode */
        ye = state->camera->y_resolution;
   }
   for (; y < ye; y++)
        /* same as before */

   return(miTRUE);
}
```

The declaration can now be changed to include the `parallel` keyword:

```
code "out_depthfade.c"
declare shader
    "out_depthfade" (scalar "near", scalar "far")
    parallel
    version 1
end declare
```

Note that the version number does not have to be changed — it refers to the shader interface, its return type and parameters, but not its implementation. Never specify the `parallel` flag in declarations of shaders that do not actually support parallelism because each call to the shader would not just write its assigned scanline block but the entire image.

3.18 Displacement Shaders

Displacement shaders are called during geometry tessellation if the material of a polygonal or free-form surface object specifies a `displace` shader. Whenever the tessellator introduces or copies a vertex, the displacement shader is called and expected to return a scalar value that tells the tessellator to move the vertex by this distance along its normal vector. If 0 is returned, the vertex remains unchanged. If the object specifies displacement approximations, curvature introduced by displacement can lead to further subdivision. Here is an example:

```
#include <stdio.h>
#include <mi/shader.h>

struct mydisplace {
   miTag             tex;
   miScalar          factor;
};

int mydisplace_version(void) {return(1);}

miBoolean mydisplace(
   miScalar          *result,
   miState           *state,
   struct mydisplace *paras)
{
   miColor           color;

   mi_lookup_color_texture(&color, state,
                            *mi_eval_tag(&paras->tex),
                            &state->tex_list[0]);

   *result += (color.r + color.g + color.b) / 3 *
                       *mi_eval_scalar(&paras->factor);
   return(miTRUE);
}
```

Note that the shader adds its displacement to the result instead of storing it. This allows chaining displacement shaders in shader lists. Shaders in shader lists get called in sequence, each adding its contribution to the result of the previous. mental ray calls the first displacement shader of the list with a result that is initialized to 0.

Displacement shaders may also change the vector *state* $\rightarrow$ *normal* along which the displacement will take place, or change *state* $\rightarrow$ *point*, which is the original vertex position that the displacement is added to. However, note that mental ray does not check that surfaces resulting from such arbitrary displacements are free of self-intersections.

3.19 Geometry Shaders

Geometry shaders are functions that procedurally create geometric objects. They are different from most of the shaders described here because they do not return a color, but a `miTag` reference to the object or instance group created by the shader. The geometry shader is called with a `miState` containing valid fields for camera, options, current shader, and version. The shader parameters are passed as the third argument. The geometry shader is expected to return the tag of the object or instance group it creates.

Here is a simple example for a geometry shader that creates a single triangle. A more robust shader would check the return values of all function calls made here. Geometry shaders use a special set of shader interface functions to create geometry. All these functions begin with *mi_api_*.

```
#include <mi/shader.h>

typedef struct {
   miTag      mtl;
} GeoTriangle;

static void
add_vector(miScalar x, miScalar y, miScalar z)
{
   miVector v;
   v.x = x; v.y = y; v.z = z;
   mi_api_vector_xyz_add(&v);
}

int geotriangle_version(void) {return(1);}

miBoolean geotriangle(
   miTag              *result,
   miState            *state,
   GeoTriangle        *paras)
{
   miObject        *obj;

   obj = mi_api_object_begin(NULL);
   obj->visible = obj->shadow = obj->trace = miTRUE;
   mi_api_basis_list_clear();
   mi_api_object_group_begin(0.0);

   add_vector(-1., 0., 0.);
   add_vector( 1., 0., 0.);
   add_vector( 0., 0., 1.);
```

```
    mi_api_vertex_add(0);
    mi_api_vertex_add(1);
    mi_api_vertex_add(2);

    mi_api_poly_begin_tag(1, *mi_eval_tag(&paras->mtl));
    mi_api_poly_index_add(0);
    mi_api_poly_index_add(1);
    mi_api_poly_index_add(2);
    mi_api_poly_end();

    mi_api_object_group_end();
    return(mi_geoshader_add_result(result,
                                   mi_api_object_end()));
}
```

In this example an unnamed object is created with the flags visible, shadow and trace set to `miTRUE`, a caustic mode set to `0`, and a label `0`. In the mandatory object group a triangle is constructed with API calls. The material of the triangle is assigned from the shader parameters. The object group definition is finalized with the polygonal information argument set to `miTRUE`.

3.20 Contours

The use of flexible, user-defined contour shaders opens up the possibility of many new effects. User-specified functions and shaders determine where the contours should be and compute contour colors and widths. These computations can be based on any information about the geometry, illumination, and materials of the scene, for example Z depth, Z depth difference, orientation, curvature, light source directions, material color, fog, etc.

The list of possible contour shaders is endless. A few ideas for contour shaders are: different styles of contour lines such as hand-drawn pencil, chalk, calligraphic pen, brush, wiggly lines, dashed lines, etc; contours between areas in shadow and areas not in shadow; contour parameters depending on motion information; highlights on contours to indicate curving edges.

The following is a detailed description of how contours are computed, and how the contour store shader, the contour contrast shader, and the contour shaders are called. Note that contour shaders do not follow the normal shader argument conventions. They do support initialization and exit shaders with standard init/exit shader prototypes and semantics.

3.20.1 Contour Computation

A regular color image is created by recursively sampling the scene, that is, casting rays into the geometry. The same samples are used to generate the contours. With each sample, some user-specified information is stored by the user-specified *contour store function*, information that is used later for determining the locations, colors, and widths of the contours. The contour store function is called right after the material shader and saves information such as ray intersection point, the normal at the intersection point, object tag, material color, refraction level, etc.

During recursive sampling, the decision whether to take additional samples is based on the comparison of two adjacent samples. New samples are taken if the color contrast is sufficiently large (as defined by the regular `contrast` and `time contrast` settings), or if a user-specified *contour contrast shader* returns `miTRUE`. The contour contrast shader can base its decision on any information that was stored by the contour store function for the two sample points. For example, the contour contrast function could return `miTRUE` if their depths or orientations differ much.

When two samples are at minimum distance (according to the value of the `max samples` parameter), and their contour contrast is still high (that is, the contour contrast shader returns `miTRUE`), mental ray assumes that a contour must be drawn between the two samples and calls a user-specified *contour shader*. The contour shader computes the contour color and width depending on, for example, curvature (orientation difference), Z depth, Z depth difference, material color, or some other information saved by the contour store shader. The contour shader of the object closest to the camera is used. If no contour shader is specified for the material, it does not get a contour. The computed contour point data (contour color, width, etc.) for each point on the contour is stored in a temporary data structure. mental ray merges these contour points into straight contour line segments, each represented by its two endpoints.

These contour line segments are received by a contour output shader in a postprocessing step. The contour output shader reads the contour segment endpoints and generates, for example, an image or a PostScript file.

3.20.2 Contour Store Function

The contour store shader stores various information needed for contour computations. The input is the regular *state* after ray intersection and the call of material shader, and the color resulting from the material shader call. The output is the information the user deems necessary to compute contours, and the size of this information. There is only one global contour store shader for a scene. The contour store function's job is to collect all information that the contour contrast function needs to decide where to put contours and that the contour shaders need to draw a contour.

To give an example of a contour store shader, assume you have decided that to compute contours, you need the ray intersection point, the normal vector, the material, and the color at that point as computed by the material shader (which means the color is not just the color of the material with the given illumination; it also includes reflected and refracted light). Then define the data type `MyInfo` as

```
typedef struct MyInfo {
    miVector   point;      /* ray intersection point */
    miVector   normal;     /* ray intersection normal */
    miTag      material;   /* material tag */
    miColor    color;      /* from material shader */
```

```
} MyInfo;
```

Here is a contour store shader that fills in these fields of `MyInfo`:

```
miBoolean my_contour_store_function(
    void      *info_void,
    int       *info_size,
    miState   *state,
    miColor   *color)
{
    struct MyInfo *info = (MyInfo *)info_void;

    info->point    = state->point;
    info->normal   = state->normal;
    info->material = state->material;
    info->color    = *color;

    *info_size = sizeof(MyInfo);

    return(miTRUE);
}
```

mental ray will store a `MyInfo` data structure with every sample until the contour contrast shader is called. The number of stored `MyInfo` data structures grows up to the number of samples taken in an image task (typically a 32×32 pixel block).

3.20.3 Contour Contrast Function

The contour contrast shader decides where the contours should be. For example, it might decide that there should be a contour when the difference in depth or orientation is large. The decision is based on the contour information for two points (the information saved by the contour store shader), the reflection or refraction level of the two points, the state, and the parameters of the contour contrast function. The output is a Boolean value indicating whether there should be a contour between the two points. If the returned value is `miTRUE`, one of two things can happen: If the distance between the two points corresponds to `max samples`, a contour will be placed between the two points (getting contour width, color, etc. by calling the material's contour shader). If not, mental ray will take some additional samples to get a more precise position of the contour. There is only one contour contrast shader for the scene.

As an example of a user-defined contour contrast shader, consider the following function with parameters `zdelta` and `ndelta`:

```
miBoolean my_contour_contrast_function(
    MyInfo                          *info1,
    MyInfo                          *info2,
    int                              level,
```

```
    miState                          *state,
    My_Contour_Contrast_Parameters   *paras)
{
    /*
     * Contour if one ray intersected an object and one
     * ray hit background
     */
    if (!info1 || !info2)
        return(miTRUE);

    /*
     * Contour if sufficiently large difference in depth
     */
    if (fabs(info1->point.z - info2->point.z) >
                                      paras->zdelta)
        return(miTRUE);

    /*
     * Contour if sufficiently large change in normal
     */
    if (mi_vector_dot(&info1->normal, &info2->normal) <
                        cos(paras->ndelta * M_PI/180.0))
        return(miTRUE);

    /*
     * No contour otherwise
     */
    return(miFALSE);
}
```

3.20.4 Contour Shaders

The contour shaders compute contour color and width (and optionally object label, material tag, motion, and normal). Their input is two contour information blocks for two adjacent samples on each side of a contour (as stored by the contour store shader), the state, and shader parameters. Each material can have a separate contour shader. If no contour shader is specified for a material, that material does not get a contour.

The contour shader to call is selected based on which object is in front. If the difference in depth is small, the selection is based on which object faces the camera the most. (This is necessary to avoid "randomly" mixing contours along an edge between two different materials.)

As an example, consider the following very simple contour shader. It makes the contours white and half a percent (of the image X resolution) wide:

```
miBoolean my_first_contour_shader(
    miContour_endpoint  *result,
    MyInfo              *info_near,
```

```
    MyInfo              *info_far,
    miState             *state,
    void                *paras)
{
    result->color.r = result->color.g =
    result->color.b = result->color.a = 1.0;
    result->width = 0.5;
    return(miTRUE);
}
```

The type of the result is

```
typedef struct {
    miVector  point;
    miColor   color;
    float     width;
    miVector  motion;
    miVector  normal;
    miTag     material;
    int       label;
} miContour_endpoint;
```

The `point` is automatically filled in, the contour shader does not have to do that. `point.x` and `point.y` are in screen coordinates, while `point.z` is in camera coordinates.

An example of a slightly more complex shader, where the contour color is a factor of the material color and the width is a parameter, is

```
miBoolean my_colordependent_contour_shader(
    miContour_endpoint      *result,
    MyInfo                  *info_near,
    MyInfo                  *info_far,
    miState                 *state,
    Factorcolor_Parameters  *paras)
{
    /*
     * Set contour color to a factor times material
     * color. The opacity color->a is set to 1.0,
     * otherwise the material will shine through the
     * contour.
     */
    float f = paras->factor;
    result->color.r = f * info_near->color.r;
    result->color.g = f * info_near->color.g;
    result->color.b = f * info_near->color.b;
    result->color.a = 1.0;

    /*
     * Contour width given by a parameter
```

```
    */
    result->width = paras->width;

    return(miTRUE);
}
```

An appropriate data type must be defined for a contour shader. In this case, the data type of the parameters, `Factorcolor_Parameters`, contains the fields `factor` and `width`.

3.20.5 Contour Output Shaders

Output shaders are called after the image has been computed. An output shader can use the function *mi_get_contour_line* to get endpoints of a contour. When *mi_get_contour_line* returns `miFALSE`, there are no more contour lines.

Here is a very simple output shader that prints the screen-space coordinates of the contour endpoints.

```
miBoolean my_contour_output_shader(
    miColor  *result,    /* unused */
    miState  *state)
    /* no parameters */
{
    miContour_endpoint p1;
    miContour_endpoint p2;

    mi_info("Contour endpoints:");

    /* Get and write the contour endpoints */
    while (mi_get_contour_line(&p1, &p2))
         mi_info("%f %f --- %f %f",
                       p1.point.x, p1.point.y,
                       p2.point.x, p2.point.y);
    return(miTRUE);
}
```

3.21 Functions for Shaders

mental ray makes a range of functions available to shaders that can be used to access data, cast rays, looking up images, and perform standard mathematical computations. The functions are grouped by the module that supplies them. The shader writer may also use C library functions, but it is **mandatory** to include <`stdio.h`> and <`math.h`> if printing functions such as *fprintf* (use *mi_info* or similar for console debugging messages) or math functions such as *sin* are used. Not including these headers may abort rendering at runtime, even though the compiler did not complain. All shaders must include the standard mental ray header file, `shader.h`.

All functions and features supported only by mental ray 2.1 and later but not by 2.0 are marked "2.1".

Here is a summary of functions provided by mental ray. Section 3.21.15 shows which functions can be used in which shaders.

Shader Calls

type	*name*	*arguments*
miBoolean	mi_call_shader	*result, type, *state, tag
miBoolean	mi_call_shader_x	*result, type, *state, tag, *arg
miBoolean	mi_call_material	*result, *state
miBoolean	mi_call_photon_material	*result, *state
void *	mi_eval	*state, *param
miBoolean *	mi_eval_boolean	*param
miInteger *	mi_eval_integer	*param
miScalar *	mi_eval_scalar	*param
miVector *	mi_eval_vector	*param
miScalar *	mi_eval_transform	*param
miColor *	mi_eval_color	*param
miTag *	mi_eval_tag	*param
void	mi_flush_cache	*state

DB

type	*name*	*arguments*
int	mi_db_type	tag
int	mi_db_size	tag
void *	mi_db_access	tag
void	mi_db_unpin	tag
void	mi_db_flush	tag

RC Functions

type	*name*	*arguments*
miBoolean	mi_trace_eye	*result, *state, *org, *dir
miBoolean	mi_trace_reflection	*result, *state, *dir
miBoolean	mi_trace_refraction	*result, *state, *dir
miBoolean	mi_trace_transparent	*result, *state
miBoolean	mi_trace_environment	*result, *state, *dir
miBoolean	mi_trace_probe[2.1]	*state, *dir, *org
miBoolean	mi_trace_light	*result, *dir, *nl, *st, i
miBoolean	mi_sample_light	*result, *dir, *nl, *st,i,*s
miBoolean	mi_trace_shadow	*result, *state
miBoolean	mi_trace_shadow_seg	*result, *state
miBoolean	mi_compute_irradiance	*result, *state
miBoolean	mi_compute_volume_irradiance	*result, *state
miBoolean	mi_sample[2.1]	*sample, *i, *state, dim, *n

RC Photon Functions

type	*name*	*arguments*
miBoolean	mi_photon_light	*energy, *state
miBoolean	mi_photon_reflection_specular	*energy, *state, *dir
miBoolean	mi_photon_reflection_glossy[2.1]	*energy, *state, *dir
miBoolean	mi_photon_reflection_diffuse[2.1]	*energy, *state, *dir
miBoolean	mi_photon_transmission_specular	*energy, *state, *dir
miBoolean	mi_photon_transmission_glossy[2.1]	*energy, *state, *dir
miBoolean	mi_photon_transmission_diffuse[2.1]	*energy, *state, *dir
miBoolean	mi_photon_transparent	*energy, *state
miBoolean	mi_photon_volume_scattering	*energy, *state, *dir
void	mi_store_photon	*energy, *state
void	mi_store_volume_photon	*energy, *state

RC Direction Functions

type	*name*	*arguments*
void	mi_reflection_dir	dir, state
void	mi_reflection_dir_specular	*dir, *state
void	mi_reflection_dir_glossy	*dir, *state, shiny
void	mi_reflection_dir_anisglossy	*dir, *state, u, v, shiny_u, shiny_v
void	mi_reflection_dir_diffuse	*dir, *state
miBoolean	mi_refraction_dir	dir, state, ior_in, ior_out
miBoolean	mi_transmission_dir_specular	*dir, *state, *in, *out
miBoolean	mi_transmission_dir_glossy	*dir, *state, *in, *out, shiny
miBoolean	mi_transmission_dir_anisglossy	*dir, *state, *in, *out, u, v, shiny_u, shiny_v
void	mi_transmission_dir_diffuse	*dir, *state
void	mi_scattering_dir_diffuse	*dir, *state
void	mi_scattering_dir_directional	*dir, *state, directionality
miScalar	mi_scattering_pathlength	*state, density

IMG Functions

type	*name*	*arguments*
void	mi_img_put_color	*image, *color, x, y
void	mi_img_get_color	*image, *color, x, y
void	mi_img_put_scalar	*image, scalar, x, y
void	mi_img_get_scalar	*image, *scalar, x, y
void	mi_img_put_vector	*image, *vector, x, y
void	mi_img_get_vector	*image, *vector, x, y
void	mi_img_put_depth	*image, depth, x, y
void	mi_img_get_depth	*image, *depth, x, y
void	mi_img_put_normal	*image, *normal, x, y
void	mi_img_get_normal	*image, *normal, x, y
void	mi_img_put_label	*image, label, x, y
void	mi_img_get_label	*image, *label, x, y

Vector and Matrix Math Functions

type	*name*	*arguments*
void	mi_vector_neg	*r
void	mi_vector_add	*r, *a, *b
void	mi_vector_sub	*r, *a, *b
void	mi_vector_mul	*r, f
void	mi_vector_div	*r, f
void	mi_vector_prod	*r, *a, *b
miScalar	mi_vector_dot	*a, *b
miScalar	mi_vector_norm	*a
void	mi_vector_normalize	*r
void	mi_vector_min	*r, *a, *b
void	mi_vector_max	*r, *a, *b
miScalar	mi_vector_det	*a, *b, *c
miScalar	mi_vector_dist	*a, *b
void	mi_matrix_null	r
void	mi_matrix_ident	r
miBoolean	mi_matrix_isident	a
void	mi_matrix_copy	r, a
miBoolean	mi_matrix_invert	r, a
void	mi_matrix_prod	r, a, b
void	mi_matrix_rot_det	a
void	mi_matrix_rotate	a, x, y, z
void	mi_matrix_rotate_axis	a, *v, r

Transformation Math Functions

type	*name*	*arguments*
void	mi_point_transform	*r, *v, m
void	mi_vector_transform	*r, *v, m
void	mi_vector_transform_T	*r, *v, m
void	mi_point_to_world	*state, *r, *v
void	mi_point_to_camera	*state, *r, *v
void	mi_point_to_object	*state, *r, *v
void	mi_point_to_light[2.1]	*state, *r, *v
void	mi_point_to_raster	*state, *r, *v
void	mi_point_from_world	*state, *r, *v
void	mi_point_from_camera	*state, *r, *v
void	mi_point_from_object	*state, *r, *v
void	mi_point_from_light[2.1]	*state, *r, *v
void	mi_vector_to_world	*state, *r, *v
void	mi_vector_to_camera	*state, *r, *v
void	mi_vector_to_object	*state, *r, *v
void	mi_vector_to_light[2.1]	*state, *r, *v
void	mi_vector_from_world	*state, *r, *v
void	mi_vector_from_camera	*state, *r, *v
void	mi_vector_from_object	*state, *r, *v
void	mi_vector_from_light[2.1]	*state, *r, *v
void	mi_normal_to_world	*state, *r, *v
void	mi_normal_to_camera	*state, *r, *v
void	mi_normal_to_object	*state, *r, *v
void	mi_normal_to_light[2.1]	*state, *r, *v
void	mi_normal_from_world	*state, *r, *v
void	mi_normal_from_camera	*state, *r, *v
void	mi_normal_from_object	*state, *r, *v
void	mi_normal_from_light[2.1]	*state, *r, *v

Noise Functions

type	*name*	*arguments*
miScalar	mi_random	
miScalar	mi_srandom	seed
miScalar	mi_erandom	seed[3]
double	mi_par_random	*state
miScalar	mi_spline	t, n, *ctl
miScalar	mi_noise_1d	p
miScalar	mi_noise_2d	u, v
miScalar	mi_noise_3d	*p
miScalar	mi_noise_1d_grad	p, *g
miScalar	mi_noise_2d_grad	u, v, *gu, *gv
miScalar	mi_noise_3d_grad	*p, *g
miScalar	mi_unoise_1d	p
miScalar	mi_unoise_2d	u, v
miScalar	mi_unoise_3d	*p
miScalar	mi_unoise_1d_grad	p, *g
miScalar	mi_unoise_2d_grad	u, v, *gu, *gv
miScalar	mi_unoise_3d_grad	*p, *g

Auxiliary Functions

type	*name*	*arguments*
miScalar	mi_fresnel	n1, n2, t1, t2
miScalar	mi_fresnel_reflection	*state, *i, *o
miScalar	mi_phong_specular	spec, *state, *dir
void	mi_fresnel_specular	*ns, *ks, s, *st, *dir, *in, *out
miScalar	mi_blinn_specular	spec, *state, *dir
miScalar	mi_blong_specular	spec, *state, *dir
miBoolean	mi_cooktorr_specular	*result, *di, *dr, *n, roughness, *ior
miScalar	mi_ward_glossy	*di, *dr, *n, shiny
miScalar	mi_ward_anisglossy	*di, *dr, *n, *u, *v, shiny_u, shiny_v
miScalar	mi_schlick_scatter	*di, *dr, directionality
miRay_type	mi_choose_scatter_type	*state, transp, *specular, *glossy, *diffuse
miInteger	mi_choose_lobe	*state, r
miBoolean	mi_lookup_color_texture	*col, *state, tag, *v
miBoolean	mi_lookup_scalar_texture	*scal, *state, tag, *v
miBoolean	mi_lookup_vector_texture	*vec, *state, tag, *v
miBoolean	mi_lookup_filter_color_texture	*col, *state, tag, *paras, ST
miBoolean	mi_texture_filter_project	p[3], t[3], *state, disc_r, space
miBoolean	mi_texture_filter_transform	ST, p[3], t[3]
miBoolean	mi_tri_vectors	*state, wh, nt, **a, **b, **c
miBoolean	mi_query	query, *state, tag, *result, ...
miBoolean	mi_fb_put[2.1]	*state, fb, *data
miBoolean	mi_fb_get[2.1]	*state, fb, *data
miBoolean	mi_geoshader_add_result	query, *state, tag, *result, ...
miBoolean	mi_geoshader_tesselate	*state, *leaves, source
miBoolean	mi_geoshader_tesselate_end	leaves
char *	mi_string_substitute[2.1]	*new, *old, size

Obsolete Auxiliary Functions

These functions are obsolete; use *mi_query* for future implementations.

type	*name*	*arguments*
void	mi_light_info	tag, *org, *dir, **paras
int	mi_global_lights_info	**tag
void	mi_texture_info	tag, *xres, *yres, **paras
void *	mi_shader_info	*state
int	mi_instance_info	*state, **paras, **p1, **p2, **p3

Contour Functions

miBoolean	mi_get_contour_line	*p1, *p2
void	mi_add_contour_lines	p1[], p2[], n

Memory Allocation

type	*name*	*arguments*
void *	mi_mem_allocate	size
void *	mi_mem_reallocate	mem, size
void	mi_mem_release	mem
void	mi_mem_check	
void	mi_mem_dump	mod

Thread Parallelism and Locks

type	*name*	*arguments*
void	mi_init_lock	*lock
void	mi_delete_lock	*lock
void	mi_lock	lock
void	mi_unlock	lock
int	mi_par_localvpu	
int	mi_par_nthreads	
int	mi_par_aborted	

Messages and Errors

type	*name*	*arguments*
void	mi_fatal	*message, ...
void	mi_error	*message, ...
void	mi_warning	*message, ...
void	mi_info	*message, ...
void	mi_progress	*message, ...
void	mi_debug	*message, ...
void	mi_vdebug	*message, ...

Shader Calls

Shaders can be called either explicitly, or implicitly by evaluating a shader parameter that may be assigned to the output of another shader.

```
miBoolean mi_call_shader(
```

```
        miColor * const result,
        miShader_type   type,
        miState * const state,
        miTag           shader)
```

```
    miBoolean mi_call_shader_x(
        miColor * const result,
        miShader_type   type,
        miState * const state,
        miTag           shader,
        void            *arg)
```

These functions call the shader specified by the tag *shader*. The extended version passes the *arg* parameter as a fourth argument to the shader. The other version passes a null pointer as fourth argument to the shader. *mi_call_shader_x* is slightly more efficient than *mi_call_shader*.

The tag is normally a texture shader or light shader or some other type of shader found in the calling shader's parameter list. The caller must pass its own state and the shader type, which must be one of `miSHADER_LENS`, `miSHADER_MATERIAL`, `miSHADER_LIGHT`, `miSHADER_SHADOW` `miSHADER_ENVIRONMENT` `miSHADER_VOLUME`, and `miSHADER_TEXTURE`. The sequence of operations is:

1. *shader* is written into *state* → *shader*.
2. If the called shader is dynamically loaded and has an init shader that has not been called yet, it is called now, with *state* as its only argument.
3. The shader referenced by *shader* is called with three arguments: the *result* pointer, the given *state*, and the shader parameters retrieved from *shader*.
4. After the shader returns, *state* → *shader* is restored to its old value.

The return value of the shader is returned. If the shader expects a result argument of a type other than `miColor`, the pointer must be cast to `miColor` when passed to *mi_call_shader*. Note that the *shader* tag references an entire function call including shader parameters as defined in the .mi file with a `texture`, `light`, or some other statement combining shading function and shader parameters; `shader` is not just a simple pointer or reference to a C function.

```
    miBoolean mi_call_material(
        miColor         *result,
        miState         *state);
```

Call the material shader in *state* → *material*.

```
miBoolean mi_call_photon_material(
    miColor         *result,
    miState         *state);
```

Call the photon shader in *state* → *material*. This is intended for photon volume shaders.

```
void *mi_eval(
    miState         *state,
    void            *param)

miBoolean *mi_eval_boolean(
    miBoolean       *param)

miInteger *mi_eval_integer(
    miInteger       *param)

miScalar *mi_eval_scalar(
    miScalar        *param)

miVector *mi_eval_vector(
    miVector        *param)

miScalar *mi_eval_transform(
    miScalar        *param)

miColor *mi_eval_color(
    miColor         *param)

miTag *mi_eval_tag(
    miTag           *param)
```

Return the value of a shader parameter. If the shader parameter value is a constant, *mi_eval* returns its argument. If the parameter is assigned to another shader, call that shader and return a pointer to its return value (or the cached return value if it has been called recently). If the parameter is assigned to a phenomenon interface, return a pointer to the value in the interface. The latter two cases let shaders operate in the contexts of shader assignments and phenomena without needing knowledge of the context, which is automatically handled. The pointer remains valid until the shader returns, which avoids the need to copy a large returned data structure such as a color or array to temporary variables. Shaders should always access their parameters with *mi_eval*. If parameters are accessed without *mi_eval* and the parameter is assigned to another shader or an interface, the shader will see garbage.

The typed variants of *mi_eval* are implemented as macros for the convenience of shader writers. They cast their argument to a void pointer, call *mi_eval*, and recast the returned pointer to the appropriate type. They all make the assumption that the shader has a local variable *state* of type `miState *` in scope. Experience has shown that the typed variants make source code look much cleaner. Note that there is only one macro *mi_eval_tag* that can be used for parameters of type shader, color texture, vector texture, scalar texture, light, material, and geometry. All typed variants have been designed to return the same type they accept as an argument.

Always use the correct simple type. For example, if the parameter has type color, it must be evaluated as a single color (probably using *mi_eval_color*). It is not possible to use four scalar evaluations to access the R, G, B, and A components separately. Also, by convention, arrays should be evaluated as a unit, evaluating two integers for the `i_` index, the `n_` member count, and the array itself. However, structures are not evaluated as a unit; a separate evaluation is necessary for every simple member it contains.

```
void mi_flush_cache(
    miState          *state)
```

Prevents the cache from being used by future calls to *mi_eval*. If mi_eval calls another shader, the result is stored in a special cache in that other shader, which is normally flushed only when the entire shader graph returns. This means that the other shader will only ever be called once during the evaluation of a shader graph, and all *mi_eval*s are satisified from the cache. Notice that flushing applies to the entire sub-graph of shaders evaluated by this and future *mi_evals*; there is no way to flush the cache of a single shader because that would leave its sub-shaders in a funny state. The result cache is still active for shaders which call *mi_flush_cache*.

This is useful if the code calls a another shader more than once, such as a texture shader to sample a texture at three different locations to compute bump mapping gradients. Although the shader, if called with *mi_call_shader* or *mi_lookup_color_texture*, will get called each time, its sub-shaders inside the same phenomenon will not if these subshaders are called as the result of *mi_eval*. (Remember that *mi_eval* results are cached.) However, if *mi_flush_cache* is used before the second and every subsequent shader call, the called shader's *mi_eval* calls will cause a fresh subshader call.

3.21.1 DB Functions

Database access functions can be used to convert pointers into tags, and to get the type of a tag. The scene database contains only tags and no pointers at all, because pointers are not valid on other machines. A tag is a 32-bit integer value that uniquely identifies a piece of data in mental ray's virtual shared database. It acts like a pointer except that it is valid across all machines on the network.

```
int mi_db_type(
    const miTag tag)
```

Return the type of a database item. The tag must exist. Valid types that are of interest in shaders are:

`miSCENE_FUNCTION`	Function to call, such as a shading function
`miSCENE_MATERIAL`	Material containing shaders and flags
`miSCENE_LIGHT`	Light source
`miSCENE_IMAGE`	Image in memory

The most important are functions and images, because general-purpose texture shaders need to distinguish procedural and image textures. See the texture shader example on page 174.

```
int mi_db_size(
    const miTag tag)
```

[2.1]Return the size of a database item in bytes. The tag must exist. This function should be avoided if possible because it has poor performance and can lead to inefficient execution orders in mental ray 3.0 in certain situations.

```
void *mi_db_access(
    const miTag tag)
```

Look up the tag in the database, pin it, and return a pointer to the referenced item. Pinning means that the database item is guaranteed to stay in memory at the same location until the item is explicitly unpinned. Rendering aborts if the given *tag* does not exist. *mi_db_access* always returns a valid pointer. If an item is accessed twice, it must be unpinned twice; *pinned* is a counter, not a flag. The maximum number of simultaneous pins on a single database element is 65535.

```
void mi_db_unpin(
    const miTag tag)
```

Every tag that was accessed with *mi_db_access* must be unpinned with this function when the pointer is no longer needed. Failure to unpin can cause a pin overflow, which may abort rendering. After unpinning, the pointer may not be used any more.

```
void mi_db_flush(
    const miTag tag)
```

Normally, a shader does not use a pointer obtained with *mi_db_access* to write to a database item. If it does, other hosts on the network may still hold stale copies, which must explicitly be deleted by calling this function. This function must be used with great care; it is an error to flush an item that another shader has pinned. For this reason, it is not generally possible to pass information back and forth between shaders or hosts by writing into database items and then flushing them. Geometry shaders are normally the only place where database entries are written, and there are more powerful function libraries available for geometry shaders that do not require *mi_db_flush*.

3.21.2 RC Functions

These are the functions supplied by the render modules of mental ray, RC*. All following trace functions return `miTRUE` if any subsequent call of a shader returned `miTRUE` to indicate presence of illumination. Otherwise no illumination is present and `miFALSE` is returned. All trace functions derive the state of the ray to be cast from the given state of the parent ray. This state becomes the "child state" that is passed to subsequent shaders that are called by the trace function. The state is always copied, and the given state is not modified except for the state fields *label*, *point*, *normal*, *dist* and *motion*. These fields are copied from the child state so that the lens shader can access them in the state modified by *mi_trace_eye*. After the trace function returns, the caller may examine the child state (but not the grandchild, which is gone if it ever existed). Volume shaders get the same state as the previous (material) shader. Note that all point and direction vectors passed as arguments to tracing functions must be in internal space.

```
miBoolean mi_trace_eye(
    miColor         *result,
    miState         *state,
    miVector        *origin,
    miVector        *direction)
```

casts an eye ray from *origin* in *direction*, or calls the next lens shader. The allowed *origin* and *direction* values are restricted when using the ray classification rendering algorithm (not recommended, it exists only for backwards compatibility). If scanline rendering is turned on and *state→scanline* is not zero, *origin* and *direction* must be the same as in the initial call of *mi_trace_eye*, and the lens shader may not modify them. Lens shaders that depend on modifying ray origin and direction should be declared with the `trace on` option. Origin and direction must be given in internal space. This function may be used only in lens shaders. Note that *mi_trace_eye* stores *origin* and *direction* in *state → org* and *state → dir*, respectively, overwriting the previous values.

```
miBoolean mi_trace_reflection(
    miColor         *result,
    miState         *state,
    miVector        *direction)
```

casts a reflection ray from *state→point* to *direction*. It returns `miFALSE` if the trace depth has been exhausted. If no intersection is found, the optional environment shader is called. The direction must be given in internal space. This function may be used only in shaders called during image rendering, but not in displacement, geometry, photon, or output shaders.

```
miBoolean mi_trace_refraction(
    miColor         *result,
    miState         *state,
    miVector        *direction)
```

casts a refraction ray from *state→point* to *direction*. It returns `miFALSE` if the trace depth has been exhausted. If no intersection is found, the optional environment shader is called. Before this functions casts the refraction ray, after copying the state, it copies *state→refraction_volume* to *state→volume* because the ray is now assumed to be "inside" the object, so the volume shader that describes the inside should be used to modify the ray while traveling inside the object. It is the caller's responsibility to set *state→refraction_volume* to the camera's volume shader *state→camera→volume* or some other volume shader if it determines that the ray is now leaving the object. The direction must be given in internal space.

If ray tracing has been disabled, *mi_trace_refraction* cannot modify the ray direction and operates like *mi_trace_transparent*. This function may be used only in shaders called during image rendering, but not in displacement, geometry, photon, or output shaders.

```
miBoolean mi_trace_transparent(
     miColor          *result,
     miState          *state)
```

does the same as *mi_trace_refraction* with *dir* == *state→dir* (that is, no change in the ray direction) but may be executed faster if the parent ray is an eye ray. It also works when ray tracing is turned off. If the ray direction does not change (because no index of refraction or similar modification is applied), it is more efficient to cast a transparency ray than a refraction ray. Like *mi_trace_refraction*, this function copies the refraction volume shader to the volume shader because the ray is now assumed to be inside the object. This function may be used only in shaders called during image rendering, but not in displacement, geometry, photon, or output shaders.

```
miBoolean mi_trace_environment(
     miColor          *result,
     miState          *state,
     miVector         *direction)
```

casts a ray into the environment. The trace depth is not incremented or checked. The environment shader in the state is called to compute the color to be returned. The direction must be given in internal space.

```
miBoolean mi_trace_probe(
     miState          *state,
     miVector         *direction,
     miVector         *org)
```

[2.1]casts a ray into the scene, starting at *org* with the direction *direction*, both in internal space coordinates. If nothing is hit, `miFALSE` is returned. If the ray hits another object, `miTRUE` is returned and *state → child* is set to the state that the material shader of the hit object would have seen. However, unlike all other *mi_trace_** functions, no shader is called. Note that the state *state → child* does not itself have a state, so it cannot be used to call a material shader at the hit object directly. This requires setting up an artificial "grandchild" state:

```
        if (mi_trace_probe(state, &dir, &org)) {
                miState grandchild;
                state->child->child = &grandchild;
                if (mi_call_material(&result, state->child))
                        /* use the result */
        }
```

This sequence works roughly like *mi_trace_reflection*, except that no ray levels are tested, no environment is sampled, and no volume shaders are called. Note that *mi_trace_probe* will always return `miFALSE` if ray tracing is disabled.

```
    miBoolean mi_sample_light(
        miColor         *result,
        miVector        *dir,
        miScalar        *dot_nl,
        miState         *state,
        miTag           light_inst,
        miInteger       *samples)
```

casts a light ray from the light source to the intersection point, causing the light source's light shader to be called. The light shader may then calculate shadows by casting a shadow ray to the intersection point. This may cause shadow shaders of occluding objects to be called, and will also cause the volume shader of the state to be called, if there is one. Before the light is sampled, the direction from the current intersection point in the state to the light and the dot product of this direction and the normal in the state are calculated and returned in *dir* and *dot_nl* if these pointers are nonzero. The direction is returned in internal space. The light instance to sample must be given in *light_inst*. *samples* must point to an integer that is initialized to `0`. *mi_sample_light* must be called in a loop until it returns `miFALSE`. **samples* will then contain the total number of light samples taken; it may be larger than 1 for area light sources.

For every call in the loop, a different *dir* and *dot_nl* is returned because the rays go to different points on the area light source. The caller is expected to use these variables, the returned color, and other variables such as diffuse and specular colors from the shader parameters to compute a color. These colors are accumulated until *mi_sample_light* returns `miFALSE` and the loop terminates. The caller then divides the accumulated color by the number of samples (**samples*) if it is greater than `0`, effectively averaging all the intermediate results. See page 167 for an example of a shader using *mi_sample_light*.

When casting light rays with *mi_sample_light*, mental ray may check whether the primitive's normal is pointing away from the light and ignore the light in this case. For this reason some shaders, such as ray-marching volume shaders, should assign `0` to *state→pri* first, and restore it before returning. Some *mi_query* modes do not work if *pri* has been modified.

Light instance tags to call this function with can be found either in shader parameters of type `light` or `array light`, or in the global light list obtained from *mi_query*.

```
    miBoolean mi_trace_light(
```

```
        miColor         *result,
        miVector        *dir,
        miScalar        *dot_nl,
        miState         *state,
        miTag           light_inst)
```

is a simpler variation of *mi_sample_light* that does not keep a sample counter, and is not called in a loop. It is equivalent to *mi_sample_light* except for area light sources. Area light sources must be sampled multiple times with different directions, which is not supported accurately by this function because it can only return a single direction and *dot_nl*. This function is provided for backwards compatibility with mental ray 1.9 only, do not use it for new projects.

```
    miBoolean mi_trace_shadow(
        miColor * const result,
        miState * const state)
```

computes shadows for the given light ray by casting shadow rays. This function is normally called from a light shader to take occluding objects that prevent some or all of the light emitted by the light source to reach the illuminated point (whose material shader has probably called the light shader). The *result* color is modified by the shadow shaders that are called if occluding objects are found. Note that light shaders can improve performance by tracing shadow rays only if the contribution from the light is greater than some threshold, for example because distance or angle attenuation has left so little of the light color (less than 1/256, for example) that applying shadow occlusion to this value is not going to make any difference. This function returns `miFALSE` if full occlusion is detected, that is, *result* is black.

```
    miBoolean mi_trace_shadow_seg(
        miColor * const result,
        miState * const state)
```

recursively calls the shadow shader for the next shadow segment and returns its result, or the result of the light shader if there is no more shadow intersection. It does nothing if shadow segments are turned off. It is used by shadow shaders only; light shaders always use *mi_trace_shadow*. See the introduction to shader types and the shadow shader explanation for details on shadow modes. This function returns `miFALSE` if full occlusion is detected, that is, *result* is black.

```
    miBoolean mi_compute_irradiance(
        miColor   *result,
        miState   *state)
```

mi_compute_irradiance computes the irradiance corresponding to indirect diffuse illumination at the intersection point given in state ($state \rightarrow point$). This function is used in material shaders to add indirect illumination such as caustics or color bleeding[2.1]. If $state \rightarrow pri$ is zero, miFALSE is returned.

```
miBoolean mi_compute_volume_irradiance(
    miColor    *result,
    miState    *state)
```

mi_compute_volume_irradiance computes the irradiance corresponding to indirect diffuse illumination at the point given in state (*state* → *point*). This function is used in volume shaders to add indirect illumination such as multiply scattered light[2.1]or volume caustics.

3.21.3 Sampling with mi_sample

```
miBoolean mi_sample(
    double   *sample,
    int      *instance,
    miState  *state,
    miUshort dimension,
    miUint   *n)
```

[2.1]This is mental ray's primary generic sampling function. It can be used to sample arbitrary functions for evaluating integrals by deterministic sample points, which converge faster than their random counterparts and thus reduce rendering time. The *mi_sample* function is a high-level easy-to-use interface hiding all mathematical details of advanced quasi-Monte Carlo integration from the shader writer. *sample* is an array with *dimension* members that the new sample point will be stored into. Sample results are uniformly distributed in the range $[0, 1)^{dim}$. *instance* is the current sample number; it must point to an integer that is initialized to 0 before the first loop iteration. If there is no loop, a null pointer may be passed. *state* is the current shader state. *dimension* is the dimension of the sample, such as 3 for XYZ vectors. *n* must point to an integer that specifies the number of samples to take. If only a single sample is taken, *n* may be a null pointer. The body of the *mi_sample* loop may not write to **sample* or **n* or vary *dimension* between any subsequent calls in the same loop because *mi_sample* computes the next sample incrementally from the previous.

mi_sample has three main applications:

1. generating single samples, which can be used in photon and other shaders for deciding on the kind of physical interaction like glossy, specular, or diffuse scattering, and then selecting a new quasi-random direction. This is the classical case of implementing random walk simulations with the von-Neumann-Ulam scheme.

2. controlling an adaptive sampling loop, where the number of samples is not known in advance and the sampling loop will be terminated adaptively by the caller. This is the only mode where the caller may and must decide when to break from the loop.

3. controlling a finite sampling loop. This is the classical case of quasi-Monte Carlo integration, where *n* samples are drawn and averaged. This can be used for sampling area light sources or depth of field shaders. The advantage of knowning the number of samples *n* in advance is an increased convergence speed.

Note that the returned sample point *sample* must be used as *one* point. This means that several one dimensional samples must not be assembled to yield a multidimensional sample, and that a multidimensional sample must not be used in order to simulate consecutive events. If, for example, 3D sampling vectors are computed with *mi_sample*, a single loop with *dimension* 3 must be used, rather than a higher dimension to obtain other sampling values at the same time, or fewer to compute the X, Y, and Z direction separately. Samples from *mi_sample* must be used consecutively. The sequence should not be terminated prematurely, nor should samples be dropped, since rejection sampling will result in biased approximations.

A call to `mi_sample` in single sample mode looks like:

```
void a_single_sample(···, miState *state, ···)
{
    double sample[2];

    mi_sample(sample, 0, state, 2, 0);
    /* use sample[0] and sample[1] */
}
```

The sampling dimension in this example is 2. Since only a single sample is required, no sample counting is indicated by passing a null pointer as `*instance` counter and to the required number of samples n. After the call to `mi_sample`, the array `x` holds a two-dimensional sample point of $[0, 1)^2$. The function call always returns `miFALSE` in single sample mode.

In the adaptive sampling mode, the number of samples to be taken is not known in advance, and the code must decide when to break from the loop (which it may not in the other two modes, where *mi_sample* returns `miFALSE`). *mi_sample* is then used the following way:

```
void adaptive_sampling(···, miState *state, ···)
{
    double sample[5];
    int sample_number = 0;

    while (mi_sample(sample, &sample_number, state, 5, 0)) {
        /* use sample[0], ..., sample[4] */
        if (enough samples taken)
            break;
    }
}
```

Adaptive sampling is indicated to *mi_sample* by passing a null pointer as the number of samples n. The `while` loop is then controlled by the *mi_sample* call, which always returns `miTRUE` in adaptive sampling mode. The current sample number starting with 1 for the first sample is kept in *sample_number*. This variable must be initialized to zero in order to force initialization in *mi_sample*. Note that in deterministic sampling, adaptive sampling (here, the `break` condition) cannot be controlled by the calculation of variance as in Monte Carlo context. This will result in biased approximations. Adaptive sampling here could be based on contrast calculations, for example. *sample* holds a sample point in the five-dimensional unit cube $[0, 1)^5$.

In the classical case, where the number of samples is known in advance, the deterministic sampling controlled by *mi_sample* very much resembles a Monte Carlo quadrature:

```
void finite_sampling(···, miState *state, ···)
{
    const miUint samples = 16;
    double sample[2];
    int sample_number = 0;

    while (mi_sample(sample, &sample_number, state, 2, &samples)) {
        /* use sample[0], sample[1] */
    }
}
```

Here, all arguments of `mi_sample` are used. Unlike the previous adaptive sampling case, the number of samples is passed explicitly to *mi_sample*. Again the integer variable *sample_number* is initialized to zero and passed by reference to *instance*. **state* is the current state of the shader. *mi_sample* returns `miTRUE` for *samples* iterations of the loop, until finally `miFALSE` is returned to terminate the loop. The loop *should not* be terminated with a `break` or `return` statement, because then the internal state of *state* does not guarantee convergence of rendering any longer (that is, *state* → *qmc_instance* and *state* → *qmc_component* are wrong until the shader terminates). In the loop, **instance* provides the current sample number, starting at 1, until *samples* is reached. The loop controls a two-dimensional integration, where *sample* is an array of `doubles` with two elements. The vector *sample* is the sample point in the two-dimensional unit cube $[0, 1)^2$. The finite sampling mode exposes a faster convergence than the adaptive sampling mode. Exceptional convergence can be achieved if the number of samples is

$$samples = \prod_{i=1}^{dimension-1} p_i^{k_i},$$

where p_i are the prime numbers, i.e. $p_1 = 2$, $p_2 = 3$, etc., and $k_i \in I\!N$ is a (positive) natural number. In two dimensions, i.e. *dimension* `==` 2, *samples* should be a power of 2. In the special case of *dimension* `== 1`, any number of samples can be used in order to achieve optimal convergence.

3.21.4 RC Photon Functions

The functions in this section implement *photon tracing*. They are to be used in photon shaders. If caustics or global illumination[2.1] are enabled, rendering distinguishes two phases: photon tracing and scanline rendering/ray tracing. Photon tracing is done first. It sends photons from certain light sources into the scene. When a photon hits an object, the object's photon shader is called, which then gets the opportunity to absorb the photon or use one of the *mi_photon_** functions to let the photon continue. The photon functions can be used only in photon shaders. Photon shaders may not use regular ray tracing functions such as *mi_trace_reflection*.

There are three main categories of photon tracing: specular, glossy, and diffuse. These terms define the distribution of the secondary photons in terms of the amount of scattering. Polished surfaces like chrome or clear glass are specular; unpolished surfaces such as aluminum or lightly frosted glass are glossy, and surfaces with no directional reflection or refraction such as paper are diffuse.

Photon tracing and ray tracing are similar in many respects, and use similar function calls. Although the operation underneath is quite different (tracing photons vs. tracing rays), a table of the operations in each phase shows the similarity as far as the shaders are concerned:

photons	rays
emanate from light sources	emanate from the camera
call photon material shaders	call material shaders
call photon volume shaders	call volume shaders
call photon emission shaders	call light shaders
—	call lens shaders
—	call environment shaders
mi_photon_light	*mi_trace_eye*
mi_reflection_dir_specular	*mi_reflection_dir*
mi_reflection_dir_glossy	—
mi_reflection_dir_anisglossy	—
mi_reflection_dir_diffuse	—
mi_transmission_dir_specular	*mi_refraction_dir*
mi_transmission_dir_glossy	—
mi_transmission_dir_anisglossy	—
mi_transmission_dir_diffuse	—
mi_scattering_dir_diffuse	—
mi_scattering_dir_directional	—
mi_scattering_pathlength	—
mi_photon_reflection_specular	*mi_trace_reflection*
mi_photon_reflection_glossy[2.1]	—
mi_photon_reflection_diffuse[2.1]	—
mi_photon_transmission_specular	*mi_trace_refraction*
mi_photon_transmission_glossy[2.1]	—
mi_photon_transmission_diffuse[2.1]	—
mi_photon_transparent	*mi_trace_transparent*
mi_photon_volume_scattering	—
mi_store_photon	*mi_compute_irradiance*
mi_store_volume_photon	*mi_compute_volume_irradiance*

There are three *mi_photon_reflection_** functions and three *mi_photon_refraction_** functions (as well as a function for transparency and one for volume scattering). Why not just one reflection function and one transmission function, similar to *mi_trace_reflection* and *mi_trace_refraction*?

The reason is that mental ray needs to know what type of reflections and transmissions the photon has undergone (its "path history") to determine which photon map to store it in, when not to store the photon, and when to terminate the photon path.

The photon reflection and transmission functions all follow the same pattern: first they check whether the intersected object is a caustic generator, if tracing caustic photons. If the object is not a caustic generator, the photon is not traced further and `miFALSE` is returned. A similar check is made for global illumination generating objects if tracing global illumination photons. Then a new state is set up with the appropriate ray type, reflection and refraction level, origin and direction (and the volume in the transmission case).

Photon shaders, photon volume shaders, and photon emission shaders are optional; if one is missing mental ray uses built-in defaults. The default photon shader absorbs all photons, the default photon volume shader behaves like empty space, and the default photon emission shader behaves like a point light source emitting photons uniformly in all directions (that have a chance of contributing illumination — but this is only an optimization).

Photon shaders can use the function *mi_choose_scatter_type* to select which type of reflection or transmission the photon should undergo next. *mi_choose_scatter_type* chooses a scatter type (reflection or transmission, diffuse, glossy, or specular) or absorption. The choice is made with probabilities depending on the scattering coefficients and the transparency. The scattering type with the highest scattering coefficients has the highest probability.

In the following, d denotes diffuse, g denotes glossy, and s denotes specular, and the indices r, g, and b mean red, green, and blue, respectively. Each of the nine scattering coefficients (specular R, G, B, glossy R, G, B, diffuse R, G, B) and the transparency must be in the range [0...1]. Furthermore, the scattering coefficients must satisfy the following conditions:

$$d_r + g_r + s_r \le 1$$
$$d_g + g_g + s_g \le 1$$
$$d_b + g_b + s_b \le 1$$

If these conditions are not met, the coefficients are adjusted so that they are met, and a warning is given (once). The probability for scattering (that is, choosing one of the six types of reflection or transmission) is

$$P = max(d_r + g_r + s_r,\ d_g + g_g + s_g,\ d_b + g_b + s_b).$$

The probability for absorption is

$$1 - P.$$

The probability for diffuse reflection[2.1] is

$$P \cdot (1 - t) \cdot \frac{d_r + d_g + d_b}{d_r + d_g + d_b + g_r + g_g + g_b + s_r + s_g + s_b}$$

while the probability for diffuse transmission[2.1] is

$$P \cdot t \cdot \frac{d_r + d_g + d_b}{d_r + d_g + d_b + g_r + g_g + g_b + s_r + s_g + s_b}.$$

Similar for glossy and specular reflection and transmission. If a certain scattering type is chosen, the three scattering coefficients (r, g, b) for that type of scattering are adjusted following the "Russian roulette" method. Note that glossy and diffuse scattering[2.1] will not be chosen if caustics are being simulated — only specular scattering (or absorption) is possible then.

The connection between the photon tracing and ray tracing phases is the *mi_compute_irradiance* function. It allows material shaders (during image rendering) to get the caustic or global illumination[2.1]color using the photons that were stored in the photon tracing phase. The function *mi_compute_volume_irradiance* is similar, but computes irradiance in a volume using the photons stored in the volume.

This distinction is still valid if ray tracing is disabled and mental ray is reduced to scanline rendering in the second phase. For the purposes of photon tracing, scanline rendering can be considered a "ray tracing emulation" mode that achieves similar effects but never actually traces a ray, at the cost of not being able to control the ray direction. For example, if the `trace off` statement or `-trace off` command-line option is specified, it is still possible to generate a caustic, but the second phase will be unable to compute raytraced reflections and refractions.

```
void mi_photon_light(
    miColor          *energy,
    miState          *state)
```

traces a photon from a light source into the scene. The photon origin is *state* → *org* and the direction is *state* → *dir*. This function should be used only in photon emitting shaders.

```
miBoolean mi_photon_reflection_specular(
    miColor          *energy,
    miState          *state,
    miVector         *direction)
```

traces a specularly reflected photon with *energy* in direction *direction*. This function may be used only in photon shaders.

```
miBoolean mi_photon_reflection_glossy(
    miColor          *energy,
    miState          *state,
    miVector         *direction)
```

[2.1]traces a glossily reflected photon with *energy* in direction *direction*. This function may be used only in photon shaders.

```
miBoolean mi_photon_reflection_diffuse(
    miColor        *energy,
    miState        *state,
    miVector       *direction)
```

[2.1]traces a diffusely reflected photon with *energy* in direction *direction*. This function may be used only in photon shaders.

```
miBoolean mi_photon_transmission_specular(
    miColor        *energy,
    miState        *state,
    miVector       *direction)
```

traces a specularly transmitted photon with *energy* in direction *direction*. This function may be used only in photon shaders.

```
miBoolean mi_photon_transmission_glossy(
    miColor        *energy,
    miState        *state,
    miVector       *direction)
```

[2.1]traces a glossily transmitted photon with *energy* in direction *direction*. This function may be used only in photon shaders.

```
miBoolean mi_photon_transmission_diffuse(
    miColor        *energy,
    miState        *state,
    miVector       *direction)
```

[2.1]traces a diffusely transmitted photon with *energy* in direction *direction*. This function may be used only in photon shaders.

```
miBoolean mi_photon_transparent(
    miColor        *energy,
    miState        *state)
```

traces a specularly transmitted photon with *energy* in the direction indicated by the state (the same direction as the previous direction). This function may be used only in photon shaders.

```
miBoolean mi_photon_volume_scattering(
    miColor        *energy,
    miState        *state,
    miVector       *dir);
```

traces a photon, scattered by a volume, with *energy* in direction *direction*. This function may be used only in photon shaders.

```
void mi_store_photon(
    miColor          *energy,
    miState          *state)
```

mi_store_photon stores a photon with the given *energy* in the photon map at the intersection point given in state *state* $\rightarrow$ *point*). Only photons with non-zero energy are stored. Photons should only be stored at surfaces which have a diffuse component in order to limit the storage costs and reduce the rendering time. This function may be used only in photon shaders.

```
void mi_store_volume_photon(
    miColor          *energy,
    miState          *state)
```

This function is equivalent to the previous, except that it is used to store a photon in a volume instead of on a surface. It is used for volume caustics and volume scattering (such as volumic light beams and clouds).

3.21.5 RC Direction Functions

The functions in this section compute ray or photon directions. In both photon and ray tracing, shaders normally first compute a direction for secondary photons or rays using one of the functions with *_dir* in the name, and then call the corresponding photon or ray tracing function with the resulting direction.

The functions *mi_choose_scatter_type*, *mi_reflection_dir_**, *mi_transmission_dir_**, and *mi_scattering_dir_** can also be used in other contexts than photon tracing, but they are listed in the photon tracing column above because they are most often used for that purpose. However, the glossy direction functions, for example, can just as well be used for ray tracing if the rendering quality setting (contrast and sampling limits) are high enough to avoid noisy images. Using diffuse directions for ray tracing is unlikely to produce acceptable results due to noise.

```
void mi_reflection_dir(
    miVector         *dir,
    miState          *state);
```

Calculate the reflection direction based on the *dir*, *normal*, and *normal_geom* state variables. The returned direction *dir* can be passed to *mi_trace_reflect*. It is returned in internal space.

```
void mi_reflection_dir_specular(
```

```
    miVector          *dir,
    miState           *state);
```

Same as *mi_reflection_dir*: computes the mirror direction. Created for symmetry with the similar functions for glossy and diffuse reflection.

```
void mi_reflection_dir_glossy(
    miVector          *dir,
    miState           *state,
    miScalar          shiny);
```

Choose a direction near the direction of ideal specular reflection (mirror direction). If *shiny* is low (for example 5), a wide distribution of directions results; if *shiny* is high (for example 100), a narrow distribution results.

```
void mi_reflection_dir_anisglossy(
    miVector          *dir,
    miState           *state,
    miVector          *u,
    miVector          *v,
    miScalar          shiny_u,
    miScalar          shiny_v);
```

Like *mi_reflection_dir_glossy*, but with different shinynesses in different directions. The *u* and *v* vectors specify the local surface orientation.

```
void mi_reflection_dir_diffuse(
    miVector          *dir,
    miState           *state)
```

Choose a direction with a distribution according to Lambert's cosine law for diffuse reflection.

```
miBoolean mi_refraction_dir(
    miVector          *dir,
    miState           *state,
    miScalar          ior_in,
    miScalar          ior_out);
```

Calculate the refraction direction in internal space based on the interior and exterior indices of refraction *ior_in* and *ior_out*, and on *dir*, *normal*, and *normal_geom* state variables. The returned direction *dir* can be passed to *mi_trace_refract*. Returns `miFALSE` and leaves **dir* undefined in case of total internal reflection.

```
miBoolean mi_transmission_dir_specular(
    miVector        *dir,
    miState         *state,
    miScalar        ior_in,
    miScalar        ior_out);
```

Same as *mi_refraction_dir*, since specular transmission occurs in the refraction direction. Created for symmetry with the similar functions for glossy and diffuse transmission.

```
miBoolean mi_transmission_dir_glossy(
    miVector        *dir,
    miState         *state,
    miScalar        ior_in,
    miScalar        ior_out,
    miScalar        shiny);
```

Choose a direction near the direction of ideal specular transmission (the refraction direction). If *shiny* is low, a very wide distribution of directions results; if *shiny* is high a narrow distribution results.

```
miBoolean mi_transmission_dir_anisglossy(
    miVector  *dir,
    miState   *state,
    miScalar  ior_in,
    miScalar  ior_out,
    miVector  *u,
    miVector  *v,
    miScalar  shiny_u,
    miScalar  shiny_v);
```

Choose a direction for anisotropic glossy transmission. The u and v vectors specify the local surface orientation.

```
void mi_transmission_dir_diffuse(
    miVector        *dir,
    miState         *state)
```

Choose a direction with a distribution according to Lambert's cosine law for diffuse transmission (also known as "diffuse translucency").

```
void mi_scattering_dir_diffuse(
    miVector        *dir,
    miState         *state)
```

Choose a direction with a uniform probability over the whole sphere. This is useful for volume scattering.

```
void mi_scattering_dir_directional(
    miVector        *dir,
    miState         *state
    miScalar        directionality)
```

Choose a direction with a probability determined by *directionality*. For values between -1 and 0 it models volume backscattering (with -1 being the most directional), for a value of 0 it models diffuse (isotropic) volume scattering, and for values between 0 and 1 it models forward volume scattering.

```
miScalar mi_scattering_pathlength(
    miState  *state,
    miScalar k);
```

Based on probability and exponential falloff, select a path length for a photon in a participating medium[2.1] with density k.

3.21.6 IMG Functions

The IMG module of mental ray provides functions that deal with images. There are functions to read and write image files in various formats, and to access in-core frame buffers such as image textures. First, the functions that access frame buffers are listed. These functions are typically used by texture shaders, which can obtain an image pointer by calling *mi_db_access* with the image tag as an argument. All these functions do nothing or return defaults if the *image* pointer is 0, or if the x or y coordinate is out of bounds. They do not check whether the frame buffer has the correct data type. All these functions are available in all shaders, including displacement, geometry, and output shaders.

```
void mi_img_put_color(
    miImg_image *image,
    miColor     *color,
    int         x,
    int         y)
```

Store the color *color* in the color frame buffer *image* at coordinate x y, after performing desaturation or color clipping, gamma correction, compensating for premultiplication, and dithering. Not all of these steps may be performed, and the behavior is dependent on the options *colorclip*[2.1], *premultiply*, *desaturate*, *gamma*, and *dither* as given on the command line or in the .mi file. This function works with 1, 2, or 4 components per pixel, and with 8, 16, or 32 (float) bits per component. The normal range for the R, G, B, and A color components is $[0, 1]$ inclusive. For 32 bit (float) frame buffers only compensation for premultiplication is done.

```
void mi_img_get_color(
    miImg_image *image,
    miColor     *color,
    int          x,
    int          y)
```

This is the reverse function to *mi_img_put_color*. It returns the color stored in a frame buffer at the specified coordinates. Gamma compensation and premultiplication, if enabled by *mi_img_mode*, are applied in reverse. The returned color may differ from the original color given to *mi_img_put_color* because of color clipping and color quantization.

```
void mi_img_put_scalar (
    miImg_image *image,
    float        scalar,
    int          x,
    int          y)
```

Store the scalar *scalar* in the scalar frame buffer *image* at coordinate x y, after clipping to the range $[0, 1]$. Scalars are stored as 8-bit or 16-bit unsigned values. This function is intended for scalar texture files of type `miIMG_S` or `miIMG_S_16`.

```
void mi_img_get_scalar (
    miImg_image *image,
    float       *scalar,
    int          x,
    int          y)
```

This is the reverse function to *mi_img_put_scalar*. It returns the scalar stored in a frame buffer at the specified coordinates, converted to a scalar in the range $[0, 1]$. If the frame buffer pointer is 0, or if the x or y coordinate is out of bounds, the scalar is set to 0.

```
void mi_img_put_vector (
    miImg_image *image,
    miVector    *vector,
    int          x,
    int          y)
```

Store the X and Y components of the vector *vector* in the vector frame buffer *image* at coordinate x y, after clipping to the range $[-1, 1]$. Vectors are stored as 16-bit signed values. This function is intended for vector texture files of type miIMG_VTA or miIMG_VTS.

```
void mi_img_get_vector (
```

```
    miImg_image *image,
    miVector    *vector,
    int         x,
    int         y)
```

This is the reverse function to *mi_img_put_vector*. It returns the UV vector stored in a frame buffer at the specified coordinates, with coordinates converted to the range $[-1, 1]$. The Z component of the vector is always set to 0. If the frame buffer pointer is 0, or if the x or y coordinate is out of bounds, all components are set to 0.

```
void mi_img_put_depth(
    miImg_image *image,
    float       depth,
    int         x,
    int         y)
```

Store the depth value *depth* in the frame buffer *image* at the coordinates x y. The depth value is not changed in any way. The standard interpretation of the depth is the (positive) Z distance of objects relative to the camera. mental ray uses this function internally to store $-state \rightarrow point.z$ (in camera space) if the depth frame buffer is enabled with an appropriate `output` statement. By convention, the value 0.0 signifies infinite distance.

```
void mi_img_get_depth(
    miImg_image *image,
    float       *depth,
    int         x,
    int         y)
```

Read the depth value to the float pointed to by *depth* from frame buffer *image* at the coordinates x y. If the image pointer is 0, or if the x or y coordinate is out of bounds, return the `MAX_FLT` constant from limits.h.

```
void mi_img_put_normal(
    miImg_image *image,
    miVector    *normal,
    int         x,
    int         y)
```

Store the normal vector *normal* in the frame buffer *image* at the coordinates x y. The normal vector is not changed in any way. This function can also be used for the motion vector frame buffer.

```
void mi_img_get_normal(
```

```
    miImg_image *image,
    miVector    *normal,
    int         x,
    int         y)
```

Read the normal vector *normal* from frame buffer *image* at the coordinates *x y*. If the image pointer is 0, or if the *x* or *y* coordinate is out of bounds, return a null vector. This function can also be used for the motion vector frame buffer.

```
void mi_img_put_label(
    miImg_image *image,
    miUint      label,
    int         x,
    int         y)
```

Store the label value *label* in the label frame buffer *image* at the coordinates *x y*. The label value is not changed in any way.

```
void mi_img_get_label(
    miImg_image *image,
    miUint      *label,
    int         x,
    int         y)
```

Read the label value to the unsigned integer pointed to by *label* from frame buffer *image* at the coordinates *x y*. If the image pointer is 0, or if the *x* or *y* coordinate is out of bounds, return 0.

3.21.7 Math Functions

Math functions include common vector and matrix operations. More specific noise and rendering functions can be found in the next two sections, Noise Functions and Auxiliary Functions.

```
void mi_vector_neg(
    miVector    *r)
```

$\vec{r} := -\vec{r}$

```
void mi_vector_add(
    miVector    *r,
    miVector    *a,
    miVector    *b)
```

$\vec{r} := \vec{a} + \vec{b}$

```
void mi_vector_sub(
    miVector    *r,
    miVector    *a,
    miVector    *b)
```

$\vec{r} := \vec{a} - \vec{b}$

```
void mi_vector_mul(
    miVector    *r,
    miScalar    f)
```

$\vec{r} := \vec{r} \cdot f$

```
void mi_vector_div(
    miVector    *r,
    miScalar    f)
```

$\vec{r} := \vec{r} \cdot \frac{1}{f}$ (If f is zero, leave $\vec{r}$ unchanged.)

```
void mi_vector_prod(
    miVector    *r,
    miVector    *a,
    miVector    *b)
```

$\vec{r} := \vec{a} \times \vec{b}$

```
miScalar mi_vector_dot(
    miVector    *a,
    miVector    *b)
```

$\vec{a} \cdot \vec{b}$

```
miScalar mi_vector_norm(
    miVector    *a)
```

$||\vec{a}||$

```
void mi_vector_normalize(
    miVector    *r)
```

$\vec{r} := \frac{\vec{r}}{||\vec{r}||}$ (If $\vec{r}$ is a null vector, leave $\vec{r}$ unchanged.)

```
void mi_vector_min(
    miVector    *r,
    miVector    *a,
    miVector    *b)
```

$$\vec{r} := \begin{pmatrix} a_x < b_x & ? & a_x & : & b_x \\ a_y < b_y & ? & a_y & : & b_y \\ a_z < b_z & ? & a_z & : & b_z \end{pmatrix}$$

```
void mi_vector_max(
    miVector    *r,
    miVector    *a,
    miVector    *b)
```

$$\vec{r} := \begin{pmatrix} a_x > b_x & ? & a_x & : & b_x \\ a_y > b_y & ? & a_y & : & b_y \\ a_z > b_z & ? & a_z & : & b_z \end{pmatrix}$$

```
miScalar mi_vector_det(
    miVector    *a,
    miVector    *b,
    miVector    *c)
```

$$\begin{vmatrix} a_x & b_x & c_x \\ a_y & b_y & c_y \\ a_z & b_z & c_z \end{vmatrix}$$

```
miScalar mi_vector_dist(
    miVector    *a,
    miVector    *b)
```

$||\vec{a} - \vec{b}||$

```
void mi_matrix_null(
    miMatrix      r)
```

$$R := \begin{pmatrix} 0 & 0 & 0 & 0 \\ 0 & 0 & 0 & 0 \\ 0 & 0 & 0 & 0 \\ 0 & 0 & 0 & 0 \end{pmatrix}$$

```
void mi_matrix_ident(
    miMatrix      r)
```

$$R := \begin{pmatrix} 1 & 0 & 0 & 0 \\ 0 & 1 & 0 & 0 \\ 0 & 0 & 1 & 0 \\ 0 & 0 & 0 & 1 \end{pmatrix}$$

```
miBoolean mi_matrix_isident(
    miMatrix      a)
```

Return `miTRUE` if a is the identity matrix, and `miFALSE` otherwise.

```
void mi_matrix_copy(
    miMatrix      r,
    miMatrix      a)
```

$R := A$

```
miBoolean mi_matrix_invert(
    miMatrix      r,
    miMatrix      a)
```

$R := A^{-1}$ (Returns miFALSE if the matrix cannot be inverted.)

```
void mi_matrix_prod(
    miMatrix      r,
    miMatrix      a,
    miMatrix      b)
```

$R := A \times B$

```
void mi_matrix_rotate(
    miMatrix         a,
    const miScalar   xrot,
    const miScalar   yrot,
    const miScalar   zrot)
```

Create a rotation matrix *a* rotating by *xrot*, then *yrot*, then *zrot*, in radians.

```
void mi_matrix_rotate_axis(
    miMatrix          a,
    miVector const   *v,
    miScalar const    r)
```

This function is similar to the previous, except that the rotation is specified with an axis and an angle. The resulting matrix will rotate a point *r* radians about the axis *v* according to the right-hand rule. *v* must have unit length, otherwise the result is undefined.

All the following transformation functions may be called with identical pointers *r* and *v*. The vector is transformed in-place in this case. If the matrix *m* is a null pointer, no transformation is done and *v* is copied to *r*. If the result of a transformation is a point in homogeneous coordinates with a *w* component that is not equal to 1.0, the result vector's *x*, *y*, and *z* components are divided by *w*. For point transformations, a *w* component of 1.0 is implicitly appended to the *v* vector at the vector-matrix multiplication. For vector transformations the *w* component is implicitly zero. Note the distinction between object and light transformations — both sets deal with object space, but the former uses the current object's object space and the latter uses the current light's object space.

```
float mi_matrix_rot_det(
    miMatrix         a)
```

Return the determinant of the 3×3 rotation part of matrix *a*.

```
void mi_point_transform(
    miVector    *r,
    miVector    *v,
    miMatrix     m)
```

$\vec{r} := \vec{v} \cdot M$

```
void mi_vector_transform(
```

```
    miVector    *r,
    miVector    *v,
    miMatrix     m)
```

$\vec{r} := \vec{v} \cdot M$ Only the upper left 3-by-3 submatrix is used since this is a vector transform. The translation row in the matrix is ignored as w is implicitly assumed to be 0.

```
void mi_vector_transform_T(
    miVector    *r,
    miVector    *v,
    miMatrix     m)
```

$\vec{r} := \vec{v} \cdot M^T$ The transpose of the upper left 3-by-3 submatrix is used for the vector transformation. The w component of v is implicitly assumed to be 0. This function is required for transformation of normals.

```
void mi_point_to_world(
    miState  * const  state,
    miVector * const  r,
    miVector * const  v)
```

Convert internal point v in the state to world space, r.

```
void mi_point_to_camera(
    miState  * const  state,
    miVector * const  r,
    miVector * const  v)
```

Convert internal point v in the state to camera space, r.

```
void mi_point_to_object(
    miState  * const  state,
    miVector * const  r,
    miVector * const  v)
```

Convert internal point v to the object space of the current object (illuminated point), r.

```
void mi_point_to_light(
    miState  * const  state,
    miVector * const  r,
    miVector * const  v)
```

[2.1]Convert internal point v in the state to the object space of the current light. This function (and the other five light transformation functions described below) are similar to the corresponding object transformation functions except that they use *state* $\rightarrow$ *light_instance* instead of *state* $\rightarrow$ *instance* to locate the correct object space transformation matrices.

```
void mi_point_to_raster(
    miState  * const  state,
    miVector * const  r,
    miVector * const  v)
```

Convert internal point v in the state to 2D raster space, r. Raster space dimension is defined by the camera resolution.

```
void mi_point_from_world(
    miState  * const  state,
    miVector * const  r,
    miVector * const  v)
```

Convert point v in world space to internal space, r.

```
void mi_point_from_camera(
    miState  * const  state,
    miVector * const  r,
    miVector * const  v)
```

Convert point in camera space v to internal space, r.

```
void mi_point_from_object(
    miState  * const  state,
    miVector * const  r,
    miVector * const  v)
```

Convert point v in the object space of the current object (illuminated point) to internal space, r.

```
void mi_point_from_light(
    miState  * const  state,
    miVector * const  r,
    miVector * const  v)
```

[2.1]Convert point v in the object space of the current light as found in *state* $\rightarrow$ *light_instance* to internal space, r.

```
void mi_vector_to_world(
    miState  * const  state,
    miVector * const  r,
    miVector * const  v)
```

Convert internal vector v in the state to world space, r. Vector transformations work like point transformations, except that the translation row of the transformation matrix is ignored. The resulting vector is not renormalized. Vector transformations transform normals correctly only if there is no scaling. For correct transformation of normals use the normal transformations described below.

```
void mi_vector_to_camera(
    miState  * const  state,
    miVector * const  r,
    miVector * const  v)
```

Convert internal vector v in the state to camera space, r.

```
void mi_vector_to_object(
    miState  * const  state,
    miVector * const  r,
    miVector * const  v)
```

Convert internal vector v to the object space of the current object (illuminated point), r.

```
void mi_vector_to_light(
    miState  * const  state,
    miVector * const  r,
    miVector * const  v)
```

[2.1]Convert internal vector v in the state to object space of the current light as found in $state \rightarrow light\_instance$, r.

```
void mi_vector_from_world(
    miState  * const  state,
    miVector * const  r,
    miVector * const  v)
```

Convert vector v in world space to internal space, r.

```
void mi_vector_from_camera(
```

```
    miState  * const  state,
    miVector * const  r,
    miVector * const  v)
```

Convert vector in camera space v to internal space, r.

```
void mi_vector_from_object(
    miState  * const  state,
    miVector * const  r,
    miVector * const  v)
```

Convert vector v in the object space of the current object (illuminated point) to internal space, r.

```
void mi_vector_from_light(
    miState  * const  state,
    miVector * const  r,
    miVector * const  v)
```

[2.1]Convert vector v in object space of the current light as found in $state \rightarrow light\_instance$ to internal space, r.

```
void mi_normal_to_world(
    miState  * const  state,
    miVector * const  r,
    miVector * const  v)
```

Convert internal normal v in the state to world space, r. Normal transformations work like vector transformations, except that the transpose of the inverse transformation matrix used. The resulting vector is not renormalized. This ensures that if a vector and a normal are orthogonal in one coordinate system they remain orthogonal after they have been transformed to a different coordinate system. This holds for arbitrary, not necessarily orthogonal transformations. The vector transformations described above transform normals correctly only if there is no scaling.

```
void mi_normal_to_camera(
    miState  * const  state,
    miVector * const  r,
    miVector * const  v)
```

Convert internal normal v in the state to camera space, r.

```
void mi_normal_to_object(
```

```
    miState  * const  state,
    miVector * const  r,
    miVector * const  v)
```

Convert internal normal v to the object space of the current object (illuminated point), r.

```
void mi_normal_to_light(
    miState  * const  state,
    miVector * const  r,
    miVector * const  v)
```

2.1Convert internal normal v in the state to object space of the current light as found in *state* → *light_instance*, r.

```
void mi_normal_from_world(
    miState  * const  state,
    miVector * const  r,
    miVector * const  v)
```

Convert normal v in world space to internal space, r.

```
void mi_normal_from_camera(
    miState  * const  state,
    miVector * const  r,
    miVector * const  v)
```

Convert normal in camera space v to internal space, r.

```
void mi_normal_from_object(
    miState  * const  state,
    miVector * const  r,
    miVector * const  v)
```

Convert normal v in the object space of the current object (illuminated point) to internal space, r.

```
void mi_normal_from_light(
    miState  * const  state,
    miVector * const  r,
    miVector * const  v)
```

2.1Convert normal v in object space of the current light as found in *state* → *light_instance* to internal space, r.

3.21.8 Noise Functions

The functions in this group provide pseudo-random numbers, quasi-Monte Carlo numbers (using low-discrepancy sequences that converge faster than pseudo-random numbers), and deterministic Perlin noise.

```
miScalar mi_random(void)
```

Return a random number in the range [0, 1). This is similar to *drand48* in the standard Unix libraries, but it is available on all platforms including Windows NT, which does not support *drand48*.

```
miScalar mi_srandom(
    long            seed)
```

Begin a new random number sequence for *mi_random*. This is equivalent to the standard Unix library function *srand48*.

```
miScalar mi_erandom(
    unsigned short  seed[3])
```

Return a random number in the range [0, 1), based on the given *seed*. This allows shaders to create private random number generators by initializing a private *seed* array to some arbitrary but constant values, and passing it to *mi_erandom* without the chance of other functions or threads disturbing the sequence by "stealing" random numbers (assuming they do not have access to the private seed). This is equivalent to the standard Unix library function *erand48*.

```
miScalar mi_par_random(
    miState         *state)
```

Return a parallel-safe random number in the range [0, 1). Parallel-safe random numbers can be used in parallel rendering to produce consistent results that do not change when the number of machines or threads changes, or when the execution order changes. All shaders that use this function share the same internal seed value. This function should not be used in geometry shaders, displacement shaders, photon shaders, output shaders, or *_init* functions of shaders because the initial seed of the random number sequence is undefined in these cases.

```
miScalar mi_spline(
    miScalar         t,
    const int        n,
    miScalar * const ctl)
```

This function calculates a one-dimensional cardinal spline at location *t*. The *t* parameter must be in the range 0 ... 1. The spline is defined by *n* control points specified in the array *ctl*. There must be at least two control points. To calculate multi-dimensional splines, this function must be called once for each dimension. For example, *spline* can be used three times to interpolate colors smoothly.

```
miScalar mi_noise_1d(
    const miScalar   p)
```

Return a one-dimensional coherent noise function of *p*. All six noise functions compute a modified Perlin noise function from the given one, two, or three dimension parameters such that the noise changes gradually with changing parameters. The modification of the classical algorithm avoids large-scale periodical behavior at lattice points, such that the noise is smooth on all levels. (This makes the algorithm perform slower than classical Perlin noise.) The returned values are in the range 0 ... 1, with a bell-shaped distribution centered at 0.5 and falling off to both sides. This means that 0.5 is returned most often, and values of less than 0.0 and more than 1.0 are never returned. See [Perlin 85].

```
miScalar mi_noise_2d(
    const miScalar   u,
    const miScalar   v)
```

Return a two-dimensional noise function of *u*, *v*.

```
miScalar mi_noise_3d(
    miVector * const p)
```

Return a three-dimensional noise function of the vector *p*. This is probably the most useful noise function; a simple procedural texture shader can be written that converts a copy of the *state→point* vector to object space, passes it to *mi_noise_3d*, and assigns the returned value to the red, green, and blue components of the result color. The average feature size of the texture will be approximately one unit in space.

```
miScalar mi_noise_1d_grad(
    const miScalar   p,
    miScalar * const g)
```

Return a one-dimensional noise function of *p*. The gradient of the computed texture at the location *p* is assigned to *g. Gradients are not normalized.

```
miScalar mi_noise_2d_grad(
```

```
    const miScalar    u,
    const miScalar    v,
    miScalar * const gu,
    miScalar * const gv)
```

Return a two-dimensional noise function of u, v. The gradient is assigned to $*gu$ and $*gv$.

```
miScalar mi_noise_3d_grad(
    miVector * const p,
    miVector * const g)
```

Return a three-dimensional noise function of the vector p. The gradient is assigned to the vector g.

```
miScalar mi_unoise_1d()
miScalar mi_unoise_2d()
miScalar mi_unoise_3d()
miScalar mi_unoise_1d_grad()
miScalar mi_unoise_2d_grad()
miScalar mi_unoise_3d_grad()
```

These functions are similar to the regular noise functions, except that the returned distribution is uniform. All returned values are roughly equally likely.

3.21.9 Auxiliary Functions

The following functions are provided for support of shaders, to simplify common mathematical operations required in shaders:

```
miScalar mi_fresnel(
    miScalar        ior_in,
    miScalar        ior_out,
    miScalar        factor1,
    miScalar        factor2);
```

Compute the reflected intensity according to Fresnel:

$$\frac{1}{2}\left(\frac{i_{in}\cdot f_2 - i_{out}\cdot f_1}{i_{in}\cdot f_2 + i_{out}\cdot f_1}\right)^2 + \left(\frac{i_{in}\cdot f_1 - i_{out}\cdot f_2}{i_{in}\cdot f_1 + i_{out}\cdot f_2}\right)^2$$

```
miScalar mi_fresnel_reflection(
    miState         *state,
    miScalar        ior_in,
    miScalar        ior_out);
```

Call *mi_fresnel* with parameters appropriate for the given indices of refraction *ior_in* and *ior_out*, and for the *dot_nd* state variable.

```
miScalar mi_phong_specular(
    miScalar        spec_exp,
    miState         *state,
    miVector        *dir);
```

Calculate the Phong factor based on the direction of illumination *dir*, the specular exponent *spec_exp*, and the state variables *normal* and *dir*. The direction must be given in internal space.

```
void mi_fresnel_specular(
    miScalar        *ns,
    miScalar        *ks,
    miScalar        spec_exp,
    miState         *state,
    miVector        *dir,
    miScalar        ior_in,
    miScalar        iot_out);
```

Calculate the specular factor *ns* based on the illumination direction *dir*, the specular exponent *spec_exp*, the inside and outside indices of refraction *ior_in* and *ior_out*, and the state variables *normal* and *dir*. *ks* is the value returned by *mi_fresnel*, which is called by *mi_fresnel_specular*. The direction must be given in internal space.

```
miBoolean mi_cooktorr_specular(
    miColor         *result,
    miVector        *dir_in,
    miVector        *dir_out,
    miVector        *normal,
    miScalar        roughness,
    miColor         *ior);
```

Calculate the specular color *result* according to the Cook-Torrance reflection model for incident direction *dir_in*, reflection direction *dir_out* at a surface with normal *normal*. The *roughness* is the average slope of surface microfacets. *ior* is the relative index of refraction for three wavelengths (ior_out/ior_in for red, green, and blue). All indices must be 1.0 or greater; if not they are clamped to 1.0. See [Foley 90].

```
miScalar mi_blinn_specular(
    miVector        *dir_in,
    miVector        *dir_out,
    miVector        *normal,
    miScalar        roughness,
    miScalar        ior);
```

Like *mi_cooktorr_specular*, but only for one wavelength. Only one index of refraction *ior* is needed, and the result is a scalar. If *ior* is less than 1.0, it is clamped to 1.0. See [Foley 90].

```
miScalar mi_blong_specular(
    miVector        *dir_in,
    miVector        *dir_out,
    miVector        *normal,
    miScalar        roughness,
    miScalar        ior);
```

This is similar to *mi_blinn_specular*, but implements a hybrid of Blinn and Phong shading instead of true Blinn shading. It is included separately to support the Softimage Blinn shading model.

```
miScalar mi_ward_glossy(
    miVector        *dir_in,
    miVector        *dir_out,
    miVector        *normal,
    miScalar        shiny);
```

Calculate the value of the isotropic Ward glossy reflection model for incident direction *dir_in*, reflection direction *dir_out* at a surface with normal *normal* and shinyness *shiny*. *dir_in* should point towards the point, while *dir_out* and *normal* should point away from the point. Shiny should be low (for example 5) for wide glossy reflection, and high (for example 100) for narrow glossy (nearly specular) reflection.

```
miScalar mi_ward_anisglossy(
    miVector        *dir_in,
    miVector        *dir_out,
    miVector        *normal,
    miVector        *u,
    miVector        *v,
    miScalar        shiny_u,
    miScalar        shiny_v);
```

Calculate the value of the anisotropic Ward glossy reflection model for incident direction *dir_in*, reflection direction *dir_out*, surface normal *normal*, and the anisotropic orientation determined by two perpendicular vectors *u* and *v*. The shinyness in the u and v direction is *shiny_u* and *shiny_v*, respectively. *dir_in* should point towards the point, while *dir_out* and *normal* should point away from the point. *u* and *v* should be perpendicular, and also perpendicular to the normal.

```
miScalar mi_schlick_scatter(
    miVector        *dir_in,
    miVector        *dir_out,
    miScalar        directionality);
```

Calculate the value of the Schlick volume scattering model for incident direction *dir_in*, scattering direction *dir_out*, and directionality *directionality*. *dir_in* should point towards the point, while *dir_out* should point away from the point. *directionality* must be between -1 and 1. For values between -1 and 0 it models backscattering (with -1 being the most directional), for a value of 0 it models diffuse (isotropic) scattering, and for values between 0 and 1 it models forward scattering.

```
miRay_type mi_choose_scatter_type(
    miState         *state,
    float           transp,
    miColor         *diffuse,
    miColor         *glossy,
    miColor         *specular)
```

In photon shaders it is generally important (although not required) to generate only one photon per photon interaction. To make this happen this function can be used to select one of several new photon types. The function returns: `miPHOTON_REFLECT_SPECULAR`, `miPHOTON_REFLECT_GLOSSY`, `miPHOTON_REFLECT_DIFFUSE`, `miPHOTON_TRANSMIT_SPECULAR`, `miPHOTON_TRANSMIT_GLOSSY`, `miPHOTON_TRANSMIT_DIFFUSE` or `miPHOTON_ABSORBED`. The return type is based on incoming coefficients and chosen in such a way that the most important component is chosen most often. Notice that for caustic simulations the diffuse and glossy components are ignored. Also note that the sum of the diffuse, glossy and specular coefficients should be less than or equal to one within each of the red, green, and blue color bands, and that *mi_choose_scatter_type* modifies the input coefficients and scales them correctly based on the probability of generating a photon of that type. To obtain a correct result the shader must use the modified coefficients in the computations performed after *mi_choose_scatter_type* has been used. The probability for reflection is $1 - transp$. See page 228 for a more detailed explanation.

```
int mi_choose_lobe(
    miState         *state,
    miScalar        r);
```

In a two-lobed volume scattering model, choose lobe 1 or 2 based on the probability *r* of the first lobe.

```
miBoolean mi_lookup_color_texture(
    miColor          *color,
    miState          *state,
    miTag            tag,
    miVector         *coord)
```

tag is assumed to be a texture as taken from a color texture parameter of a shader. This function checks whether the tag refers to a shader (procedural texture) or an image, depending on which type of `color texture` statement was used in the .mi file. If *tag* is a shader, *coord* is stored in *state→tex*, the referenced texture shader is called, and its return value is returned. If *tag* is an image, *coord* is brought into the range (0..1, 0..1) by removing the integer part, the image is looked up at the resulting 2D coordinate, and `miTRUE` is returned. If the texture is marked with the `filter` keyword, multi-level pyramid filtering is performed, a procedure related to classical mip-mapping. In both cases, the color resulting from the lookup is stored in **color*.

```
typedef struct {
    miScalar         eccmax;
    miScalar         max_minor;
    miScalar         circle_radius;
    miBoolean        bilinear;
    miScalar         spare[10];
} miTexfilter;

miBoolean mi_lookup_filter_color_texture(
    miColor          *color,
    miState          *state,
    miTag            tag,
    miTexfilter      *paras,
    miMatrix         ST)
```

This function provides higher quality filtering than the multi-level pyramid filtering of *mi_lookup_color_texture* described above using a transformation *ST* which transforms the coordinate system centered in the current raster position in screen space to texture space. The functions *mi_texture_filter_project* and *mi_texture_filter_transform* are provided for helping to calculate this transformation matrix.

This function expects that *tag* does not refer to a texture shader, that is, it works only on texture images. It will return `miFALSE` when used with incorrect parameters or if a projection failed.

In the filtering algorithm a circle around the current raster position is projected to an ellipse in texture space, and returns the average color of all texture pixels inside the ellipse. If the texture defined by *tag* is a pyramid texture, multi-level lookup of the texture pixels is performed to speed up the filtering. In the algorithm the level calculation is based on the minor radius of the ellipse.

The filtering can be controlled by choosing different values in *paras*. If *paras* is a null, default values for medium filter quality are used.

The *eccmax* field in `miTexfilter` specifies the maximum allowed eccentricity of the ellipse. The eccentricity is defined by the ratio of the major and minor radius. Under severe projective distortion the ellipse can have a very large eccentricity and too many texture pixels would be covered by the elliptical area, resulting in long rendering times. In order to limit the filtering time in these cases, the eccentricity threshold can be specified. If the eccentricity is greater than this value, the minor radius of the ellipse is made larger allowing for a potentially higher level in the texture image pyramid since the level calculation is based on the minor radius.

In this calculation a level is selected where the minor radius of the ellipse has a maximum length of *max_minor* texture pixels. In each successive level in the image pyramid the radius is divided by two, and there are fewer pixels inside the elliptical area. The useful range for *eccmax* is approximately 10 to 30, higher values will result in better antialiasing. For *max_minor* the range should be 3 to 8. Higher values result in better antialiasing.

The size of the projected screen-space circle can be modified with the *circle_radius* parameter. Larger values will result in more blurring since the elliptical area is also made larger. Smaller values will increase the aliasing. The useful range for this field is 0.4 to 1.0.

When a magnification area is detected, that is, an area in which the pixels are not compressed (the elliptical area is smaller than a texture pixel), bilinear texture pixel interpolation can be switched on by setting the *bilinear* field to `miTRUE`, and resulting in a more blurry image.

See page 177 for an example.

```
miBoolean mi_lookup_scalar_texture(
    miScalar        *scalar,
    miState         *state,
    miTag           tag,
    miVector        *coord)
```

This function is equivalent to *mi_lookup_color_texture*, except that *tag* is assumed to refer to a scalar texture shader or scalar image, as defined in the .mi file with a `scalar texture` statement, and a scalar is looked up returned in **scalar*.

```
miBoolean mi_lookup_vector_texture(
    miVector        *vector,
    miState         *state,
    miTag           tag,
    miVector        *coord)
```

This function is also equivalent to *mi_lookup_color_texture*, except that *tag* is assumed to refer to a vector texture shader or vector image, as defined in the .mi file with a `vector texture` statement, and a vector is looked up returned in **vector*.

```
miBoolean mi_texture_filter_project(
```

```
        miVector          p[3],
        miVector          t[3],
        miState *const    state,
        miScalar          disc_r,
        miUint            space)
```

This function helps in calculating the screen to texture space transformation matrix required by *mi_lookup_filter_color_texture*. It projects three points including the current raster position onto the current intersection primitive (state→pri) plane and calculates the texture coordinates in the intersections. If state→pri is null, or if the projection fails, `miFALSE` is returned.

This function assumes that the current intersected object has a texture space associated and uses *space* as an index into the texture space. The three screen space points are returned in *p*, the corresponding two dimensional texture space points are put into *t*. The first point in the array is always the central raster position (0,0), the others are inside a disc with radius of *disc_r* from this central position. Note that the points are relative to the central position, absolute screen space coordinates are not used. The value of *disc_r* should be set to 0.5 in most cases, since the full pixel is projected to texture space. However, when there are highly curved objects in the scene, a smaller value can effectively remove projection problems where the projected points are far outside the hit triangle primitive. In texture filtering example an example is given using this function.

```
    miBoolean mi_texture_filter_transform(
        miMatrix          ST,
        miVector          p[3],
        miVector          t[3])
```

This function helps in calculating the screen to texture space transformation matrix required by *mi_lookup_filter_color_texture*. The three two dimensional screen space points in *p* and the corresponding three two dimensional texture space points form a linear equation which is solved for the transformation matrix. See page 177 for an example. This function returns `miFALSE` if the linear equation mentioned above has no solution.

```
    void mi_tri_vectors(
        miState           *state,
        int               which,
        int               ntex,
        miVector          **a,
        miVector          **b,
        miVector          **c)
```

All the information in the state pertains to the interpolated intersection point in a triangle. This function can be used to obtain information about the uninterpolated triangle vertices. Together with the barycentric coordinates in the state, parameters retrieved with *mi_tri_vectors* may be interpolated differently by the shader. The *which* argument is a character that controls which triple of vectors is to be retrieved:

which	vector
'p'	the points in space
'n'	the normal vectors
'm'	the motion vectors
't'	the texture coordinates of texture space *ntex*
'u'	the U bump basis vectors
'v'	the V bump basis vectors
'U'	the first surface derivative in U ($d\vec{P}du$)
'V'	the first surface derivative in U ($d\vec{P}dv$)
'X'	the second surface derivative $d^2\vec{P}du^2$
'Y'	the second surface derivative $d^2\vec{P}dv^2$
'Z'	the second surface derivative $d^2\vec{P}dudv$
'*'	the user vectors

A pointer to the vectors is stored in $*a$, $*b$, and $*c$. The shader may not modify these vectors. They are stored in the space used when the scene was created (either object space or camera space depending on *state* → *options* → *render_space*); the original data is accessed without implicit transformation to internal space. If the requested triple is not available, `miFALSE` is returned. This function relies on *state* → *pri*; it only works if the shader has not modified this variable, as some ray-marching volume shaders do.

```
miBoolean mi_query(
    const miQ_type  query,
    miState *const  state,
    miTag           tag,
    void * const    result,
    ...)
```

Return various pieces of information about the current state of mental ray. *query* is the request code specifying what piece of information to query; *state* is the shader state, *tag* is the tag of the DB element to query, if any, and *result* is a pointer to the variable to store the results in. Some queries do not require a tag; in this case `miNULLTAG` must be passed as *tag*. Some queries require extra arguments in addition to the four standard arguments. *mi_query* returns `miFALSE` if the queried value is not available or an unknown type code is used.

The following *query* codes are available:

query code	*state*	*tag*	*result*	*purpose*
`miQ_VERSION`	○	○	char *	mental ray version string
`miQ_DATE`	○	○	char *	mental ray compilation date
`miQ_NUM_GLOBAL_LIGHTS`	○	○	int	number of global lights
`miQ_GLOBAL_LIGHTS`	○	○	miTag *	array with global light tags
`miQ_NUM_TEXTURES`	●	○	int *	# of textures in state->tex_list
`miQ_GEO_LABEL`	○	○	miUint	translator-defined triangle label
`miQ_GEO_DATA`	○	○	miTag	user data block of current object

(continued on next page)

(continued from previous page) query code	state	tag	result	purpose
miQ_PRI_BBOX_MIN	•	○	miVector	bounding box of intersected primitive
miQ_PRI_BBOX_MAX	•	○	miVector	bounding box of intersected primitive
miQ_TILE_PIXELS	•	○	int[4]	lower left and upper right tile pixel coord
miQ_TILE_SAMPLES	•	○	int[4]	same but including filter source margin
miQ_INST_FUNCTION	○	•	miTag	optional procedural transformation
miQ_INST_GLOBAL_TO_LOCAL	○	•	miMatrix *	instance transformation
miQ_INST_LOCAL_TO_GLOBAL	○	•	miMatrix *	inverse instance transformation
miQ_INST_IDENTITY	○	•	miBoolean	miTRUE if identity transformation
miQ_INST_ITEM	○	•	miTag	instanced scene element
miQ_INST_PARENT	○	•	miTag	leaf instance parent (0 otherwise)
miQ_INST_HIDE	○	•	miBoolean	instance is inactive
miQ_INST_VISIBLE	○	•	miUint	visible to primary rays
miQ_INST_TRACE	○	•	miUint	visible to secondary rays
miQ_INST_SHADOW	○	•	miUint	invisible to shadow rays
miQ_INST_CAUSTIC	○	•	miUint	bitmap: 1=enable casting, 2=enable receiving, 3=disable casting, 4=disable receiving
miQ_INST_DECL	○	•	miTag	inherited parameter declaration
miQ_INST_PARAM_SIZE	○	•	int	inherited parameter size
miQ_INST_PARAM	○	•	void *	inherited parameters
miQ_INST_MATERIAL	○	•	miTag	inherited material
miQ_INST_LABEL	○	•	miUint	translator-defined instance label
miQ_INST_DATA	○	•	miTag	user data block
miQ_TRANS_INTERNAL_TO_WORLD	•	○	miMatrix *	internal to world space transformation
miQ_TRANS_INTERNAL_TO_CAMERA	•	○	miMatrix *	internal to camera space transformation
miQ_TRANS_INTERNAL_TO_OBJECT	•	○	miMatrix *	internal to object space transformation
miQ_TRANS_WORLD_TO_INTERNAL	•	○	miMatrix *	world to internal space transformation
miQ_TRANS_CAMERA_TO_INTERNAL	•	○	miMatrix *	camera to internal space transformation
miQ_TRANS_OBJECT_TO_INTERNAL	•	○	miMatrix *	object to internal space transformation
miQ_TRANS_WORLD_TO_CAMERA	•	○	miMatrix *	world to camera space transformation
miQ_TRANS_WORLD_TO_OBJECT	•	○	miMatrix *	internal to world space transformation
miQ_TRANS_CAMERA_TO_WORLD	•	○	miMatrix *	camera to world space transformation
miQ_TRANS_OBJECT_TO_WORLD	•	○	miMatrix *	object to world space transformation
miQ_GROUP_MERGE_GROUP	○	•	miBoolean	miTRUE if merged or connected
miQ_GROUP_NKIDS	○	•	int	number of child instances
miQ_GROUP_KID	○	•	miTag	*n*th child (*n* is fifth argument)
miQ_GROUP_LABEL	○	•	miUint	translator-defined group label
miQ_GROUP_DATA	○	•	miTag	user data block
miQ_OBJ_TYPE	○	•	int	0=polygonal, 1=surfaces

(continued on next page)

(continued from previous page) query code	state	tag	result	purpose
miQ_OBJ_VISIBLE	○	•	miBoolean	visible to primary rays
miQ_OBJ_TRACE	○	•	miBoolean	visible to secondary rays
miQ_OBJ_SHADOW	○	•	miBoolean	invisible to shadow rays
miQ_OBJ_VIEW_DEPENDENT	○	•	miBoolean	contains view-dependent surfaces
miQ_OBJ_CAUSTIC	○	•	miUint	0=none, 1=casts, 2=receives, 3=both
miQ_OBJ_LABEL	○	•	miUint	translator-defined object label
miQ_OBJ_DATA	○	•	miTag	user data block
miQ_LIGHT_TYPE	○	•	int	0=point, 1=directional, 2=spot
miQ_LIGHT_AREA	○	•	int	0=none, 1=rectangle, 2=disc, 3=sphere
miQ_LIGHT_EXPONENT	○	•	miScalar	distance falloff, n in $\frac{1}{r^n}$
miQ_LIGHT_CAUSTIC_PHOTONS	○	•	int	number of caustic photons
miQ_LIGHT_GLOBAL_PHOTONS	○	•	miColor	number of globillum photons
miQ_LIGHT_ENERGY	○	•	miTag	energy for caustics and globillum
miQ_LIGHT_SHADER	○	•	miTag	tag of light shader
miQ_LIGHT_EMITTER	○	•	miVector	tag of light photon emitter shader
miQ_LIGHT_ORIGIN	○	•	miVector	light position
miQ_LIGHT_DIRECTION	○	•	miVector	light direction
miQ_LIGHT_AREA_R_EDGE_U	○	•	miVector	U size of rectangular area light
miQ_LIGHT_AREA_R_EDGE_V	○	•	miVector	V size of rectangular area light
miQ_LIGHT_AREA_D_NORMAL	○	•	miVector	normal vector of disc area light
miQ_LIGHT_AREA_D_RADIUS	○	•	miScalar	radius of disc area light
miQ_LIGHT_AREA_S_RADIUS	○	•	miScalar	radius of spherical area light
miQ_LIGHT_AREA_C_RADIUS	○	•	miScalar	radius of cylinder area light
miQ_LIGHT_AREA_C_AXIS	○	•	miVector	axis of cylinder area light
miQ_LIGHT_AREA_SAMPLES_U	○	•	int	number of samples in U direction
miQ_LIGHT_AREA_SAMPLES_V	○	•	int	number of samples in V direction
miQ_LIGHT_SPREAD	○	•	miScalar	outer cone angle of spot light
miQ_LIGHT_USE_SHADOWMAP	○	•	miBoolean	light has a shadow map
miQ_LIGHT_LABEL	○	•	int	light label
miQ_LIGHT_DATA	○	•	miTag	user data block
miQ_MTL_OPAQUE	○	•	miBoolean	material is opaque to shadow rays
miQ_MTL_SHADER	○	•	miTag	material shader
miQ_MTL_DISPLACE	○	•	miTag	displacement shader
miQ_MTL_SHADOW	○	•	miTag	shadow shader
miQ_MTL_VOLUME	○	•	miTag	volume shader
miQ_MTL_ENVIRONMENT	○	•	miTag	environment shader
miQ_MTL_CONTOUR	○	•	miTag	contour shader
miQ_MTL_PHOTON	○	•	miTag	photon shader
miQ_MTL_PHOTONVOL	○	•	miTag	photon volume shader
miQ_FUNC_USERPTR	○	•	void *	user pointer in shader instance

(continued on next page)

(continued from previous page) query code	state	tag	result	purpose
miQ_FUNC_LOCK	○	•	miLock *	local shader instance lock
miQ_FUNC_TYPE	○	•	int	0=C/C++, 1=phen., 2=output file
miQ_FUNC_DECL	○	•	miTag	tag of shader declaration
miQ_FUNC_NEXT	○	•	miTag	next shader in shader list
miQ_FUNC_INDIRECT	○	•	miTag	take params from this shader
miQ_FUNC_PARAM_SIZE	○	•	int	size of shader parameters in bytes
miQ_FUNC_RESULT_SIZE	○	•	int	shader result size in bytes
miQ_FUNC_PARAM	○	•	void *	shader parameters
miQ_FUNC_*	•	○	*see above*	same for *state → shader*
miQ_DECL_LOCK	○	•	miLock *	shared by all shader instances
miQ_DECL_TYPE	○	•	int	*miTYPE_** result type
miQ_DECL_RESULT_SIZE	○	•	int	result size, 4 unless struct
miQ_DECL_NAME	○	•	char *	shader name
miQ_DECL_PARAM	○	•	char *	ascii-encoded parameter declaration
miQ_DECL_VERSION	○	•	int	shader declaration version
miQ_DECL_*	•	○	*see above*	same for *state → shader*
miQ_IMAGE_WIDTH	○	•	int	width of image in pixels
miQ_IMAGE_HEIGHT	○	•	int	height of image in pixels
miQ_IMAGE_BITS	○	•	int	num of bits per component (8,16,32)
miQ_IMAGE_COMP	○	•	int	num of components (1,2,3,4)
miQ_IMAGE_FILTER	○	•	miBoolean	image allows filtering
miQ_IMAGE_DESATURATE	○	○	miBoolean	color frame buffer desaturation mode
miQ_IMAGE_DITHER	○	○	miBoolean	color frame buffer dithering mode
miQ_IMAGE_NOPREMULT	○	○	miBoolean	color frame buffer premultiplication mode
miQ_IMAGE_GAMMA	○	○	double	color frame buffer gamma factor
miQ_DATA_PARAM	○	•	char *	user data contents
miQ_DATA_DECL	○	•	miTag	user data declaration if any, or 0
miQ_DATA_NEXT	○	•	miTag	next user data block in chain, or 0
miQ_DATA_LABEL	○	•	miUint	translator-defined user data label
miQ_DATA_PARAM_SIZE	○	•	int	size of user data block in bytes
miQ_DATA_NEEDSWAP	○	•	miBoolean	requires byte-swapping by shader

The "○" symbol in the *state* column indicates that the state is not used. The "○" symbol in the *tag* column means that `miNULLTAG` must be passed. Some queries can specify a state instead of a tag. Their query codes are indicated with a *, which stands for any of the preceding codes whose names begin with the same prefix; in this case *mi_query* will take the current shader (*state → shader*) instead of an arbitrary tag. This is slightly faster than passing a tag.

The *result* type in the table indicates the type of the variable that *mi_query* accepts a pointer to: to obtain an integer result from *mi_query* (the table lists an "int"), a pointer to an integer must be passed as the fourth argument ("int *"). For *mi_query*, "function" is synonymous with "shader".

The result of the miQ_INST_VISIBLE, miQ_INST_SHADOW, miQ_INST_TRACE, and miQ_INST_CAUSTIC queries depend on whether a scene DAG or leaf instance tag is passed. A scene DAG instance contains the flags specified by the scene description language when the instance was created. A leaf instance contains the effective instance flags for rendering, that is, with instance inheritance and object flags taken into account. The miQ_INST_VISIBLE etc. modes should be used instead of the miQ_OBJ_VISIBLE etc. modes because they return the same modes that mental ray uses when rendering.

The result vectors of the miQ_LIGHT_ORIGIN and miQ_LIGHT_DIRECTION queries are defined in internal space if the light instance tag is passed, otherwise the vectors are defined in local space.

The miQ_TILE_* codes are supported by mental ray 2.1.34.107 or later. They describe the location and size of the currently rendered image tile. The returned values are in the order *xlow xhigh ylow yhigh*. The sampled area may be larger than the tile due to filtering and jittering.

The query codes miQ_NUM_TEXTURES and miQ_GEO_LABEL may only be used if *state* → *pri* has not been modified by the shader or calling shader. Ray-marching volume shaders sometimes clear this state variable. Both are not supported in displacement shaders. miQ_GEO_LABEL also returns miFALSE if the object is not marked *tagged* and no polygon/surface labels exist.

Note that a return type of miMatrix * means that the address of a pointer must be passed, not the address of a matrix. This reduces the number of bytes that *mi_query* has to copy from 64 (sixteen floats) to only four (or eight, on some CPU architectures).

```
miBoolean mi_fb_put(
    miState          *state,
    int              fb,
    void             *data)
```

[2.1]Store *data* into the sample so that it gets filtered and stored in user frame buffer *fb* later. The type of the data to copy from **data* is determined by the frame buffer type as defined in the options block. The frame buffer number *fb* must be in the range 0...7. If this frame buffer was not defined, this function has no effect and returns miFALSE. The data is stored in the current sample (i.e., the current location for which the primary ray was cast), and is filtered to create frame buffer pixels after all samples in the region have been taken. There is no way to store user frame buffer data in arbitrary locations with this function. It should be called for all samples and all defined user frame buffers to avoid leaving holes; if user frame buffer data is left undefined in a sample because *mi_fb_put* was not called, the data defaults to zero and is filtered as such. Output shaders may not use this function because there is no notion of "samples" during output shading; instead, they must use the standard *mi_img_put_** functions with an offset of miRC_IMAGE_USER + *fb*. Shaders may get the data type of a frame buffer *n* by inspecting *state* → *options* → *image_types*[*n*].

```
miBoolean mi_fb_get(
    miState          *state,
    int              fb,
    void             *data)
```

[2.1]Retrieve *data* from user frame buffer *fb*. The type of the data copied to **data* is determined by the frame buffer type as defined in the options block. It will never be larger than 16 bytes (the size of a `miColor`). The frame buffer number *fb* must be in the range 0...7. If this frame buffer was not defined, this function returns `miFALSE`, and no data is stored. This function is intended to let shaders retrieve data that may have been stored by shaders called in later ray generations, but like *mi_fb_put* it is limited to the current sample. Again, output shaders may not use this function because there is no notion of "samples" during output shading; instead, they must use the standard *mi_img_get_** functions with an offset of `miRC_IMAGE_USER + ` *fb*.

```
miBoolean mi_geoshader_add_result(
    miTag           *result,
    const miTag     item)
```

This function should be called from geometry shaders for adding a scene element to the result. If *result* or *item* are null, `miFALSE` is returned. If *result* refers to a null tag, an instance group is created and returned in *result*. If *result* is non-null but does not refer to an instance group, an instance group is created, the *result* element is put into this group and the group is returned in *result*. Now that this function has enforced that an instance group element is always returned, the *item* element is put into the returned group. See page 201 for an example.

```
miBoolean mi_geoshader_tesselate(
    miState         *state,
    miTag           *leaves,
    miTag           source)
```

This function should be called from geometry shaders only. It builds a list of instances that describes the object, instance group, or instance *source*. If *source* contains more than one object, there will be multiple instances in the *leaves* list. The *leaves* argument is set to the tag of the first instance; the others are chained to one another with the *next* field in each instance. The last instance in the list has a null *next* field.

The tessellation function also tessellates the geometry described by each instance, and attaches the triangles resulting from the tessellation to the *boxes* field of the instance. Triangles are stored in boxes, which are data structures consisting of a header, a vector list, a vertex list, and a triangle list. Boxes have a maximum size; if an object does not fit into one box more are generated and chained using the *next_box* tag in each box. See chapter 4 for more detail.

```
miBoolean mi_geoshader_tesselate_end(
    miTag           leaves)
```

Release all memory allocated by *mi_geoshader_tesselate*. This function releases all instances and boxes attached to the instance chain *leaves*, which was created by *mi_geoshader_tesselate*. Multiple instance lists can exist at the same time; it is not necessary to release one before creating the next but since memory demands may be substantial if the tessellated geometry is large, it is recommended to not keep instance lists longer than necessary.

```
miBoolean mi_string_substitute(
    char            *newname,
    char            *name,
    long            size)
```

This function[2] performs substitutions on the file path *name*, and returns the substituted path in *newname*, which must point to a char buffer of sufficient size (`miPATHSIZE` is recommended). The size of the buffer must be passed as *size* to prevent buffer overruns. Substitutions are taken from the `MI_RAY_SUBSTITUTE` environment variable, the mental ray registry mechanism, and the (obsolete) Softimage Linktab mechanism. For details on the first two refer to [Driemeyer 99].

```
miBoolean mi_inclusive_lightlist(
    int         *n_lights,
    miTag       **lights,
    miState     *state)
```

This function accepts a list of light source instances, and returns a modified list that includes all other instances of the instanced lights as well. If a light is instanced three times in the scene, and one (or more) of them appears in **lights*, then **lights* will contain all three after this call. *n_lights* points to an integer containing the original list size, and *lights* points to a pointer to the original list. After the function returns, the integer holds the new list length, and the pointer points to a new list. Both the integer and the pointer should be on the stack and should be initialized from the shader parameters using *mi_eval* to avoid overwriting the actual shader parameters, which should remain intact for the next shader call.

The new list is a copy of the global light list (see *mi_query*) with only those lights that match the passed original list included. The returned list remains valid until the next call to *mi_inclusive_lightlist* or *mi_exclusive_lightlist*. Note that this function involves a loop over all lights, and may be a good candidate for calling once in the init shader instead of once every time the shader is called, if **lights* is known to be constant during the frame.

```
miBoolean mi_exclusive_lightlist(
    int         *n_lights,
    miTag       **lights,
    miState     *state)
```

This function is similar to the previous, but returns all global light instances *except* those whose instanced light match a light instanced in the given list. Both functions return mutually exclusive lists when called with the same argument list. *n_lights* points to an integer containing the original list size, and *lights* points to a pointer to the original list. After the function returns, the integer holds the new list length, and the pointer points to a new list. Both the integer and the pointer should be on the stack and should be initialized from the shader parameters using *mi_eval* to avoid overwriting the actual shader parameters, which should remain intact for the next shader call.

[2]This function was introduced in mental ray 2.1.36.

The new list is a copy of the global light list (see *mi_query*) with the matches with the original list removed. This function is slightly slower than the previous. The returned list remains valid until the next call to *mi_inclusive_lightlist* or *mi_exclusive_lightlist*.

3.21.10 Obsolete Auxiliary Functions

These functions are obsolete; use *mi_query* for future implementations.

```
void mi_light_info(
    miTag           tag,
    miVector        *org,
    miVector        *dir,
    void            **paras)
```

tag is assumed to be a light source instance as found in a light parameter of a shader, or returned by *mi_query*. It is looked up, and its origin (location in internal space) is stored in **org*, and its direction (also in internal space) is stored in **dir*. If *tag* refers to a light source instead of the instance, both vectors are defined in local space. Since light sources can only have one or the other but not both, the unused vector is set to a null vector. This can be used to distinguish directional (infinite) light sources; their *org* vector is set to (0, 0, 0). The *paras* pointer is set to the shader parameters of the referenced light shader; if properly cast by the caller, it can extract information such as whether a non-directional light source is a point or a spot light, and its color and attenuation parameters. (mental ray considers a spot light to be a point light with directional attenuation.) Any of the three pointers *org*, *dir*, and *paras* can be a null pointer.

```
int mi_global_lights_info(
    miTag           **tag)
```

Returns the address of an array containing all global light leaf instances. The tags in this array can be used like light shader parameters for calls to *mi_sample_light* and *mi_light_info*. One important difference between shader light parameters and global lights is that global lights are the result of instancing, so if a light is transformed and/or multiply instanced it will appear transformed and/or more than once in the global light list, while shader parameters will be accessed as stored in the scene with no instancing applied. It is recommended that translators that support multiple light instancing use material shaders that use the global light list instead of a light array in the shader parameter list (which, however, may still be useful as an argument for *mi_inclusive_lightlist* and *mi_exclusive_lightlist*).

```
void mi_texture_info(
    miTag           tag,
    int             *xres,
    int             *yres,
    void            **paras)
```

tag is assumed to be a texture as found in a texture parameter of a shader. If *tag* refers to a procedural texture shader, **xres* and **yres* are set to 0 and **paras* is set to the shader parameters of the texture shader. If *tag* is an image texture, **xres* and **yres* are set to the image resolution in pixels, and **paras* is set to 0. Any of the three pointers can be a null pointer.

```
void *mi_shader_info(
    miState          *state)
```

Returns a pointer to the user pointer of the current shader in the state, $state \rightarrow shader$. This is useful for shader that allocate memory during startup (in the instance init shader) and need a place to store the pointer to the initialized data in a place where shader instances can pick it up. A unique user pointer is returned for each shader instance (each unique function/parameters pair).

```
int mi_instance_info(
    miState          *state,
    void ** const    paraspp,
    void ** const    spare1,
    void ** const    spare2,
    void ** const    spare3)
```

Returns the size of and a pointer to the inherited instance parameters. Instance parameters are attached to the instances of the scene DAG, and are combined in a scene DAG traversal step during scene preprocessing, before rendering begins. The structure of the inherited data is determined by the inheritance function, not by the shader, and is generally under control of the translator that generated the scene. Typically, all instances contain either no parameters at all (size 0), or they all use the same data structure. The instance being checked is $state \rightarrow instance$. The *spare* pointers must be passed as 0.

3.21.11 Contour Functions

```
miBoolean mi_get_contour_line(
    miContour_endpoint *p1,
    miContour_endpoint *p2);
```

This function can be used by a contour output shader to get end points of a contour line segment. When *mi_get_contour_line* returns miFALSE, there are no more contour lines.

```
void mi_add_contour_lines(
    miContour_endpoint p1[],
    miContour_endpoint p2[],
    int                n);
```

This is another function available to contour output shaders. It adds extra contour lines to the ones that were found during rendering. *p1* is the list of first endpoints, *p2* is the list of second endpoints, and *n* is the number of contour lines to be added (the number of elements in the lists). This can for example be used by a combination of two contour output shaders: the first one adds some extra contour lines, and the second one renders all contour lines (both the contour lines found during rendering and the extra contour lines added using *mi_add_contour_lines*). Or, as another example, the first contour output shader can read all contour lines, analyze them, and write back a subset of them (or even some altogether different contours) with *mi_add_contour_lines*.

3.21.12 Memory Allocation

mental ray's memory allocation functions replace the standard *malloc* packages found on most systems. They have built-in functions for memory leak tracing and consistency checks, and handle errors automatically. Shaders should always use these functions and not *malloc* or similar libc functions directly.

```
void *mi_mem_allocate(
    const int      size)
```

Accepts one argument specifying the size of the memory to allocate. A pointer to the allocated memory is returned. If the allocation fails, an error is reported automatically, and mental ray tries to recover memory or aborts if this fails. This call is guaranteed to return a valid pointer, or not to return at all. The allocated memory is zeroed. This and most other *mem_** functions use locking and should therefore not be used in time-critical places to prevent multithreading efficiency from dropping through the floor. See page 267 for details on the effect of locks on efficiency. A good place for memory allocation is init shaders.

```
void *mi_mem_reallocate(
    void * const  mem,
    const int     size)
```

Change the size of an allocated block of memory. There are two arguments: a pointer to the old block of memory, and the requested new size of that block. A pointer to the new block is returned, which may be different from the pointer to the old block. If the old pointer was a null pointer, *mi_mem_reallocate* behaves like *mi_mem_allocate*. If the new size is zero, *mi_mem_reallocate* behaves like *mi_mem_release*, and returns a null pointer. If there is an allocation error, an error is reported and raylib is aborted. Like *mi_mem_alloc*, *mi_mem_reallocate* never returns if the re-allocation fails. If the block grows, the extra bytes are zeroed.

```
void mi_mem_release(
    void * const  mem)
```

Frees a block of memory. There is one argument: the address of the block. If a null pointer is passed, nothing is done. There is no return value. After releasing memory it may no longer be accessed.

3.21.13 Thread Parallelism and Locks

In addition to network parallelism, *mental ray* also supports shared memory parallelism through threads. Network parallelism is a form of distributed memory parallelism where processes cooperate by exchanging messages. Messages are used to exchange data as well as to synchronize. With shared memory data can easily be exchanged, a process must only access the common memory to do so. A different mechanism has to be used for synchronization. This is usually done by *locking*. Basically what has to be done is one process has to tell the other that it is waiting to access data, and another process can signal that it has finished working with it, so that any other process may now access it.

By default threads are used on shared memory multiprocessor machines. Threads are sometimes also called lightweight processes. Threads behave like processes running on a common shared memory.

Since memory is shared between two threads, both can write to memory at the same time. It can also happen that one thread writes while another reads the same memory. Both these cases can lead to surprising unwanted results. Therefore – to guard against these surprises – when using threads certain precautions have to be observed. Care has to be taken when using heap memory such as global or static data, as any thread may potentially modify it. To prevent corrupting any data (or reading corrupted data), locking must be used when it is not otherwise guaranteed that concurrent accesses will not occur. The stack, however, is always safe because every thread has its own stack that is not shared with any other thread.

In addition to making sure that write accesses to data are performed when no other thread accesses the data, it is important to use only so-called concurrency safe libraries and calls. If a call to a nonreentrant function is done, locking should be used. A function is called *reentrant* if it can be executed by multiple threads at the same time without adverse effects. (Reentrancy and concurrency safety are related, but the terms stem from different historical contexts, and reentrancy also implies the ability to recurse safely.) Details and examples are explained below.

For example, static data on a shared memory multiprocessor can be modified by more than one processor at a time. Consider this test:

```
static miBoolean is_init = miFALSE;
...
if (!is_init) {
    is_init = miTRUE;
    initialize();
}
```

This does not guarantee that *initialize* is called only once. The reason is that all threads share the *is_init* flag, so two threads may simultaneously examine the flag. It is possible that both will find that it has not been set, and enter the *if* body. Next, both will set the flag to `miTRUE`, and then both will call the *initialize* function. This situation is called a *race condition*. The example is contrived because initialization and termination should be done with init and exit shaders as described in the next section, but this problem can occur with any heap variable. Even incrementing global or static variables with "++" is not safe – the time window that leads to errors may be small, but that makes such mistakes all the more difficult to find. In general, all threads on a host share all data except local `auto` variables on the stack.

The behavior described above could also occur if more than one thread is used on a single processor, but by default *mental ray* does not create more threads than there are processors.

There are two methods for guarding against race conditions. One is to guarantee that only one thread executes certain code at a time. Such code surrounded by lock and unlock operations is called a *critical section*. Code inside of critical sections may access global or static data or call any function that does so (as long as all is protected by the same lock). The lock used in this example is assumed to have been created and initialized with a call to *mi_init_lock* before it used here. (See below how locks are initialized.) Here is an example of how a critical section may be used:

```
miLock lock;

mi_lock(lock);
if (!is_init) {
    is_init = miTRUE;
    initialize();
}
mi_unlock(lock);
```

The other method is to use separate variables for each thread. This is done by allocating an array with one entry for each thread, and indexing this array with the current thread number (which can be found in *state* → *thread*). Allocation is done in the shader's initialization function (which has the same name as the shader with `_init` appended). No locking is required because it is called only once. The termination function (which also has the same name but with `_exit` appended) must release the array.

Locks reduce multithreading efficiency and should be used only when absolutely necessary. The probability of one thread blocking because another has locked a section of code grows very quickly with the number of threads, and a thread that is blocked is not available to do useful work. Efficiency describes the degree of parallelism: if n threads increase the speed by a factor m, then the efficiency is $\frac{m}{n}$. If two threads have an efficiency of 0.95, then 32 threads have an efficiency of only $0.95^{32} \approx 0.19$, so over 80% of all CPU cycles are wasted! Efficiency drops surprisingly quickly, so careful attention to locks is required. Note that memory allocation and releasing functions (*mi_mem_allocate* et. al.) contain a lock.

mental ray provides two locks for general use: *state*→*global_lock* is a lock shared by all threads and all shaders. No two critical sections protected by this lock can execute simultaneously on this host. The second is *state*→*shader*→*lock*, which is local to all instances of the current shader. The lock is tied to the shader, not the particular call with particular shader parameters. Every shader in mental ray, built-in or dynamically linked, has exactly one such lock. mental ray internally uses this lock and the global lock to guarantee that the init and exit shaders of a shader do not execute concurrently. Therefore, they must not be used in these functions.

The relevant functions provided by the parallelism modules are:

```
void mi_init_lock(
    miLock * const  lock)
```

Before a lock can be used by one of the other locking functions, it must be initialized with this function. Note that the lock variable must be static or global. Shaders will normally use this function in their *_init* function. Shaders should not initialize (or delete) *state* $\rightarrow$ *global_lock* or the local shader lock; they are pre-initialized by mental ray.

```
void mi_delete_lock(
    miLock * const  lock)
```

Destroy a lock. This should be done when it is no longer needed. The code should use lock and immediately unlock the lock first to make sure that no other thread is in or waiting for a critical section protected by this lock. Shaders will normally use this function in their exit shader. Do not delete the predefined locks.

```
void mi_lock(
    const miLock    lock)
```

Check if any other code holds the lock. If so, block; otherwise set the lock and proceed. This is done in a parallel-safe way so only one critical section locked can execute at a time. Note that locking the same lock twice in a row without anyone unlocking it will block the thread forever, effectively freezing mental ray, because the second lock can never succeed.

```
void mi_unlock(
    const miLock    lock)
```

Release a lock. If another thread was blocked attempting to set the lock, it can proceed now. Locks and unlocks must always be paired, and the code between locking and unlocking must be as short and as fast as possible to avoid defeating parallelism. There is no fairness guarantee that ensures that the thread that has been blocked for the longest time is unblocked first.

```
miVpu mi_par_localvpu(void)
    int   miTHREAD(miVpu vpu)
    int   miHOST(miVpu vpu)
    miVpu miVPU(int host, int thread)
```

The term *VPU* stands for Virtual Processing Unit. All threads on the network have a unique VPU number. *mi_par_localvpu* returns the VPU number of the VPU this thread is running on. VPUs are a concatenation of the host number and the thread number, both numbered from 0 to the number of hosts or threads, respectively, minus 1. (Future versions of mental ray may use noncontiguous host numbers, but not noncontiguous thread numbers.)

The miTHREAD macro extracts a thread number from a VPU, and the miHOST macro extracts the host number from a VPU. Thread 0 is called the client thread; host 0 is called the client host. Thread 0 on host 0 is normally running the translator that controls the entire operation. The miVPU macro puts a host and thread number together to form a VPU number. The *mi_par_localvpu* function returns the VPU of the current thread on the local host.

In a shader the fastest way of finding the current thread number is $state \rightarrow thread$.

```
int mi_par_nthreads(void)
```

Returns the number of threads on the local host. This is normally 1 on a single-processor system. This number can be used to allocate an array of per-thread variables in the shader initialization code. The array can then be indexed by the shader with $state \rightarrow thread$.

```
int mi_par_aborted(void)
```

Return a nonzero value if mental ray has been aborted, and the shader should stop what it is doing, clean up, and return. This is only of interest in output shaders because they can run for a long time. This allows the user to press on an abort button, which causes calls to *mi_pat_aborted* to return nonzero, and have the shader return as soon as possible. For example, the shader might call this function in its scanline loop (not for every pixel to avoid slowing it down), and skip the remaining lines. The shader must still clean up, for example releasing memory that it has allocated.

3.21.14 Messages and Errors

Shaders may print messages and errors. They are printed in the same format as rendering (RC) messages. Options given to the translator determine which messages are printed and which are suppressed. All message routines have the same parameters as *printf(3)*. All append a newline to the message. Messages are printed in the form

RC *host.thread level: message*

with the module name, e.g. `RC`, the host number *host* if available, the thread number *thread* with a leading dot if available, the message type *level* (fatal, error, warning etc), and the message given in the function call. In a networked environment, the messages of servers are usually transferred to the client rendering host and printed in the order they were received. Messages resulting from connection problems and those that were dropped to avoid a network overload may be found in a local file (`/tmp/raylib.log`). Newlines in the message are replaced with blanks.

```
void mi_fatal(
    const char * const message,
    ...)
```

An unrecoverable error has occurred. Unlike all others, this call will not return; it will attempt to recover mental ray and return to the top-level translator. Recovering may involve aborting all operations in progress and clearing the entire database. Fatal messages can be suppressed, but mental ray is always exited. This function should never be used in a shader because it may also exit any application that mental ray is embedded in, without giving the user a chance to save his work!

```
void mi_error(
    const char * const message,
    ...)
```

An unrecoverable error has occurred. The caller then aborts the current operation gracefully and returns.

```
void mi_warning(
    const char * const message,
    ...)
```

A recoverable error occurred. The current operation proceeds.

```
void mi_info(
    const char * const message,
    ...)
```

Prints information about the current operation such as the number of triangles and timing information. Infos should be used sparingly; do not print information for every intersection point or shader call except during debugging, especially on Windows NT 4.x with its slow and nonparallel I/O system.

```
void mi_progress(
    const char * const message,
    ...)
```

Prints progress reports such as rendering percentages.

```
void mi_debug(
    const char * const message,
    ...)
```

Prints debugging information useful only for shader development.

```
void mi_vdebug(
    const char * const message,
    ...)
```

Prints more debugging information useful only for shader development. Messages that are likely to be useful only in rare circumstances, or that generate a very large number of lines should be printed with this function.

Note that all these functions incur some runtime overhead even if the verbosity level is set such that no message is printed. It is often a good idea to enclose shader debugging messages that occur frequently in `ifdef DEBUG` statements to make sure they are omitted in production versions of the shader.

3.21.15 Callable Functions by Shader Type

The following table describes which shader interface functions are available in which types of shaders:

G	geometry shader
D	displacement shader
P	photon shader and photon volume shader
E	photon emitter shader
Le	lens shader
M	material shader and texture shader
T	texture shader
V	volume shader
Lg	light shader
S	shadow shader
Cs	contour store shader
C	contour contrast shader and contour shader
O	output shader

The rules for init shaders and exit shaders are the same as for the main shader they apply to.

In the following table, "•" means that the function may be used, "○" means that it may not be used, and "▪" means that it is available but is not normally useful. Asterisks "*" denotes omission unless an earlier more specific table row overrides it. For example, mi_eval* means all functions beginning with mi_eval, including mi_eval itself, mi_eval_boolean, and so on.

function	G	D	P	E	Le	M	V	Lg	S	Cs	C	O
Shader Calls												
(continued on next page)												

(continued from previous page) function	G	D	P	E	Le	M	V	Lg	S	Cs	C	O
mi_call_shader*	●	●	●	●	●	●	●	●	●	●	●	●
mi_call_material	○	○	○	○	○	●	○	○	○	○	○	○
mi_call_photon_material	○	○	●	○	○	○	○	○	○	○	○	○
mi_eval*	○	●	●	●	○	●	●	●	●	●	○	○
mi_flush_cache	○	●	●	●	○	●	●	●	●	●	○	○
DB												
mi_db_*	●	●	●	●	●	●	●	●	●	●	●	●
RC Functions												
mi_trace_eye	○	○	○	○	●	○	○	○	○	■	■	○
mi_trace_reflection	○	○	●	●	●	●	●	●	●	■	■	○
mi_trace_refraction	○	○	●	●	●	●	●	●	●	■	■	○
mi_trace_transparent	○	○	●	●	●	●	●	●	●	■	■	○
mi_trace_environment	○	○	●	●	●	●	●	●	●	■	■	○
mi_trace_probe[2.1]	○	○	●	●	●	●	●	●	●	■	■	○
mi_trace_light	○	○	●	●	●	●	●	○	○	■	■	○
mi_sample_light	○	○	●	●	●	●	●	○	○	■	■	○
mi_trace_shadow	○	○	○	○	○	○	○	●	○	○	○	○
mi_trace_shadow_seg	○	○	○	○	○	○	○	○	●	○	○	○
mi_compute_irradiance	○	○	○	○	●	●	●	●	●	●	○	○
mi_compute_volume_irradiance	○	○	○	○	●	●	●	●	●	●	○	○
mi_sample[2.1]	○	○	●	●	●	●	●	●	●	●	●	●
RC Photon Functions												
mi_photon_light	○	○	●	○	○	○	○	○	○	○	○	○
mi_photon_reflection_specular	○	○	●	○	○	○	○	○	○	○	○	○
mi_photon_reflection_glossy[2.1]	○	○	●	○	○	○	○	○	○	○	○	○
mi_photon_reflection_diffuse[2.1]	○	○	●	○	○	○	○	○	○	○	○	○
mi_photon_transmission_specular	○	○	●	○	○	○	○	○	○	○	○	○
mi_photon_transmission_glossy[2.1]	○	○	●	○	○	○	○	○	○	○	○	○
mi_photon_transmission_diffuse[2.1]	○	○	●	○	○	○	○	○	○	○	○	○
mi_photon_transparent	○	○	●	○	○	○	○	○	○	○	○	○
mi_photon_volume_scattering	○	○	●	○	○	○	○	○	○	○	○	○
mi_store_photon	○	○	●	○	○	○	○	○	○	○	○	○
mi_store_volume_photon	○	○	●	○	○	○	○	○	○	○	○	○
RC Direction Functions												
mi_reflection_dir	■	●	●	●	●	●	●	●	●	●	●	■
mi_reflection_dir_specular	■	●	●	●	●	●	●	●	●	●	●	■
mi_reflection_dir_glossy	■	●	●	●	●	●	●	●	●	●	●	■
mi_reflection_dir_anisglossy	■	●	●	●	●	●	●	●	●	●	●	■
mi_reflection_dir_diffuse	■	●	●	●	●	●	●	●	●	●	●	■
mi_refraction_dir	■	●	●	●	●	●	●	●	●	●	●	■
mi_transmission_dir_specular	■	●	●	●	●	●	●	●	●	●	●	■
mi_transmission_dir_glossy	■	●	●	●	●	●	●	●	●	●	●	■
mi_transmission_dir_anisglossy	■	●	●	●	●	●	●	●	●	●	●	■

(continued on next page)

(continued from previous page)

function	G	D	P	E	Le	M	V	Lg	S	Cs	C	O
mi_transmission_dir_diffuse	■	●	●	●	●	●	●	●	●	●	●	■
mi_scattering_dir_diffuse	■	●	●	●	●	●	●	●	●	●	●	■
mi_scattering_dir_directional	■	●	●	●	●	●	●	●	●	●	●	■
mi_scattering_pathlength	■	●	●	●	●	●	●	●	●	●	●	■
IMG Functions												
mi_img_put_*	●	●	●	●	●	●	●	●	●	●	●	●
mi_img_get_*	●	●	●	●	●	●	●	●	●	●	●	●
Math Functions												
mi_point_to_*	○	●	●	●	●	●	●	●	●	●	●	○
mi_point_from_*	○	●	●	●	●	●	●	●	●	●	●	○
mi_vector_to_*	○	●	●	●	●	●	●	●	●	●	●	○
mi_vector_from_*	○	●	●	●	●	●	●	●	●	●	●	○
mi_normal_to_*	○	●	●	●	●	●	●	●	●	●	●	○
mi_normal_from_*	○	●	●	●	●	●	●	●	●	●	●	○
mi_vector_*	●	●	●	●	●	●	●	●	●	●	●	●
mi_matrix_*	●	●	●	●	●	●	●	●	●	●	●	●
mi_point_*	●	●	●	●	●	●	●	●	●	●	●	●
Noise Functions												
mi_par_random	○	○	○	○	●	●	●	●	●	●	●	○
mi_*random	●	●	●	●	●	●	●	●	●	●	●	●
mi_spline	●	●	●	●	●	●	●	●	●	●	●	●
mi_noise_*	●	●	●	●	●	●	●	●	●	●	●	●
mi_unoise_*	●	●	●	●	●	●	●	●	●	●	●	●
Auxiliary Functions												
mi_fresnel	○	●	●	●	●	●	●	●	●	●	●	●
mi_fresnel_reflection	○	●	●	●	●	●	●	●	●	●	●	●
mi_phong_specular	○	●	●	●	●	●	●	●	●	●	●	●
mi_fresnel_specular	○	●	●	●	●	●	●	●	●	●	●	●
mi_blinn_specular	○	●	●	●	●	●	●	●	●	●	●	●
mi_blong_specular	○	●	●	●	●	●	●	●	●	●	●	●
mi_cooktorr_specular	○	●	●	●	●	●	●	●	●	●	●	●
mi_ward_glossy	○	●	●	●	●	●	●	●	●	●	●	●
mi_ward_anisglossy	○	●	●	●	●	●	●	●	●	●	●	●
mi_schlick_scatter	○	●	●	●	●	●	●	●	●	●	●	●
mi_choose_scatter_type	○	●	●	●	●	●	●	●	●	●	●	●
mi_choose_lobe	○	●	●	●	●	●	●	●	●	●	●	●
mi_lookup_*_texture	●	●	●	●	●	●	●	●	●	●	●	●
mi_texture_filter_project	○	●	●	●	●	●	●	●	●	●	●	●
mi_texture_filter_transform	○	●	●	●	●	●	●	●	●	●	●	●
mi_tri_vectors	○	○	●	●	○	●	●	●	●	●	●	○
mi_query	●	●	●	●	●	●	●	●	●	●	●	●
mi_fb_put[2.1]	○	○	○	○	●	●	●	●	●	●	●	○
mi_fb_get[2.1]	○	○	○	○	●	●	●	●	●	●	●	○

(continued on next page)

(continued from previous page) function	G	D	P	E	Le	M	V	Lg	S	Cs	C	O
mi_geoshader_add_result	●	○	○	○	○	○	○	○	○	○	○	○
mi_geoshader_tesselate	●	○	○	○	○	○	○	○	○	○	○	○
mi_geoshader_tesselate_end	●	○	○	○	○	○	○	○	○	○	○	○
mi_string_substitute[2.1]	●	●	●	●	●	●	●	●	●	●	●	●
Obsolete Auxiliary Functions												
mi_*_info	○	●	●	●	●	●	●	●	●	●	●	●
Contour Functions												
mi_get_contour_line	○	○	○	○	○	○	○	○	○	○	○	●
mi_add_contour_lines	○	○	○	○	○	○	○	○	○	○	○	●
Memory Allocation												
mi_mem_*	●	●	●	●	●	●	●	●	●	●	●	●
Thread Parallelism and Locks												
mi_init_lock	●	●	●	●	●	●	●	●	●	●	●	●
mi_delete_lock	●	●	●	●	●	●	●	●	●	●	●	●
mi_lock	●	●	●	●	●	●	●	●	●	●	●	●
mi_unlock	●	●	●	●	●	●	●	●	●	●	●	●
mi_par_localvpu	●	●	●	●	●	●	●	●	●	●	●	●
mi_par_nthreads	●	●	●	●	●	●	●	●	●	●	●	●
mi_par_aborted	●	●	●	●	●	●	●	●	●	●	●	●
Messages and Errors												
mi_fatal	●	●	●	●	●	●	●	●	●	●	●	●
mi_error	●	●	●	●	●	●	●	●	●	●	●	●
mi_warning	●	●	●	●	●	●	●	●	●	●	●	●
mi_info	●	●	●	●	●	●	●	●	●	●	●	●
mi_progress	●	●	●	●	●	●	●	●	●	●	●	●
mi_debug	●	●	●	●	●	●	●	●	●	●	●	●
mi_vdebug	●	●	●	●	●	●	●	●	●	●	●	●

See page 157 for a similar table listing available state variables.

3.22 Initialization and Cleanup

mental ray provides a way to define initialization and cleanup functions for each user defined function. Many shaders need to perform operations such as initializing color tables or allocating arrays before they are called for the first time. They may also need to do cleanup operations after rendering has finished, for operations like releasing storage to prevent memory leaks.

Before a shader is called for the first time, ray checks if a function of the same name with `_init` appended exists. If so, it assumes that this is an initialization function (also called *init shader*) and calls it once before the first call of the shader. The state passed to the initialization function is the same as passed to the first call of the actual shader to be initialized. Note that the order of shader calls is unpredictable because the order of pixel samples is unpredictable, so the initialization function should not rely on sample-specific state variables such as *state→point*.

The initialization function has the option of requesting *shader instance initializations* by setting the boolean variable its third argument points to to miTRUE. A shader instance is a unique pair of shader and shader parameters. For example, if the shader *soft_material* is used in two different materials it is said to have two different instances (even if the parameter values happen to be equal). When an init shader is called as part of the shader instance initialization, it receives the same parameters that the main shader will receive. As always, shaders may not write back into their shader parameters because that confuses other threads or hosts that access the shader simultaneously, because it changes the scene for the next frame, and because a shader or interface assignment may get mangled.

When rendering has finished, mental ray checks for each user provided shader that was called whether a function of the same name with _exit appended exists. If yes, it assumes that this is a cleanup function and calls it once. For example, if a shader *myshader* exists, the functions *myshader_init* and *myshader_exit* are called for initialization and cleanup if they exist.

The functions are assumed to have the following type:

```
void myshader_init(miState   *state,
                   void      *paras,
                   miBoolean *inst_init_req);

void myshader_exit(miState   *state,
                   void      *paras);
```

The -i option of the mkmishader utility automatically creates init and exit shader prototypes. Here is an example for init and exit shaders for a shader named *myshader*. When *myshader* is about to be used for the first time in a frame, the calling order is:

1. *myshader_init* with a null *paras* argument
2. *myshader_init* with non-null *paras* argument
3. *myshader* itself with the same non-null *paras* argument
4. more calls to *myshader* with the same *paras* argument, and calls to other instances of *myshader_init* and *myshader* with different *paras* arguments,
5. one *mi_shader_exit* with a non-null *paras* argument for each corresponding *myshader_init*
6. finally one *myshader_exit* with a null *paras* argument.

Steps 2 and 5 would have been omitted if *myshader_init* in step 1 had not set its third argument *inst_req* to miTRUE. Two different instances of the same shader always have different *paras* argument pointers. However, a shadow or photon shader and a material shader in the same material may share parameters as described above; in this case both shaders are called with the same *paras* argument. Most scenes are built this way, it is recommended to write material shaders so they can also be used as shadow and photon shaders to simplify scene construction.

```
DLLEXPORT void myshader_init(   /* must end with "_init" */
    miState         *state,
    struct myshader *paras,     /* valid for inst inits */
    miBoolean       *inst_req)  /* for inst init request */
{
    if (!paras) {               /* main shader init */
        *inst_req = miTRUE;     /* want inst inits too */
        ...
    } else {                    /* shader instance init */
                                /* just an example: */
        state->shader->user.p = mi_mem_allocate(...);
        ...
    }
}

DLLEXPORT void myshader_exit(   /* must end with "_exit" */
    miState         *state,
    struct myshader *paras)     /* valid for inst inits */
{
    if (!paras) {               /* main shader exit */
        ...                     /* no further inst exits
                                 * will occur */
    } else {                    /* shader instance exit */
                                /* just an example: */
        mi_mem_release(state->shader->user.p);
        ...
    }
}
```

Note that there will generally be many instance init/exits (if enabled), but only one shader init/exit. If an init/exit shader is not available, it is not called; this is not an error. Initialization and cleanup are done on every host where the function was used, but only once on shared memory parallel machines. They are done for each frame separately. Init and exit shaders will never run concurrently with each other or the actual shader on shared-memory multiprocessor machines; mental ray takes care of the appropriate locking using the shader lock. For this reason, init and exit shaders should never lock the shader lock (obtainable with the `miQ_FUNC_LOCK` mode of the *mi_query* function) because that would deadlock mental ray.

3.23 Automatic Source Generation with mkmishader

In order to write a new shader, a number of prototypes and other mechanical work must be done, such as writing prototypes, evaluation of parameters, versioning, and so on. The mkmishader utility can do this automatically. For example, the *mib_illum_lambert* shader in the base shader library has the following .mi declaration:

```
declare shader
    color "mib_illum_lambert" (
```

```
        color                "ambience",
        color                "ambient",
        color                "diffuse",
        integer              "mode",
        array light          "lights"
    )
    version 2
end declare
```

If this declaration is stored in a file, and the mkmishader utility is run with the `-i` option (which creates init and exit shaders), a new file `mib_illum_lambert.c` is created with the following content:

```
#include <stdio.h>
#include <math.h>
#include <shader.h>

typedef struct {
   miColor         ambience;
   miColor         ambient;
   miColor         diffuse;
   miInteger       mode;
   int             i_lights;
   int             n_lights;
   miTag           lights[1];
} mib_illum_lambert_t;

DLLEXPORT int mib_illum_lambert_version(void) {return(2);}

DLLEXPORT miBoolean mib_illum_lambert_init(
   miState *state,
   mib_illum_lambert_t *param,
   miBoolean *init_req)
{
   if (!param) {
           /* shader init */
           *init_req = miTRUE; /* do instance inits */
   } else {
           /* shader instance init */
   }
   return(miTRUE);
}

DLLEXPORT miBoolean mib_illum_lambert_exit(
   miState *state,
   mib_illum_lambert_t *param)
{
```

```
    if (param) {
            /* shader instance exit */
    } else {
            /* shader exit */
    }
    return(miTRUE);
}

DLLEXPORT miBoolean mib_illum_lambert(
    miColor *result,
    miState *state,
    mib_illum_lambert_t *param)
{
    /*
     * get parameter values. It is inefficient to do this all
     * at the beginning of the code. Move the assignments here
     * to where the values are first used. You may want to use
     * pointers for colors and vectors.
     */
    miColor ambience = *mi_eval_color(&param->ambience);
    miColor ambient = *mi_eval_color(&param->ambient);
    miColor diffuse = *mi_eval_color(&param->diffuse);
    miInteger mode = *mi_eval_integer(&param->mode);
    int i_lights = *mi_eval_integer(&param->i_lights);
    int n_lights = *mi_eval_integer(&param->n_lights);
    struct lights_s *lights = (struct lights_s *)mi_eval(
                                      state, param->lights);
    /*
     * sample array loops
     */
    int i;
    for (i=0; i < n_lights; i++) {
            /* use lights[i_lights + i]; */
    }

    /*
     * set shader results. ``+='' etc. is useful for shaders
     * in shader lists but other shaders may need to simply
     * assign result variables.
     */
    result->r += 0.0;
    result->g += 0.0;
    result->b += 0.0;
    result->a += 0.0;
    return(miTRUE);
}
```

This skeleton source code can then be filled in with the implementation of the actual algorithm. It is important to move the *mi_eval* functions to the places where they are first used because if the shader does not need a variable it is faster to not access it. For example, if the light array *lights* is empty, so *n_lights* is zero, then there is no need to access *i_light*, *lights*, and *diffuse*. The functions used in this skeleton will be described later.

3.24 Shaders and Trace Functions

Trace functions are functions provided by mental ray that allow a shader to cast a ray into the scene, most of them using standard ray tracing. Not all types of tracing functions can be used in all types of shaders. Conversely, many trace functions cause shaders to be called. This chapter lists these interdependencies.

The following list shows which shaders are called from which trace functions. ○ means no, • means yes. Displacement, contour, and photon shaders are never called by any of the functions, and may not call any of them.

	lens	mtl	env	light	shad	vol
mi_trace_eye	•	•	•	○	○	•
mi_trace_reflection	○	•	•	○	○	•
mi_trace_refraction	○	•	•	○	○	•
mi_trace_transparent	○	•	•	○	○	•
mi_trace_environment	○	○	•	○	○	•
mi_trace_light	○	○	○	•	○	•
mi_sample_light	○	○	○	•	○	•
mi_trace_shadow	○	○	○	○	•	○
mi_trace_shadow_seg	○	○	○	○	•	•

Environment rays do not have entries in this tree. The data in the tree is used for acceleration and can be overridden if a shader wants to cast rays not normally allowed, by setting the state variable *state→cache* to zero. This should only be done if necessary because it reduces efficiency. The following table shows which trace functions may be called from which shaders:

	lens	mtl	env	light	shad	ray vol	light vol
mi_trace_eye	•	○	○	○	○	○	○
mi_trace_reflection	⋆⋆	•	⋆	⋆⋆	⋆⋆	•	⋆⋆
mi_trace_refraction	⋆⋆	•	⋆	⋆⋆	⋆⋆	•	⋆⋆
mi_trace_transparent	⋆⋆	•	⋆	⋆⋆	⋆⋆	•	⋆⋆
mi_trace_environment	⋆	•	•	⋆	•	•	•
mi_trace_light	⋆	•	⋆	⋆⋆	⋆⋆	•	⋆⋆
mi_sample_light	⋆	•	⋆	⋆⋆	⋆⋆	•	⋆⋆
mi_trace_shadow	○	○	○	•	○	○	•
mi_trace_shadow_seg	○	○	○	○	•	○	○

○ no

● yes

⋆ yes, if the shader generates an artificial intersection point by setting *point*, *normal*, and *normal_geom* in the state.

⋆⋆ yes, if the shader removes RC's internal ray tree data by setting *cache* in the state to NULL and generates an artificial intersection point if none is present.

3.25 Example Scene with Custom Shader

This section shows how to create a .mi file that uses a custom shader that is linked at runtime. This example uses a texture shader, but the same procedure is used to create and link any other type of shader.

Step 1: Writing the Shader Source

This texture shader operates in object space and colors the object into eight cubes that meet at the object coordinate origin. A cube mapped with this texture looks like a Rubik's cube for beginners that consists of eight subcubes, each with a different color. The brightness and saturation of the colors is determined by the shader parameters *min* and *max*.

```
#include <stdio.h>
#include <mi/shader.h>

struct mytexture { miScalar min, max; };

int mytexture_version(void) {return(1);}

miBoolean mytexture(
    miColor            *result,
    miState            *state,
    struct mytexture *paras)
{
    miVector           vec;
    miScalar           min, max;

    mi_point_to_object(state, &vec, &state->point);
    min = *mi_eval_scalar(&paras->min);
    max = *mi_eval_scalar(&paras->max);
    result->r = vec.x < 0 ? min : max;
    result->g = vec.y < 0 ? min : max;
    result->b = vec.z < 0 ? min : max;
    result->a = 1;
    return(miTRUE);
}
```

This code should be written to a file `mytexture.c`.

Step 2: Compiling and Linking

There are several ways to integrate this shader into a scene file: placing the source code directly into the .mi file with `$code` and `$end code` statements, referencing the source file with a `code` statement, or compiling the source and referencing the object code with a `link` statement. The recommended method, and also the fastest method, is to create a DSO (Dynamic Shared Object) file on Unix systems, or a DLL on Windows NT systems. To do this, the shader must be compiled and linked manually:

```
% cc -O2 -shared -o mytexture.so mytexture.c
```

This example uses SGI syntax; other compilers require different command lines. See the beginning of this chapter for the commands required for different types of systems. You may also want to specify the `-g` option for debugging, `-O` for optimization, or `-I`*directory* to tell the compiler where the directory containing the *shader.h* file can be found (refer to the compiler documentation for details). After this command, there is a *mytexture.so* DSO in the current directory; move it to a place accessible to all hosts, for example with

```
% mv mytexture.so /usr/share/local
```

Assuming a directory */usr/share/local* exists and is accessible to you. You may also choose a directory such as */usr/tmp*, but since this directory is not normally accessible from other hosts that you want to use as servers (at least not under this name), you will have to copy *mytexture.so* to */usr/tmp* on the other hosts too.

Step 3: Linking and Declaring the Shader

Now the shader needs to be linked and declared in the .mi scene file that contains the object or objects to be mapped with the new texture. Linking means that the DSO (or DLL) becomes callable by mental ray, and the declaration informs mental ray about the shader parameters:

```
link "/usr/share/local/mytexture.so"
declare shader
    color "mytexture" (scalar "min", scalar "max")
    version 1
end declare
```

It is important that the declaration matches the type and order of the C declaration in the source file, *struct mytexture*. These lines should be added near the beginning of the .mi file, before the first use and before the `frame` statement if there is one. For complicated DSOs, it is recommended to put all declarations for the library into a separate file *mytexture.mi*, and use a `$include` statement:

```
link "/usr/share/local/mytexture.so"
$include "/usr/share/local/mytexture.mi"
```

Either way, the library must be linked before the declaration is given because mental ray makes sure that a declared shader exists.

Step 4: Using the Shader

Now the shader can be used in a real .mi file. The following example puts the texture on a cube. Note the `transform` statements; they describe the camera and object transformations to allow the call to *mi_point_to_object* in the shader to work correctly.

```
verbose on
$include <base.mi>
link "base.so"
link "/usr/share/local/mytexture.so"

declare shader
    color "mytexture" (scalar "min", scalar "max")
    version 1
end declare

options "opt"
end options

camera "cam"
    output     "rgb" "demo.rgb"
    focal      1.0
    aperture   1.0
    aspect     1.0
    resolution 500 500
end camera

instance "cam_inst"
    "cam"
end instance

light "light"
    "mib_light_point" ("color" 1.0 1.0 1.0)
    origin   15.614674 14.370044 -10.951728
end light

instance "light_inst"
    "light"
end instance

color texture "tex"
    "mytexture" (
        "min" 0.3,
        "max" 1.0
```

```
    )

material "mtl" opaque
    "mib_illum_phong" (
        "ambience"  .3 .3 .3,
        "ambient"   = "tex",
        "diffuse"   = "tex",
        "specular"  1 1 1,
        "exponent"  50,
        "lights"    [ "light_inst" ]
    )
end material

object "cube" visible shadow trace
    group "mesh"
            -7.288994    -2.709234    -23.455124
            -0.695147    -7.196985    -17.423435
            -7.288994     5.313703    -17.485828
            -0.695147     0.825951    -11.454139
             0.229063     1.226829    -28.745323
             6.822910    -3.260922    -22.713634
             0.229063     9.249765    -22.776028
             6.822910     4.762013    -16.744339

            v 0   v 1   v 3   v 2
            v 1   v 5   v 7   v 3
            v 5   v 4   v 6   v 7
            v 4   v 0   v 2   v 6
            v 4   v 5   v 1   v 0
            v 2   v 3   v 7   v 6

            p "mtl"  0 1 2 3
            p        4 5 6 7
            p        8 9 10 11
            p        12 13 14 15
            p        16 17 18 19
            p        20 21 22 23
    end group
end object

instance "cube_inst" "cube"
    transform   0.751806  0.000000  0.659385 0.0
                0.393606  0.802294 -0.448775 0.0
               -0.529020  0.596930  0.603169 0.0
             -10.861954 11.174661 12.737814 1.0
end instance

instgroup "root"
    "cam_inst" "light_inst" "cube_inst"
end instgroup

render "root" "cam_inst" "opt"
```

Chapter 4

Geometry Shaders

4.1 Introduction

Geometry shaders can be used in two places: in instance definitions that reference a shader instead of an object, light, camera, or instance group:

```
instance "name"
    geometry function
    ...
end instance
```

or in phenomena, where they can be attached to the geometry root:

```
declare phenomenon
    ...
    geometry function
    ...
end declare
```

In either case, the geometry shader is evaluated during scene preprocessing before any other operation such as rendering starts. The geometry shader is expected to create an object, light, camera, or instance group and add the tag of the created element to the result. The *result* pointer passed as its first argument always has the type `miTag *`, and the shader must be declared as

```
declare shader
```

```
    geometry "shader_name" ("parameter_decl")
    ...
end declare
```

If *result* is a null tag, the created element can be returned directly using this pointer, otherwise the geometry shader must check whether the type of the item to which *result* refers is `miSCENE_GROUP`. If it refers to an instance group, the created entities can be put into this group, otherwise the shader must create the group and put the element to which *result* refers together with the entities created by the geometry shader into the instance group. The newly created instance group must be returned in *result* in this case. This ensures that geometry shaders always return either an object or an instance group, and that they can be chained such that the end result is a group. There is a shader interface function available for adding scene entities to *result* which takes all the above rules into account; refer to *mi_geoshader_add_result*.

Creation of geometry requires an altogether different set of shader interface functions. The shader is basically doing the same thing that an object or other definition expressed in the .mi language is doing, and must have the same functionality available to it. In fact, the shader interface functions for geometry shaders closely model the .mi language features: there are *begin/end* functions for most top-level entities and complex sub-entities, and various helper functions to create and attach complex information. Many of these return pointers to the created data structures that let the geometry shader store primitive data directly without the use of a shader interface function.

Geometry shaders must include `geoshader.h` after `shader.h`. Note that this file is not compatible between mental ray 2.0 and mental ray 2.1 because a number of features that were introduced in mental ray 2.1 required extra fields in data structures such as `miBox`. This means that geometry shaders compiled for mental ray 2.0 will not, in general, work with mental ray 2.1, and vice versa!

This chapter provides an example and lists all shader interface API functions and data structure declarations available to geometry shaders. It does not explain the structure and order of specific API calls needed to create a scene. Refer to the "Scene Description Language" section for the sequence of operations necessary to create a scene element, and to appendix A for the correspondence between API calls and the entities in the scene description language they create.

In any case, writing geometry shaders is far more complex than writing another type of shader. Although a geometry shader has free run of the entire scene database, and is free to alter or create any part of it, it is generally a good idea to avoid doing too much with them. Instead, it is usually preferable to pass objects, materials, and shaders as input parameters instead of creating entire graphs in geometry shaders, although this is possible and sometimes needed in geometry shaders used in phenomena. Normally, geometry shaders should not modify existing parts of the scene because this can confuse future incremental changes and scene traversal during preprocessing, which geometry shaders are part of. Instead, the element to be modified should be passed to the geometry shader as a parameter of type `geometry`, and be used as a template to create a new, modified element.

All geometry shader API calls and data structures may *only* be used in geometry shaders, not any other type of shader. Conversely, no regular shader interface function related to rendering may be used in a geometry shader because it is called before rendering begins. Geometry shaders are called during the same stage as displacement shaders, but before the displacement shaders of objects created by this geometry shader.

4.2 Examples

The following example shader creates an axis-aligned unit cube at the origin. Using unit sizes and centering objects at the origin is usually a good idea because the position, orientation, and sizes of objects are better adjusted with instances than by hardcoding them into the object. This assumes that mental ray is switched to object space mode, which is recommended for all scenes anyway (this is done in the `options` statement).

```
#include <shader.h>
#include <geoshader.h>

int geocube_version(void) {return(1);}

#define add_vector(x, y, z) \
   v.x = x; v.y = y; v.z = z;\
   mi_api_geovector_xyz_add(&v);

static int vertex_order[] = {
   0, 3, 5, 4,
   3, 2, 6, 5,
   2, 1, 7, 6,
   1, 0, 4, 7
};

miBoolean geocube(
   miTag           *result,
   miState         *state,
   miTag           *mtl)
{
   int             i, k, ix=0;
   miObject        *obj;
   miGeoVector     v;
   miTag           mtl_tag;

   mtl_tag = *mi_eval_tag(&mtl);
   obj = mi_api_object_begin(NULL);
   obj->visible = obj->shadow = obj->trace = miTRUE;
   mi_api_basis_list_clear();
   mi_api_object_group_begin(0.0);

   add_vector(-0.5., -0.5., -0.5.);
   add_vector(-0.5.,  0.5., -0.5.);
   add_vector( 0.5.,  0.5., -0.5.);
   add_vector( 0.5., -0.5., -0.5.);

   add_vector(-0.5., -0.5.,  0.5.);
```

```
        add_vector( 0.5., -0.5.,  0.5.);
        add_vector( 0.5.,  0.5.,  0.5.);
        add_vector(-0.5.,  0.5.,  0.5.);

        for (i=0; i < 4; i++)
                mi_api_vertex_add(i);

        for (i=4; i < 8; i++)
                mi_api_vertex_add(i);

        for (i=0; i < 16; i++)
                mi_api_vertex_add(vertex_order[i]);

        for (i=0; i < 6; i++) {
                mi_api_poly_begin_tag(1, mtl_tag);
                for (k=0; k < 4; k++)
                        mi_api_poly_index_add(ix++);
                mi_api_poly_end();
        }
        mi_api_object_group_end();
        return(mi_geoshader_add_result(result,
                                       mi_api_object_end()));

}
```

The next example creates a trimmed B-Spline free-form surface. There is one trimming curve defined which is used as a hole curve to cut a square hole out of the surface. It also shows how a texture surface can be added to a surface.

```
#include <shader.h>
#include <geoshader.h>

int bspline_surface_version(void) { return 1; }

miBoolean bspline_surface(
   miTag           *result,
   miState         *state,
   void            *paras)
{
   int             i, k;
   miObject        *obj;
   miGeoScalar     knot;
   miDlist         *params, *uparams, *vparams;
   miGeoRange      range;
   miApprox        approx;
   miTag           otag;
   miVector cp[] = {
           /* ----- 16 surface control points */
           {0, 2, 0}, {1, 2, 0}, {2, 2, 0}, {3, 2, 0},
           {0, 3, 0}, {1, 3, 1}, {2, 3, 1}, {3, 3, 0},
           {0, 4, 0}, {1, 4, 1}, {2, 4, 1}, {3, 4, 0},
```

```
        {0, 5, 0}, {1, 5, 0}, {2, 5, 0}, {3, 5, 0},
        /* ----- 4 (2d) curve control points */
        {0.4, 0.4, 0}, {0.6, 0.4, 0},
        {0.6, 0.6, 0}, {0.4, 0.6, 0},
        /* ----- 4 (3d) texture surface control points */
        {0,0,0},{1,0,0},{0,1,0},{1,1,0}};
miGeoScalar curve_knots[] = {0, 1, 2, 3, 4};
miUint curve_v[] = {16, 17, 18, 19, 16}; /*closed loop*/
miUint texsurf_v[] = {20,21,22,23};
miGeoScalar tex_uknots[] = {0.0, 1.0};
miGeoScalar tex_vknots[] = {0.0, 1.0};

/* ************ create object ************ */
obj = mi_api_object_begin(NULL);
obj->visible = obj->shadow = obj->trace = miTRUE;

mi_api_basis_list_clear();
mi_api_basis_add(mi_mem_strdup("bspline_3"),
        miFALSE, miBASIS_BSPLINE, 3, 0, 0);
mi_api_basis_add(mi_mem_strdup("bezier_1"),
        miFALSE, miBASIS_BEZIER, 1, 0, 0);

mi_api_object_group_begin(0.0);

/* control points and references */
for(i=0; i < 24; i++)
        mi_api_vector_xyz_add(&cp[i]);
for(i=0; i < 24; i++)
        mi_api_vertex_add(i);

/* ************ create trim-curve ************ */
mi_api_curve_begin(mi_mem_strdup("curve_0"),
        mi_mem_strdup("bezier_1"), miFALSE);

/* curve knot sequence */
params = mi_api_dlist_create(miDLIST_GEOSCALAR);
for(i=0; i < 5; i++)
        mi_api_dlist_add(params, &curve_knots[i]);

/* curve control point references,
   non-rational (w=1) */
for(i=0; i < 5; i++)
        mi_api_vertex_ref_add(curve_v[i], 1.0);

mi_api_curve_end(params);

/* ********** create free-form surface ********** */
mi_api_surface_begin_tag(mi_mem_strdup("surf_0"), 0);

/* create the uv knot vectors for the
   (bezier) surface */
for (k=0; k < 2; k++) {
        params = mi_api_dlist_create(
```

```
                                    miDLIST_GEOSCALAR);
        knot = 0.0;
        for(i=0; i < 4; i++)
                mi_api_dlist_add(params, &knot);
        knot = 1.0;
        for(i=0; i < 4; i++)
                mi_api_dlist_add(params, &knot);
        mi_api_surface_params(k == 0 ? miU : miV,
                mi_mem_strdup("bspline_3"),
                           0., 1., params, miFALSE);
}

/* control point references, nonrational(w=1) */
for(i=0; i < 16; i++)
        mi_api_vertex_ref_add(i, 1.0);

/* ************ add a texture surface *********** */
uparams = mi_api_dlist_create(miDLIST_GEOSCALAR);
for (i=0; i < 2; i++)
        mi_api_dlist_add(uparams, &tex_uknots[i]);
vparams = mi_api_dlist_create(miDLIST_GEOSCALAR);
for (i=0; i < 2; i++)
        mi_api_dlist_add(vparams, &tex_vknots[i]);
mi_api_surface_texture_begin(miFALSE,/* is_volume */
                         miFALSE,   /* is_bump */
                         mi_mem_strdup("bezier_1"),
                         uparams,
                         miFALSE,   /* v_rational */
                         mi_mem_strdup("bezier_1"),
                         vparams,
                         miFALSE);  /* v_rational */
/* texture surface control point references, nonrational */
for(i=0; i < 4; i++)
        mi_api_vertex_ref_add(texsurf_v[i], 1.0);

/* define one hole curve on the surface */
range.min = 0.0;
range.max = 4.0;
mi_api_surface_curveseg(miTRUE,         /* newloop */
                        miCURVE_HOLE,
                        mi_mem_strdup("curve_0"),
                        &range);

mi_api_surface_end();

/* set approximation method for the surface */
miAPPROX_DEFAULT(approx);
approx.method = miAPPROX_CURVATURE;
approx.cnst[miCNST_DISTANCE] = 0.01;
mi_api_surface_approx(mi_mem_strdup("surf_0"),
                      &approx);

/* set approximation method for the curve */
```

```
        miAPPROX_DEFAULT(approx);
        approx.method = miAPPROX_PARAMETRIC;
        approx.cnst[miCNST_UPARAM] = 1;
        mi_api_curve_approx(mi_mem_strdup("curve_0"),
                            &approx);

        mi_api_object_group_end();
        otag = mi_api_object_end();
        return(mi_geoshader_add_result(result, otag);
}
```

The next example accepts an object as input, and creates a new object based on the input object. The new object is identical to the old one except that only points in space are copied and all normals, texture vectors, motion, and other information is ignored. Also, it deals with groups correctly only if it does not contain multiple local spaces because it ignores the transformation matrices in the instance loop.

```
#include <assert.h>
#include "shader.h"
#include "geoshader.h"

int facet_version(void) {return(1);}

static miBoolean box_to_object(
   miTag           *result,
   miBox           *box)
{
   int             i, vs = box->vert_info.sizeof_vertex;
   miObject        *obj;
   miIndex         *vert = miBOX_GET_VERTICES(box);
   miTriangle      *tri  = miBOX_GET_PRIMITIVES(box);
   miVector        norm;

   assert(box->type == miBOX_TRIANGLES);
   obj = mi_api_object_begin(NULL);
   obj->visible = obj->shadow = obj->trace = miTRUE;
   mi_api_basis_list_clear();
   mi_api_object_group_begin(0.0);

   for (i=0; i < box->vect_info.no_points; i++)
           mi_api_vector_xyz_add(box->vectors + i);

   for (i=0; i < box->no_vertices; i++, vert+=vs)
           mi_api_vertex_add(*vert);

   for (i=0; i < box->no_primitives; i++, tri++) {
           mi_api_poly_begin_tag(1, 0);
           mi_api_poly_index_add(tri->a);
           mi_api_poly_index_add(tri->b);
           mi_api_poly_index_add(tri->c);
           mi_api_poly_end();
```

```
    }
    mi_api_object_group_end();
    return(mi_geoshader_add_result(result,
                                   mi_api_object_end()));
}

miBoolean facet(
    miTag          *result,
    miState        *state,
    miTag          *param)
{
    miTag          leaves, scan, boxes, next;
    miBoolean      ret;

    ret = mi_geoshader_tesselate(state, &leaves,
                                 *mi_eval_tag(param));

    for (scan=leaves; scan; scan=next) {
            miInstance *inst = mi_db_access(scan);
            for (boxes=inst->boxes; boxes; boxes=next) {
                    miBox *box = mi_db_access(boxes);
                    ret &= box_to_object(result, box);
                    next = box->next_box;
                    mi_db_unpin(boxes);
            }
            next = inst->next;
            mi_db_unpin(scan);
    }
    mi_geoshader_tesselate_end(leaves);
    return(ret);
}
```

The main *facet* shader first tessellates the input geometry. This builds a leaf instance list containing a sequence of instances that contain both an *item* field pointing to the source geometry (which may be difficult to handle because it may include many different types of complex free-form surface and polygonal geometry), and a *boxes* field that points to triangles. Without mi_geoshader_-tesselate, the *boxes* field may be empty, and the shader would have to do its own traversal to find the instances.

The following nested loops consider all instances, and all boxes in each instance. There are multiple instances if the input object passed to the shader as its only parameter is an instance group or a merge group. An instance may contain multiple boxes if the object has too many vectors, vertices, or triangles to fit into a single box. For each box, a new object is generated by calling *box_to_object*, which is similar to the previous example except that it gets its information from a box. Every new object is appended to the result using *mi_geoshader_add_result*.

Finally, the shader calls *mi_geoshader_tesselate_end* to release the instance list, including all triangle boxes, that was created by mi_geoshader_tesselate. This is important because this list may be very large, and would introduce a large memory leak if not freed.

4.3 Geometry Shader API

The API module has been patterned after the .mi2 language, to the point where the .mi2 *yacc* grammar consists almost entirely of one or very few API calls or variable assignments for every statement and clause. To understand the correct order of API calls, refer to the .mi2 language description. The complete *yacc* grammar that parses the .mi2 language, including C code, is reprinted in the appendix of this document. For information on the syntax of a *yacc* grammar description, refer to the Unix manual page for *yacc*.

Note that all character string arguments passed to any of the API functions below are expected to have been allocated with *mi_mem_allocate* or, more commonly, *mi_mem_strdup*. All API functions release such strings using *mi_mem_release*, so the same allocated string may not be passed to API twice. Similarly, `miDlists` created with *mi_api_dlist_create* and passed as an argument to an API call are freed by API, and should not be passed to API twice. The reason for this is that API keeps most strings for extended periods of time, so allocation is almost always necessary *somewhere*, and putting the burden on the API caller avoids double allocations in cases where the caller works with allocated strings anyway (for example in *yacc* parsers). In the few cases where API could work with non-allocated strings (*mi_api_debug*, for example) allocation is required anyway to avoid requiring allocation for some strings but not others, which would invite hard-to-find bugs. Functions whose name does not begin with *mi_api_* generally do not require string allocation.

Most API functions return a boolean, a pointer, or a tag. If the function succeeds, `miTRUE`, a non-null pointer, or a non-null tag is returned, respectively. If an error occurs, `miFALSE` or a null pointer or tag is returned; this means that errors can be caught with C's "`!`" operator. The tags returned by the calls whose names end in `_end` are merely a convenience; they are not generally useful to standard name-based translators.

Note that many of these functions come in *begin* and *end* pairs, such as *mi_api_object_begin* and *mi_api_object_end*. These calls may not be interleaved in any way; there may only be one "pending" unfinished *begin* block at any time.

4.3.1 Symbol Tables

The API module identifies all entities by name. Different name spaces are provided for different purposes. In particular, the API module supports both the .mi1 and .mi2 languages, which have a different name space concept. The .mi2 module uses a shared global name space for all element types, while the .mi1 format uses separate name spaces for each element type.

Note that shader parameter names do not use a persistent name space and have no assigned symbol table. Shader parameters are stored in declarations and are not accessible in any symbol table. There are also other short-lived sub-entities such as curves or surfaces that are not stored in symbol tables.

In general, symbol tables are used by the API module internally only. There is normally no need for another module to access specific symbol tables. However, API provides lookup functions for symbol tables that return the tag for individual named entities. This can be used for accessing the tessellated renderable representation of a geometric object, or for applying low-level SCENE functions to entities created with API functions.

For example, the API module can be used to set up a small scene consisting of a single free-form surface object, which is then "rendered" using a render function that does not call any renderer, but uses the symbol table to find the object's tag, accesses the tessellated geometry, and displays a wireframe of the tessellation in a GUI window. This is a useful application of API because it visualizes the effects of user-defined approximation modes.

The following table lists the symbol tables. All except the global and variable symbol tables are used for .mi1 entities (bracketed by `frame` and `end frame` statements) only.

table	purpose
S_GLOBAL	all .mi2 entities
S_FUNCDECL	Function declarations (`declare` statements)
S_OPTIONS	Options (`options` statements)
S_CAMERA	Cameras (`camera` statements)
S_LIGHT	Lights (`light` statements)
S_OBJECT	Geometric objects (`object` statements)
S_INSTANCE	Instances (`instance` statements)
S_INSTGROUP	Instance groups (`group` statements)
S_MATERIAL	Materials (`material` statements)
S_CTEXTURE	Color textures (`color texture` statements)
S_STEXTURE	Scalar textures (`scalar texture` statements)
S_VTEXTURE	Vector textures (`vector texture` statements)
S_VARIABLE	For internal use only

It is possible to use the symbol table lookup functions defined by the LIB module (see the LIB chapter) for direct lookups. However, API defines a number of specialized functions that perform lookups required during parsing:

```
miTag mi_api_name_lookup(
    char *          name)
```

Look up the element *name* in the .mi2 element and function declaration symbol tables (`S_GLOBAL` and `S_FUNCDECL`, and return the tag if found. Otherwise, return a null tag. Other symbol tables are not searched because .mi1 elements are temporary and disappear when the current frame ends.

```
miTag mi_api_decl_lookup(
    char *          name)
```

Same thing but just for shader declarations. This is a separate function because if an object and a declaration have the same name (this is legal because they are in different name spaces), *mi_api_name_lookup* will never see the declaration and always return the other object.

```
miBoolean mi_api_variable_set(
    char            *name,     /* variable name */
    char            *value)    /* value or 0 to unset */
```

Set a variable *name* to a value *value*. If *value* is a null pointer, delete the variable. Variables can be redefined. The main purpose is to store meta-data in .mi scene files using the `set` command for variables such as author, translator, creation date, etc, whose values can be picked up by the client application or even a shader.

```
const char *mi_api_variable_lookup(
    char            *name)     /* variable name */
```

Return the value of the variable *name*, as set with a preceding *mi_api_variable_set*. If the variable is not defined, a null pointer is returned. The returned string should not be modified or released.

```
const char *mi_api_tag_lookup(
    miTag           tag)
```

This is a reverse lookup function. Given a tag, it scans all symbol tables for an element with this tag and returns its name. This function is intended for printing more helpful error messages if only a tag is known, and to allow database dumps containing names. If the tag cannot be found, a null pointer is returned. A non-null pointer should not be modified or released, it points directly into the symbol table.

```
miTag mi_api_light_lookup(
    char            *name)     /* instance to look up */
```

Look up a light by name and return its tag. If no light by this name is found, return a null tag.

```
miTag mi_api_material_lookup(
    char            *name)     /* material to look up */
```

Look up a material by name and return its tag. If no material by this name is found, return a null tag.

```
miTag mi_api_texture_lookup(
    char            *name,     /* texture to find */
    int             type)      /* 0=col, 1=scal, 2=vec */
```

Look up a texture by name and return its tag. If no texture by this name is found, return a null tag. *type* is the desired texture type: `0` for color textures, 1 for scalar textures, and 2 for vector textures.

```
miBoolean mi_api_surface_lookup(
    char            *name,      /* name of face */
    miTag           *instance, /* instance with face */
    miGeoIndex      *idx)       /* index of face */
```

Look up a surface by name and return its tag. If no surface by this name is found, return `miFALSE`, otherwise return `miTRUE`. This function can be used only while defining a geometric object group, between *mi_object_group_begin* and *mi_object_group_end*. Its purpose is finding surfaces to be connected for `connection` statements. The surface instance tag (not currently used) and the surface index (a sequential number beginning with 0 in every object that enumerates the surfaces in the object) are also returned.

```
void *mi_api_curve_lookup(
    char                *name,     /* existing curve */
    enum miCurve_type type,      /* type of curve */
    miBoolean           newloop,  /* is this a new loop */
    miGeoRange          *range,   /* range of the curve */
    int                 *no_scalars)
```

Look up a curve by name and type and return an identifying pointer. If no curve by this name is found, return a null pointer. The curve type is one of `miCURVE_TRIM`, `miCURVE_HOLE`, and `miCURVE_SPECIAL`, as defined by the SCENE module. This function is used when a surface references a curve as a trim, hole, or special curve with the given range. This function not only looks up the curve, but also creates a new curve reference entry containing the curve identifier, the *type*, whether this curve begins a new loop or continues an old one (*newloop*), and the parameter *range* of the curve to use. The number of parameters of the curve is returned in **no_scalars*. This function may only be used during the definition of a surface. Because of the side effects, this is not a true lookup function.

4.3.2 Dynamic Lists

Dynamic lists (*dlists*) are used by API to buffer certain types of data where it is not known in advance how many will be needed. They are implemented as linked lists of pages. For example, surface and curve parameter lists are sequences of numbers or number pairs that are collected in a *dlist*, which is then passed to an appropriate API function.

There are seven types of *dlists* containing different data types:

dlist type	data type	purpose
miDLIST_SCALAR	miScalar	single precision
miDLIST_GEOSCALAR	miGeoScalar	double precision
miDLIST_DOUBLE	double	double precision
miDLIST_INTEGER	int	integer
miDLIST_POINTER	void *	generic pointer
miDLIST_VREF	struct miVref	rational parameter
miDLIST_TAG	miTag	material tag list

The *miVref* structure contains an integer parameter value and a double-precision floating-point weight. It is used for parameter lists of rational curves and surfaces. Tag lists are currently used only for material arrays in instances.

```
typedef struct miVref {
    int          ref;
    miGeoScalar  w;
} miVref;
```

There are three API functions that deal with dynamic lists, one to create a list, one to append data to a list, and one to delete the list after it has been passed to another API function that expects a dynamic list:

```
miDlist *mi_api_dlist_create(
    int               type)
```

Create a dynamic list of the specified type. The *type* argument must be one of the standard dlist types such as `miDLIST_SCALAR`. The returned pointer identifies the list and is passed to the other API functions.

```
miBoolean mi_api_dlist_add(
    register miDlist *dlp,
    void              *data)
```

Append data to an existing dlist. The *elem* pointer argument must point to a data entry of the type that agrees with the type of the dlist, as listed in the second column of the dlist type table above.

```
miBoolean mi_api_dlist_delete(
    miDlist          *dlp)
```

Delete the dlist. The dlist pointer may not be used after this call. dlists passed to an API function (other than *mi_api_dlist_add* are deleted automatically, so this call is not normally needed.

```
miTag mi_api_taglist(
    miDlist          *list)
```

Convert a dlist of type `miDLIST_TAG` to a scene element of type `miSCENE_TAG`, and return the tag of the new scene element. If the dlist has the wrong type or is empty, a null tag is returned. This can be used to create a material list for instances.

4.3.3 Incremental Changes

```
miBoolean mi_api_incremental(
    miBoolean        incr)
```

Enable or disable incremental mode. Incremental mode is off by default. If turned on, the next options, camera, texture, light, material, object, instance, or instance group definition (initiated with the appropriate *begin* call listed below) is not created with fresh defaults, but with the values it was created with earlier. It is an error to request an incremental change to an element that does not exist, and to define an element that already exists without specifying incremental mode first. Incremental mode is automatically reset after the following *begin* call it applies to; it is generally unnecessary to call *mi_api_incremental* with a `miFALSE` argument.

Note that although the API module establishes all links in the scene graph with name strings, the strings are immediately converted to tags by all API functions. All internal links in the graph use tags. This means that if an element is created with a certain name, and this name is passed to another function to establish a link, the link remains intact only if all future changes to the named element are done in incremental mode. If the element were instead deleted and recreated with the same name, the same name would be associated with a new tag, and all previous links would become stale. It is therefore important to use incremental mode even when modifying elements that do not actually retain information when changed, such as instance groups.

4.3.4 Options, Cameras, and Outputs

Any scene needs at least one camera and at least one options block. In a frame block they are implicitly created at frame begin; in the .mi2 language they must be created explicitly with the following calls.

```
miOptions    *mi_api_options_begin(
    char             *name)      /* name of options */
```

Create an options element and return a pointer to it. The options element is created with default parameters. The caller may modify the defaults by writing directly into the returned structure. Any number of options entities can be created but only one of them can be named in any render operation.

```
miTag mi_api_options_end (void)
```

After modifying the default options, this function must be called to complete the options definition. If an error occurs, a null tag is returned; otherwise the tag of the new options element is returned. The type of the returned element is `miSCENE_OPTIONS`.

```
miCamera *mi_api_camera_begin(
    char              *name)      /* name of camera */
```

Create a camera element and return a pointer to it. The caller can use the pointer to modify the defaults.

```
miTag mi_api_camera_end (void)
```

Complete the definition of the camera, after all parameters have been adjusted. If an error occurs, a null tag is returned; otherwise the tag of the new camera element is returned. The type of the returned element is `miSCENE_CAMERA`.

```
miTag mi_api_output_file_def(
    miUlong           typemap,   /* data type bitmap */
    miUlong           interpmap, /* interp req bitmap */
    char              *format,   /* file type string */
    char              *fname)    /* file name */
```

Define an output file and return an output function describing the file to write. The returned function has a special type code that tells *mi_api_output_shaders* to write a file instead of calling an output shader, and has the given format and file name encoded in its parameter area. It is not a normal shading function but can be treated as one by the caller, and can be appended to the camera's *output* function list.

When the output list is evaluated after rendering, this definition will write a frame buffer to the named file *fname*, using the file format *format*. Valid formats are extension strings such as `"rgb"` or `"rla"`; refer to the user's manual for a complete list. The *typemap* is a bitmap. Valid bit numbers are defined by the `miImg_type` enum as defined by the IMG module. Each bit informs the renderer that this shader requires a frame buffer of this type; at rendering time all active bitmaps (those defined in the camera used for rendering) are OR-ed. Only one bit should be set.

The *interpmap* bitmap uses the same pattern as *typemap*. It has a bit set if the frame buffer described by the corresponding set bit in *typemap* should be interpolated.

```
miBoolean mi_api_output_file_parameter(
    miTag             function,       /* output file function */
    miInteger         code,           /* parameter value code */
    void              *value)         /* parameter value pointer */
```

2.1 Supply one parameter value identified by its code to an output file function. The *function* tag identifies the output file function returned by a call to *mi_api_output_file_def*. The output file function is able to store 8 float parameter values. The *code* determines which one of these values will be changed. The actual meaning of a parameter value is not predefined and depends on the file format used. Currently, the `miIMG_FORMAT_JPEG` format interprets the first parameter value as compression quality.

```
miTag mi_api_output_function_def(
    miUlong         typemap,      /* data type bitmap */
    miUlong         interpmap,    /* interp req bitmap */
    miTag           function)     /* output shader */
```

Define an output shader. Like output files, output shaders require a *typemap*. Unlike output files, output shaders may have multiple bits set. The *function* tag identifies the shader to be called. Shader tags are obtained during shader definition, they are returned by *mi_api_function_call_end*. The returned function tag can be appended to the camera's *output* function list by the caller.

The *interpmap* bitmap uses the same pattern as *typemap*. It has a bit set if the frame buffer described by the corresponding set bit in *typemap* should be interpolated.

```
miBoolean mi_api_output_file_override(
    char            *format,
    char            *fname)
```

Specify a file type and a file name that overrides the corresponding arguments of the next *mi_api_output_file_def* call. This call is not normally used to define a scene; it is intended for command-line option parsers that accept overrides for the file type and name specified in the scene. The override function must be called before the call to *mi_api_output_file_def* whose arguments should be overridden.

```
miBoolean mi_api_output_type_identify(
    miUlong         *typemap,     /* type bitmap */
    miUlong         *interpmap,   /* interp bitmap */
    char            *typename)    /* data type */
```

This function converts a type string to a type map as required by the output file and output shader definition functions above. A type string is a comma-separated list of types, such as `"rgba,n,contour"`. The special type `contour` is accepted also; it is the only one that is handled by RC only and not by IMG. All other types are identified in the same way as done by *mi_img_type_identify*. The type bitmap is returned in **typemap*; the bits correspond to 1 shifted left by the `miIMG_TYPE_*` code.

Types can be prefixed with '+' or '-' to turn interpolation on or off for the frame buffer, respectively. Interpolation means that unsampled pixels get a value interpolated from its neighbors, rather than becoming a copy of one of its neighbors. Interpolation is on by default for all kinds of color frame buffers and off for all others. The interpolation bitmap is returned in **interpmap*; the bit layout is the same as for **typemap*.

```
miBoolean mi_api_output_imfdisp_handle(
    miTag            camera_tag)    /* camera tag */
```

This function should be called after all output files have been defined. For every output file in the camera's output list of camera specified by *camera_tag*, a 128-byte file is created, containing the image resolution and the gamma factor from the camera, as well as information about how to open a socket to mental ray and version information. This information is understood by programs such as `imf_disp` which can connect to mental ray during rendering and show the rendered image as it is being created. Note that mental ray, when connected to in this way, will always transfer the RGBA picture regardless of the type of the file used to establish the connection.

```
miBoolean mi_api_output_list(
    miTag            cam_tag)    /* camera tag */
    miTag            opt_tag)    /* options tag */
```

This function calls mi_phen_output_list, which collects all the type maps from the output list in the given camera and places appropriate frame buffer records into the options structure specified by *tag*. This function is no longer used; RC calls *mi_phen_output_list* directly after output shaders introduced by phenomena have been added. *mi_api_output_list* may be removed in a future version of mental ray because it doesn't take phenomena into account, which means it generates incomplete frame buffer lists.

```
miBoolean mi_api_output_shaders(
    miTag            cam_inst_tag,    /* camera inst */
    miTag            opt_tag,         /* options tag */
    miTag            *images)         /* frame bufs */
```

This function is obsolete since output shaders are called from *mi_rc_render*. Therefore it prints a warning and always returns `miTRUE`. The output list remains unchanged in the process.

```
miBoolean mi_api_framebuffer(
    miOptions        *opt,            /* set framebuffer here */
    int              n,               /* frame buffer 0..7 to set */
    char             *type)           /* frame buffer type: "+rgba" etc */
```

This function sets or clears the definition of a user-defined frame buffer. There are up to eight user frame buffers numbered 0 through 7. Each can have an arbitrary user-defined type. The same types as for output statements are available, such as `+rgba`, `-z`, `m`, etc. As for output statements, "+" indicates sample interpolation and "-" indicates padding. If the type is a null pointer, the frame buffer is deleted from the options. Shaders can access these frame buffers with the *mi_fb_get* and *mi_fb_put* functions.

4.3.5 Lights, Materials, Textures

```
miLight *mi_api_light_begin(
    char                *name)        /* light name */
```

Begin the definition of a light with the specified *name*. A pointer to the light is returned; the caller may modify the structure.

```
miBoolean mi_api_light_end (void)
```

Complete the definition of a light after all parameters have been set.

```
miMaterial *mi_api_material_begin(
    char                *name)       /* material name */
```

Begin the definition of a material with the specified *name*. A pointer to the material is returned; the caller may modify the structure.

```
miTag mi_api_material_end (void)
```

Complete the definition of a material after all parameters have been set. If an error occurs, a null tag is returned; otherwise the tag of the new material element is returned. The type of the returned element is `miSCENE_MATERIAL`.

```
miTag mi_api_texture_begin(
    char                *name,       /* texture name */
    int                 type,        /* 0=col, 1=scal, 2=vec*/
    int                 flags)       /* bit0=loc, bit1=filt */
```

Begin the definition of a texture with the specified *name*. In incremental mode, the tag of the existing texture to be changed is returned; otherwise a null tag is returned. The tag is useful mainly to determine whether the previous texture was an image or a shader, using the *mi_db_type* function. The *type* of the texture and a *flags* bitmap must also be specified.

Bit 0 of the flags, if set, specifies that the texture is local. This is meaningful for image textures only, it specifies that each host on the network should read the image from its local file system instead of fetching the texture across the network. Memory-mapped textures are not flagged explicitly; they are recognized automatically at load time. Bit 1 of the flags, if set, specifies that the texture image is looked up using a filter. This flag is ignored for procedural (function) textures.

Bit 1 of the flags, if set, enables pyramid filtering, an algorithm comparable to mip-map textures. mental ray will convert the texture to pyramid format, which takes about 30% more memory but allows filtered lookups. This avoids texture aliasing, which is a problem for point-sampled non-filter textures that are far away so that each point sample hits widely spaced pixels in the texture.

This call is always the first stage of creating a texture and must be followed by one of the next three *def* calls, which complete the texture definition.

```
miTag mi_api_texture_file_def(
    char              *file)      /* file name to open */
```

The new texture is defined as a file texture, using the path *file*. The path must be valid on the local host and, if the texture is local, on all other hosts on the network. If an error occurs, a null tag is returned; otherwise the tag of the new texture element is returned. The type of the returned element is `miSCENE_IMAGE`.

```
miTag mi_api_texture_function_def(
    miTag             function)   /* function with args */
```

The new texture is defined as a procedural texture, using the texture shader *function*. Function tags are created when defining functions, and are returned by *mi_api_function_call_end*. The local flag is ignored for procedural textures. If an error occurs, a null tag is returned; otherwise the tag of the new texture element is returned. The type of the returned element is `miSCENE_FUNCTION`.

```
miBoolean mi_api_texture_array_def_begin(
    int               xres,       /* width in pixels */
    int               yres,       /* height in pixels */
    int               zres)       /* bytes/comp, 1 or 2 */
```

The final method of defining a texture is verbatim. It is equivalent to a file texture except that the pixel data is not read from a file on disk but is stored by the API caller using the texture copy calls below. This kind of texture cannot be flagged local. The texture resolution is set with the *xres* and *yres* arguments. The number of bytes per component is set with the *zres* argument. The number of components per pixel is determined by the *type* argument of the preceding call to *mi_api_texture_begin*: 4 for color textures, 1 for scalar textures, and 2 for vector textures. Vector textures always assume 4 bytes per component (one float) regardless of whether *zres* is 1 or 2. If the verbatim texture is filtered[2.1], only the highest resolution is given with *mi_api_texture_byte_copy*; the lower resolutions of the pyramid are built automatically by mental ray.

```
miBoolean mi_api_texture_byte_copy(
    int            len,       /* number of bytes */
    miUchar        *bytes)    /* from the mi file */
```

After the texture was defined the contents of the texture must be copied. A total of $xres \cdot yres \cdot zres \cdot nc$ bytes must be copied, with *zres* being 4 for vector textures and *nc* being the number of components. The copy function can be called multiple times to collect the required number of bytes, the sum of all *len* arguments must be the total required number of bytes. The byte order is big-endian (MSB first) if $zres \geq 1$. Pixels are stored in pixel scanline order: first the bottom scanline is copied in RGBARGBA... order, then the next scanline, up to the top scanline. Scalar textures have only one component, vector texture pixels are stored U first, then V.

```
miTag mi_api_texture_array_def_end (void)
```

After all texture bytes have been copied, the texture must be completed with this call. If an error occurs, a null tag is returned; otherwise the tag of the new texture element is returned. The type of the returned element is `miSCENE_IMAGE`.

4.3.6 User Data

Sometimes large amounts of opaque data must be entered into the scene that cannot be efficiently handled with shader parameters. For example, shaders may need large amounts of particle data. For this purpose, user data blocks can be defined. A user data block consists of a header describing the data block, and the data itself. User data blocks are named.

```
miUserdata *mi_api_data_begin(
    char           *name,          /* name of user data block */
    int            type,           /* 0=literal, 1=file, 2=declared */
    void           *parm)          /* type 0:size, 1:file, 2:decl */
```

Begin the definition of a user data block named *name*. Its contents can be defined in three different ways: if *type* is `0`, the data must be copied verbatim with *mi_api_data_copy* (see below); if *type* is 1, the data is read from a file; and if *type* is 2, the data is defined similar to regular shader parameters. This last mode is useful if the data block itself is not large but shared among a large number of shaders or other elements. In mode `0`, *parm* is an integer specifying the number of bytes to be stored. In mode 1, *parm* is an allocated string that specifies the file name to load from. In mode 3, *parm* is the tag of a function that the parameters will be taken from (this works exactly like the *params* argument of the *mi_api_instance_end* function except that the declaration can, but doesn't have to, be of type `miFUNCTION_DATA`). This function returns a pointer to the new user data block, which lets the caller set up the `miUserdata` header.

```
miTag mi_api_data_end(void)
```

Complete the definition of the user data block, and return its tag.

```
miTag mi_api_data_append(
    miTag           front,          /* list to append to */
    miTag           back)           /* list to append */
```

Append the *back* user data block list to the *front* user data tag list, and return the first tag of the concatenated list. Either or both lists may be empty (*front* and/or *back* is a null tag). User data block concatenation works the same way as shader list concatenation.

```
miBoolean mi_api_data_byte_copy(
    int             len,            /* number of bytes */
    miUchar         *bytes)         /* bytes from the mi file */
```

Append the given number of bytes to the user data block. The number of bytes may not exceed 1024 bytes. This must be called between *mi_api_data_begin* and *mi_api_data_end* if the *type* of the user data block is 0. It may be called zero or more times, and the sum of all *len* arguments may not exceed the user data block size specified in the begin call. If this function may not be called for type 1 or 2 blocks, it overwrites data from the file or parameters.

```
miTag mi_api_data_lookup(
    char            *name)          /* data block name to look up */
```

Look up the user data block with the given *name*, and returns its tag. If the database element with that name is not a user data block, or if the name is unknown, an error is printed and a null tag is returned.

4.3.7 Instances and Instance Groups

Instances and instance groups are used to construct the scene DAG (directed acyclic graph). Instance groups are unordered lists of one or more instances. Instances are nodes of the DAG, they reference an item to be placed into the DAG together with a space transformation, optional inheritance parameters, and various flags. Elements that can be referenced by instances are geometric objects, cameras, lights, and instance groups. If more than one instance references the same item, this is called *multiple instancing*.

```
miInstance *mi_api_instance_begin(
    char            *name)      /* instance name */
```

Begin the definition of an instance with the given *name*. In incremental mode, a pointer to the existing instance is returned; otherwise a pointer to a temporary instance is returned. It is not necessary to store the various flags and IDs in the instance transformation, this is done during preprocessing.

```
miTag mi_api_instance_end(
    char            *item,      /* item to instance */
    miTag           function,   /* geometry shader */
    miTag           params)     /* transformation func */
```

Complete the definition of the instance. If the instanced item is not a geometry shader, the item to be instanced is given by *item* and *function* must be a null tag. If the instanced item is a geometry shader, the function list is passed in *function* and *item* must be a null pointer. It is an error if both *item* and *function* are requested to be instantiated. Incremental changes from regular to geometry shader instances and vice versa are possible.

The *params* tag is either the null tag (no inheritance parameters), the numerical value `-1` (leave parameters unchanged during an incremental change), or the tag of a function containing inheritance parameters. Only the parameters are used, the function is ignored. The function should be deleted after being passed to *mi_api_instance_end*.

If an error occurs, a null tag is returned; otherwise the tag of the new instance element is returned. The type of the returned element is `miSCENE_INSTANCE`.

```
miBoolean mi_api_instgroup_begin(
    char            *name)      /* group name */
```

Begin the definition of an instance group with the given *name*. The list of elements is not cleared even if incremental mode is disabled.

```
miBoolean mi_api_instgroup_clear(void)
```

After the instance group definition was begun, all its instances references can be cleared with this call, as if *mi_api_instgroup_delitem* had been called for every one of them.

```
miBoolean mi_api_instgroup_additem(
    char            *name)      /* instance name */
```

After the instance group definition was begun, instances can be added to it. The order of the instances being added is irrelevant. Only instances can be added, never elements such as geometric objects directly.

```
miBoolean mi_api_instgroup_delitem(
    char            *name)      /* instance name */
```

After the instance group definition was begun, instances can be deleted from it.

```
miTag mi_api_instgroup_end (void)
```

After all instances have been added to the instance group, this call completes the creation of the instance group. If an error occurs, a null tag is returned; otherwise the tag of the new instance group element is returned. The type of the returned element is `miSCENE_GROUP`.

4.3.8 Geometric Objects

Geometric objects can be divided into polygonal, free-form surface, and space curve[2.1] objects. Each object contains one or more object groups that group geometry. Object groups are maintained for backwards compatibility with the .mi1 language; newer designs should use multiple objects rather than a single object with multiple object groups. Object groups are unrelated to instance groups as described above.

4.3.8.1 Objects

```
miObject *mi_api_object_begin(
    char              *name)      /* object name */
```

Begin the definition of an object with the given *name*. If the *name* parameter is zero, the object is not registered in the symbol tables, so it cannot be referenced by name. In this case the tag returned by *mi_api_object_end* must be used for referencing the object. All geometrical information is deleted regardless of incremental mode. This is the first call of the object definition sequence. After the object begin, first bases are defined if the object contains free-form surfaces. Next, the object group or groups must be defined. The returned `miObject` pointer can be used to write the `visible` and other flags into the object. Note that since the final size of the object is not known at this point, the returned pointer points to a temporary structure that does not contain geometry and that will be deleted by *mi_api_object_end*.

```
miBoolean *mi_api_object_matrix(
    miMatrix          transform)
```

This function is for backwards compatibility with the .mi1 syntax only. It stores the object's texture transformation matrix. It should not be used.

```
miBoolean mi_api_object_group_begin(
    double            merge)      /* merge epsilon */
```

The next step after the begin call is beginning an object group. If the object contains free-form geometry, and the surfaces in the group should be merged automatically (using adjacency detection), a nonzero merge epsilon must be specified. Merge epsilons in objects are a .mi1 feature that has been superseded by .mi2 merge groups; for new designs the *merge* argument should be zero.

```
miBoolean mi_api_object_group_connection(
    char          *surfname1,   /* first surface */
    char          *curvename1,  /* first curve */
    miGeoRange    *range1,      /* of first curve */
    char          *surfname2,   /* second surface */
    char          *curvename2,  /* second curve */
    miGeoRange    *range2)      /* of second curve */
```

After all surfaces in the free-form object have been defined, just before *mi_api_object_group_end* is called, this function can be used to establish connections between surfaces. Connections can only be defined along the trimming curves on the surfaces, which must exist. Untrimmed surfaces cannot be connected, but a trivial trim curve that follows the parameter boundaries such that no part is actually trimmed off is simple to create. A parameter range must be specified for both curves.

```
miBoolean mi_api_object_group_end(void)
```

After all geometry in the object group has been defined, this function completes the object group definition. Another group can be begun after ending the current one.

```
miTag mi_api_object_end (void)
```

Complete the finished object. This is the last call of the object definition sequence. If an error occurs, a null tag is returned; otherwise the tag of the new object or group element is returned. API decides whether to create and return an object or an instance group element based on the object complexity: if it has multiple object groups, or a merge epsilon, or connections, an instance group is created that has the *merge_group* flag set, and references one or more instances, each of which references an object element containing a single object group. If there is only one object group, no merge epsilon, and no connections, the object is created and returned directly without creating intermediate instances or connections. This decision is transparent to the caller; the tessellator accepts instance groups in this case as well as objects. The type of the returned element is either `miSCENE_OBJECT` or `miSCENE_GROUP`.

4.3.8.2 Bases

Objects containing free-form surfaces must contain at least one basis. A basis defines the curve type or one of the two surface parameter axis types (e.g., NURBS or Bézier), a rational flag, and the degree. All surfaces in all object groups of an object share the same basis list in the object, and reference bases by name.

```
miBoolean mi_api_basis_list_clear (void)
```

Delete all bases in the current object basis list. This function is largely obsolete because it is implicitly called when beginning and ending objects.

```
miBoolean mi_api_basis_add(
    char             *name,       /* name of basis */
    miBoolean        rational,    /* rational surface? */
    enum miBasis_type type,       /* basis type */
    miUshort         degree,      /* degree of basis */
    miUshort         stepsize,    /* opt. step size */
    miDlist          *matrix)     /* opt. basis matrix */
```

Append a basis to the basis list of the current object. The basis *name*, a *rational* flag, the basis *type*, and the *degree* must be defined. The matrix *stepsize* and the basis *matrix* must be defined only for the basis matrix type. The matrix is passed as a dlist (dynamic list, see above) because its size depends on the degree of the basis; $(degree + 1)^2$ floating-point numbers of type `miGeoScalar` are expected.

```
miGeoIndex mi_api_basis_lookup(
    char             *name,       /* basis to look up */
    miBoolean        *rational,   /* rational flag */
    miUshort         *degree)     /* returned degree */
```

This function allows basis lookups by basis name. The sequential number of the basis in the object's basis list is returned, as well as the rational flag and the degree if the second and third arguments are non-null pointers. This function is not essential for scene definition.

4.3.8.3 Polygonal Geometry

An object group can contain either polygonal or free-form surface geometry. Polygonal geometry requires the definition of three blocks of data: vectors, vertices, and polygons. Optionally, an approximation may be given which is used by the tessellator for displacement-mapped polygons.

```
miBoolean mi_api_geovector_xyz_add(
    miGeoVector      *newvec)    /* vector to append */

miBoolean mi_api_vector_xyz_add(
    miVector         *newvec)    /* vector to append */
```

After beginning the object group that should contain polygonal geometry, one call to this function for every XYZ vector to be used must be done. Vectors will be referenced by sequential number, beginning with 0 in every object group, to be used as points in space, normals, motion vectors, and various other purposes. There are restrictions of vector sharing; for example, a vector cannot be used as a point in space and a normal at the same time. Also, vectors should be listed in a certain order (points in space first, then normals, and so on) for maximum efficiency. Any other order will be re-sorted automatically.

There are two versions of this call. The first accepts single-precision vectors and the second accepts double-precision vectors. Both store the vectors in double precision. If the vector is available in double precision, always use *mi_api_geovector_xyz_add* to avoid precision loss. Both versions can be mixed, they are identical except for the argument type.

```
miBoolean mi_api_vector_lookup(
    miGeoVector     *pos,       /* vertex position */
    int             idx)        /* index of vector */
```

This function looks up a vector in the current object by index, and returns its value. This function is not essential for scene definition.

```
miBoolean mi_api_vertex_add(
    int             p)          /* point in space */

miBoolean mi_api_vertex_normal_add(
    int             n)          /* normal vector */

miBoolean mi_api_vertex_deriv_add(
    int             u,          /* dPdu derivative */
    int             v)          /* dPdv derivative */

miBoolean mi_api_vertex_deriv2_add(
    int             u,          /* d2Pdu2 derivative */
    int             v,          /* d2Pdv2 derivative */
    int             uv)         /* d2Pduv derivative */

miBoolean mi_api_vertex_tex_add(
    int             t,          /* texture parameter vector */
    int             x,          /* X basis vec or -1 */
    int             y)          /* Y basis vec or -1 */

miBoolean mi_api_vertex_motion_add(
    int             m)          /* motion vector */

miBoolean mi_api_vertex_user_add(
    int             u)          /* user vector */
```

After all vectors have been defined, vertices must be defined. Vertices must contain a point in space, defined with *mi_api_vertex_add*, optionally followed by a normal, first and second surface derivatives, one or more texture vectors with optional bump basis vectors, a motion vector, and one or more user vectors. After the initial point in space, the order of the other calls is fixed. Vectors are referenced by sequential number in the object group, with 0 being the first vector. A vector index -1 means "none," which is useful for defining texture vectors without bump basis vectors. Either no or two bump basis vector indices must be given. All *add* functions until the next call to *mi_api_vertex_add* or the end of the vertex list append to the current vertex. The next *mi_api_vertex_add* begins the next vertex.

```
miBoolean mi_api_vertex_lookup(
    miGeoVector      *pos,      /* vertex position */
    int              idx)       /* index of vertex */
```

This functions looks up the point in space of the vertex specified by the index *idx*. Vertices, like vectors, are sequentially beginning with 0 in every object group. This function is not essential for scene definition.

```
miBoolean mi_api_poly_begin(
    int              type,      /* 0=concave, 1=convex */
    char             *material) /* material name */
```

```
miBoolean mi_api_poly_begin_tag(
    int              type,       /* 0=concave, 1=convex */
    miTag            material)   /* material tag */
```

After all vectors and vertices have been defined, polygons are defined. Each polygon requires a begin call followed by at least three index add calls followed by an end call. Optionally, holes may be defined. At this time, *type* must be either 0 (concave or unknown) or 1 (convex). Specifying type 1 improves performance because the tessellator does not need to test the convexity of the polygon. The first polygon in an object group must always specify a material by either a name or a tag, therefore the two begin functions are provided. For all following polygons, a null pointer or a null tag may be passed to specify "same material as before in the same object group." This improves API performance. In the case of tagged objects, the material pointer or tag *must* be null; the label is passed as an extra index (using *mi_api_poly_index_add*) before the regular vertex indices.

```
miBoolean mi_api_poly_index_add(
    int      idx)               /* new index to append */
```

After the polygon begin call, at least three vertices must be specified by index. The first vertex in the current object group has index 0. The order is significant; polygon vertices must be defined in counter-clockwise order. Polygons (and their holes) should be planar. Small deviations are handled gracefully but very large deviations may lead to unpredictable behavior. This function is also used to store the polygon label directly after *mi_api_poly_begin* if the object is tagged.

```
miBoolean mi_api_poly_hole_add (void)
```

After the boundary loop of the polygon has been specified using index add calls, this call may be used to indicate the end of the current loop and the beginning of a hole loop. Hole loops, like boundary loops, consist of a sequence of at least three index add calls. No two loops may intersect, and a hole loop must be fully contained in the boundary loop in the plane of the polygon.

```
miBoolean mi_api_poly_end (void)
```

After all boundary and optional hole loops have been added, the polygon must be completed with this call. After the end call, a new polygon may be begun.

```
miBoolean mi_api_poly_approx(
    miApprox          *approx)       /* approx technique */
```

After the last polygon an approximation statement may be specified. It is used by the tessellator for displacement-mapped polygons only. Displacement mapping is a feature of the material assigned to polygons.

4.3.8.4 Free-Form Surface Geometry

Object groups containing free-form surfaces also consist of three sections: the vector list, the vertex list (more accurately called the control point list), and the curve and surface lists. The vector list is defined using one call to *mi_api_vector_xyz_add* for every vector. All vectors have three components X, Y, Z; weights for rational curves and surfaces are specified as part of the vertex references later.

The vertex list is defined with calls to *mi_api_vertex_add*, exactly like in the polygonal case, except that all normals, textures, and other optional vertex information except motion vectors is ignored and should not be specified. Surfaces always compute their own normals, and there are special constructs for textures and bump maps.

The curve and surface list uses the vertices defined in the first section as control points. Curves can be used as trimming curves, hole curves, and special curves. Vertices can also be used as special points on surfaces. Special points and special curves are always included in the tessellated surface.

```
miBoolean mi_api_surface_begin(
    char              *name,      /* surface name */
    char              *mtlname)   /* material name */
```

Begin the definition of a surface with the given *name*. The name is valid only inside the object group and is used for connections and approximations. The given material is assigned to the surface. The name may not be a null pointer.

```
miBoolean mi_api_surface_begin_tag(
    char              *name,      /* surface name */
    miTag             mtltag)     /* material name */
```

This function is similar to *mi_api_surface_begin*, but instead of a name a material tag must be specified. This tag may not be a null tag.

```
miBoolean mi_api_surface_params(
    int             dimen,        /* miU or muV */
    char            *basis_name, /* basis for U or V */
    miGeoScalar     range_min,    /* minimum range */
    miGeoScalar     range_max,    /* maximum range */
    miDlist         *params,      /* params for U or V */
    miBoolean       rational)     /* rational flag */
```

A surface has two parameter directions, U and V. After the surface begin call, both must be defined with this call, once with *dimen* = `miU` and once with *dimen* = `miV`. Both times, the basis name as defined at the beginning of the object definition must be given, as well as the parameter range, the surface parameter list, and the rational flag. The rational flag can either be set here or in the basis; the latter is recommended. The rational flag can be specified here for backwards compatibility with the .mi1 language.

The parameter list is a dlist (dynamic list, see above) containing the parameter vector. The length of this vector depends on the basis; refer to the .mi2 language specification in the mental ray manual for the exact numbers. The type of the dlist is `miDLIST_GEOSCALAR`, containing floating-point numbers of type `miGeoScalar`.

```
miBoolean mi_api_vertex_ref_add(
    int     ref,              /* vertex reference */
    double  w)                /* homogeneous coordinate */
```

After both surface parameter vectors have been specified, the control points must be listed. The number of control points depends on both bases and the length of their parameter vectors; again refer to the mental ray manual for details. For every control point one call to *mi_api_vertex_ref_add* is required. If both bases are non-rational, it is sufficient to specify a vertex index *ref*. As with polygons, `0` selects the first vertex in the current object group. For rational bases, a weight *w* must be given for every control point reference.

```
miBoolean mi_api_surface_curveseg(
    miBoolean           newloop,    /* new loop? */
    enum miCurve_type type,         /* type of curve */
    char                *name,      /* existing curve */
    miGeoRange          *range)     /* curve range */
```

After the surface parameters have been defined, this call can be used to attach curves to the surface. The curve must have been defined in the same object group (see below) and is referenced by *name*. The *type* of the curve is one of `miCURVE_TRIM`, `miCURVE_HOLE`, and `miCURVE_SPECIAL`. The parameter *range* specifies the piece of the curve to be used. Multiple curves or pieces of curves can be concatenated to form the final loop; curves specified by consecutive *mi_api_surface_curveseg* are concatenated to a single loop by setting *newloop* to `miTRUE` for the first call and to `miFALSE` for all following curves to be appended.

```
miBoolean mi_api_surface_specpnt(
    int     uv_index,          /* 2D point reference */
    int     v_index)           /* optional 3D point */
```

Attach a special point to a surface. A vertex index *uv_index* must be given that contains the coordinate in the surface's UV space. The tessellated surface will contain a triangle vertex at that UV coordinate. If *v_index* is not −1, the special point is assigned the XYZ coordinate contained in the indexed vertex.

```
miBoolean mi_api_surface_texture_begin(
    miBoolean       is_volume,
    miBoolean       is_bump,
    char            *ubasis_name,
    miDlist         *uparams,
    miBoolean       u_rational,
    char            *vbasis_name,
    miDlist         *vparams,
    miBoolean       v_rational)
```

This call attaches a texture surface to the most recently defined surface. A texture surface is a simplified type of surface that causes texture vectors to appear in the vertices of the triangles that result from tessellation. Whenever the tessellator creates a triangle vertex at a certain UV coordinate of the main surface, it looks up this UV coordinate in the texture surface and computes the location of the texture surface at that point, and stores that as texture vector. If *is_volume* is `miFALSE`, wrap compensation is applied before storing the texture vector; this ensures that texture lookups near the surface seam do not "rewind." Generally it should be `miFALSE` for 2D textures and `miTRUE` for 3D (volume) textures. If *is_bump* is `miTRUE`, a pair of basis vectors is created in the tessellated surface instead of a texture vector. The bases and parameters in both the U and V directions are specified in the same call; they must use the same parameter ranges as the base surface.

Note: whenever the texture on a surface looks strangely shifted, or if texture coordinates are too large by a constant of 1, the reason is usually that *is_volume* had not been set to `miTRUE` on a 3D texture.

```
miBoolean mi_api_surface_derivative(
    int             degree)      /* 1=1st, 2=2nd deriv */
```

Specify that during tessellation, first or second derivatives should be computed and stored with the vertices of the tessellated surface that was most recently begun with *mi_api_surface_begin*. If both first and second derivatives should be stored, this function must be called twice.

```
miBoolean mi_api_surface_end (void)
```

After the surface, both of its parameter directions, all its texture surfaces and its derivatives have been specified, this call must be used to complete the surface definition. After this call, the next surface can be started by repeating the sequence beginning with *mi_api_surface_begin*.

```
miBoolean mi_api_surface_approx(
    char            *name,      /* name of surface */
    miApprox        *approx)    /* approx technique */
```

After the definition of a surface is complete, an approximation can be attached to it. The default is parametric approximation. This call can be used to change the default to regular parametric, curvature-dependent or spatial approximations. This call must be used before the object group ends because at that point the surface names go out of scope.

```
miBoolean mi_api_surface_approx_displace(
    char            *name,      /* name of surface */
    miApprox        *approx)    /* approx technique */
```

In addition to *mi_api_surface_approx*, which control the approximation of the base surface, this function stores an approximation for the displaced surface. The default is parametric. This is often useful to provide a high-resolution parametric approximation for the base surface to catch small displacement map features, and a curvature dependent tessellation for the displaced surface to properly approximate the curvature introduced by the displacement.

```
miBoolean mi_api_surface_approx_trim(
    char            *name,      /* name of surface */
    miApprox        *approx)    /* approx technique */
```

This function assigns an approximation to the trimming, hole, and special curves attached to the named surface, just like the previous function assigns an approximation to the surface itself.

4.3.8.5 Curves

Curves can be used as trimming curves, hole curves, and special curves as described in the free-form surface section above. In addition, curves can be used in space curves[2.1]to represent curve objects.

This section lists the API functions to create curves. This can be done inside any object group, after the vectors and vertices are defined, in any place where a surface definition would be legal. Like surface names, curve names are in object group scope and can only be referenced in the object group they are defined in.

```
miBoolean mi_api_curve_begin(
```

```
    char            *name,      /* name of the curve */
    char            *basis,     /* name of the basis */
    miBoolean       rational)
```

Create a new curve with the given *name*, using the specified basis. Like surfaces, a *rational* flag can be set for backwards compatibility reasons. The recommended method is setting the rational flag in the basis. Curves and surfaces can share the same bases.

```
miBoolean mi_api_curve_specpnt(
    int     t_index,            /* 1D point reference */
    int     v_index)
```

Attach a special point to a curve at the parameter point *v_index* of the curve. *v_index* references the vertex to use; only the X value is used.

```
miBoolean mi_api_curve_end(
    miDlist         *dlp)       /* parameter list */
```

Complete the definition of the curve, and pass the parameter vector. The type of the dlist is either `miScalar` for the non-rational case or `miVref` for the rational case.

```
miBoolean mi_api_curve_approx(
    char            *name,      /* name of curve */
    miApprox        *approx)    /* approx technique */
```

This function assigns an approximation to the curve. Alternatively, an approximation can be assigned to all curves used in a surface at once using *mi_api_surface_approx_trim*, which overrides the approximation set with *mi_api_curve_approx*.

4.3.8.6 Space Curves[2.1]

This section lists the API functions to create space curves. Space curve objects are primarily useful in geometry shaders, they are not used for rendering. Geometry shaders can build renderable surfaces with space curve objects or use them for dynamic trimming operations on surfaces. The definition can be done inside any object group, after the vectors and vertices are specified. Like curve or surface names, space curve names are in object group scope and can only be referenced in the object group they are defined in.

```
miBoolean mi_api_spacecurve_begin(
    char            *name)      /* space curve */
```

Create a new space curve with the given *name*.

```
miBoolean mi_api_spacecurve_curveseg(
    miBoolean        newloop,    /* is this a new loop */
    char             *name,      /* curve name */
    miGeoRange       *range)     /* range of the curve */
```

This call can be used to attach curve segments to the space curve. The curve must have been defined in the same object group (see below) and is referenced by *name*. The parameter *range* specifies the piece of the curve to be used. Multiple curves or pieces of curves can be concatenated to form the final space curve; curves specified by consecutive *mi_api_spacecurve_curveseg* are concatenated to a single curve by setting *newloop* to `miTRUE` for the first call and to `miFALSE` for all following curves to be appended.

```
miBoolean mi_api_spacecurve_approx(
    char             *name,      /* name of surface */
    miApprox         *approx)    /* approx technique */
```

After the definition of a space curve is complete, an approximation can be attached to it. The default is parametric approximation. This call can be used to change the default to regular parametric, curvature-dependent or spatial approximations. This call must be used before the object group ends because at that point the space curve names go out of scope.

```
miBoolean mi_api_spacecurve_end (void)
```

This function must be called to finalize the definition of a space curve. After this call, the next space curve can be started by repeating the sequence beginning with *mi_api_spacecurve_begin*.

4.3.8.7 Subdivision Surfaces[2.1]

Object groups containing subdivision surfaces[2.1] also consist of three sections: the vector list, the vertex list, and the subdivision surface list. As before, the vector list is defined using one call to *mi_api_vector_xyz_add* for every vector, and the vertex list is defined with calls to *mi_api_vertex_add* like in the polygon case. The subdivision surface list uses the vertices as polygon vertices. Subdivision surface vertices can have flags attached, they can be added by calling:

```
typedef enum {
    miAPI_V_SMOOTH=0,
    miAPI_V_CORNER,
    miAPI_V_CONIC,
    miAPI_V_CUSP,
    miAPI_V_DART
} miApi_vertexflags;
```

```
miBoolean mi_api_vertex_flags_add(
    miApi_vertexflags flags,
    miScalar          value)
```

[2.1]This function adds a sharpness feature to the current vertex. It should be called only once for each vertex, and may be called for individual vertices. If not called for a vertex, default flags are used (miAPI_V_SMOOTH), which will lead to smooth vertex processing. *value* specifies the sharpness for conic and cusp vertices. For corner vertices zero sharpness should be passed. It is redundant to mark a vertex smooth with this call.

The call order for subdivision construction is

```
mi_api_subdivsurf_begin
   mi_api_subdivsurf_poly              (any number of times)
      mi_api_subdivsurf_mtl            (optional)
      mi_api_subdivsurf_index          (n times)
      mi_api_subdivsurf_flags          (optional, f times)
      mi_api_subdivsurf_push           (optional)
         mi_api_subdivsurf_kit
            mi_api_subdivsurf_mtl      (0..4 times)
            mi_api_subdivsurf_index    (4 times)
            mi_api_subdivsurf_flags    (optional)
            mi_api_subdivsurf_push
               mi_api_subdivsurf_kit   (0..4 times)
               ...                     (optional, same as above)
            mi_api_subdivsurf_pop
      mi_api_subdivsurf_pop
mi_api_subdivsurf_end
```

n is 3 or 4 for triangles or quads, respectively, plus either 1 (base polygon) or 4 (polygon kit) if the object is tagged, in which case the triangle/quad labels must be passed first. A "kit" consists of 3 or 4 indices that subdivide the edge of the parent polygon into four sub-polygons, each of which may have its own material (part of the kit) and each may in turn be subdivided (using up to four separate push/pop blocks). `f` is 3 or 4 for base triangles or quads, and 9 or 12 for triangle or quad kits.

```
miBoolean mi_api_subdivsurf_begin(
    char            *name)     /* name of the surface */
```

[2.1]Begin the definition of a subdivision surface with the given *name*. The name is valid only inside the object group.

```
miBoolean mi_api_subdivsurf_poly(
    int             nvert)     /* 3 or 4 */
```

2.1 Begin the definition of a triangle or quad after *mi_api_subdivsurf_begin*. The number of vertices *nvert* must be either 3 or 4 for base polygons, or 0 for subpolygons (which then remember the number of vertices from the base polygon).

```
miBoolean mi_api_subdivsurf_kit(void)
```

2.1 If a polygon has sub-polygons, this function must be called after the polygon vertex index and the optional flags have been passed, and *mi_api_subdivsurf_push* was called. It must be followed with zero to four materials, three (triangles) or four (quads) vertex indices, an optional flag string, and optionally another push/pop block. The vertex indices subdivide each edge of the parent polygon. The order of these edge vertices is the same as for the polygon vertices, each splitting the edge starting at the corresponding polygon vertex.

```
miBoolean mi_api_subdivsurf_mtl(
    char            *mtlname)  /* material name or 0 */
```

2.1 Add a material to the previous polygon or kit. A polygon may have only one material; a kit may have up to four. If only the nth sub-kit of a kit has a material, then the first $n - 1$ materials must be set to null first with this function. If the object is tagged, this function may not be used.

```
miBoolean mi_api_subdivsurf_mtl_tag(
    miTag           mtltag)    /* material tag or 0 */
```

2.1 This function is equivalent to the previous but specifies the material as a tag.

```
miBoolean mi_api_subdivsurf_index(
    int             idx)       /* poly vertex index */
```

2.1 After a polygon is begun, calls to this function provide first the polygon label if the object is tagged, and then either three or four vertex indices, depending on the *nvert* argument of the begin function. If the object is not tagged, only the three or four vertex indices but no label must be given. The definition of the polygon ends if any API function beginning with *mi_api_subdivsurf_* other than *mi_api_subdivsurf_index* is called. Polygons may also have zero indices (in the case of unspecified sub-polygons, see below); in this case the next polygon is started without any calls to *mi_api_subdivsurf_index* that specify vertex indices (if called once to specify the label if the object is tagged, it is ignored).

```
typedef enum {
    miAPI_E_CREASE=0
} miApi_edgeflags;

miBoolean mi_api_subdivsurf_flags(
    miApi_edgeflags flags,
    miScalar        value)
```

2.1 Add an edge flag definition for the previous polygon. Currently there is a possibility to tag edges as creases, which are sharp edges. *value* is the sharpness of the crease in the range 0..1. This function must be called as many times as there are edges in the current polygon or kit. If an edge should not be tagged as a crease, a 0 must be passed for the sharpness value.

```
miBoolean mi_api_subdivsurf_push(void)
```

2.1 The polygons that follow the beginning of the subdivision surface are called *base* polygons. Any polygon, base or otherwise, may have subdivision polygons that divide it into four sub-triangles or sub-quads. After the definition of a polygon, *mi_api_subdivsurf_sub* and *mi_api_subdivsurf_push* must be called as described above before the four sub-polygons are defined, and *mi_api_subdivsurf_pop* must be called after they are defined and before the next polygon on the same level can be begun.

Sometimes only some of the four sub-polygons are defined; trailing subpolygon definitions can be omitted and leading or middle polygons can be specified by beginning the unneeded polygon but not giving any indices for it.

```
miBoolean mi_api_subdivsurf_pop(void)
```

2.1 After up to four sub-polygons for a polygon were specified, the sub-polygon definition must be terminated with this function to return to the state before *mi_api_subdivsurf_push*.

```
miBoolean mi_api_subdivsurf_end(void)
```

2.1 Complete the definition of the subdivision surface started with *mi_api_subdiv_begin*.

```
miBoolean mi_api_subdivsurf_approx(
    char            *name,
    miApprox        *approx)
```

2.1 Change the default approximation of a subdivision surface with name *name* to *approx*. Currently parametric subdivision must be specified. The subdivision approximation level must be stored in the `miCNST_UPARAM` field in the approximation constant array *cnst* of *miApprox*.

4.3.9 Function Declarations

Functions are user-written C routines with parameters that are used as shaders during preprocessing, rendering, and postprocessing. Before a function can be defined (by giving its name and listing its parameter values), it must be declared so mental ray knows the complete parameter list the C function accepts, and the data type for each parameter. For a complete list of available shaders, refer to the mental ray manual.

```
miParameter *mi_api_parameter_decl(
    miParam_type    type,       /* one of miTYPE_* */
    char            *name,      /* parameter name */
    int             strlength) /* not used */
```

Before the function itself is declared, a complete description of the parameters and their types must be built. This function builds a `miParameter` structure for a single parameter to be appended to the list. The parameter , the parameter *name*, and the maximum length of the string if the type is `miTYPE_STRING`, must be specified. The string length includes the trailing null byte.

```
miParameter *mi_api_parameter_append(
    miParameter     *list,      /* list of parameters */
    miParameter     *parm)      /* new parameter */
```

Parameter structures created with the previous function must be concatenated to a list with this function. It appends a new parameter *parm* to an existing list *list*. The parameter pointer created with the definition of the first parameter, which is also the anchor of the parameter list that will be passed to *mi_api_funcdecl_end*, can be used as *list* argument, but it is more efficient to pass the parameter pointer returned by the previously appended parameter.

```
miBoolean mi_api_parameter_child(
    miParameter     *parm,      /* struct or array */
    miParameter     *child)     /* str/array to attach */
```

Function parameter lists are not necessarily linear lists. Parameters of type `miTYPE_STRUCT` and `miTYPE_ARRAY` require a sublist of parameters. Arrays always require a single parameter as subtree, which becomes the type of the array, while structures require a list as subtree that contains one parameter for every member of the structure. The sub-parameter or sub-parameter list *child* is attached to the array or structure parameter *parm* with this function.

```
miFunction_decl *mi_api_funcdecl_begin(
    miParameter     *outparms,  /* result parameters */
    char            *name,      /* function name */
    miParameter     *inparms)   /* parameter list */
```

After the parameter list (or tree, if arrays and structures are present) has been built, the function itself can be declared. The return parameter, the function name (which must agree with the name of the C function to be executed), and the anchor of the parameter list must be passed. This call completes the declaration of a function.

The result parameter list is similar to the input parameter list, but may only be either a simple type or a structure, not an array or a structure containing structures or arrays. The result parameter does not have a name (i.e. the *name* argument in the call to *mi_api_parameter_decl* that returned *outparms* was a null pointer), but if the result parameter is a structure, the structure members must be named as usual. The *outparms* pointer should be a null pointer if a structured user data block is being declared (see *mi_api_data_begin*). This function always stores the declaration type miFUNCTION_C, so if a phenomenon or user data block is being declared, the caller must modify the *type* field of the returned declaration.

Earlier versions of the API passed a miParam_type instead of a miParameter. This was changed to allow structured return types. For backward compatibility, *mi_api_funcdecl_end* still accepts miParam_type codes, but since the function prototype changed the compiler will generate an error unless a cast is applied.

```
miTag mi_api_funcdecl_end(void)
```

After the function declaration is finished, this call finishes the declaration and returns the tag of the new database element.

4.3.10 Function Definitions

Functions, also called function calls, are references to a particular C function bundled with a set of parameter values. A function definition begins with naming the desired C function, which must have been declared (see above), followed by assignments of numerical or other values to individual parameters. The order of assignments is irrelevant; it is done by parameter name. Parameters that remain unassigned have a numerical value 0 or the empty string.

```
miBoolean mi_api_function_call(
    char            *name)      /* called function */
```

Every function definition begins with this call, which references the C function by name. An error occurs if the name is not declared. This function is special in that it does not insist on *name* to be declared in the current scope (see Scopes below). Instead, it searches for the function beginning in the innermost scope and works back towards the outermost scope. This is useful because shader declarations usually appear in the form of a $include statement at the beginning of the scene file, it would be inconvenient to force a redeclaration in every scope (such as phenomenon definitions) just to have the correctly scoped names handy.

```
miBoolean mi_api_parameter_name(
    char            *name)      /* new parameter */
```

After *mi_api_function_call*, the parameter values are assigned. The first step for an assignment is this call, which specifies the name o the parameter to be assigned to. The name must be one of those specified when the function was declared. *name* is always a simple name; to access the subtrees of arrays and structs special functions (push, pop, array element) are provided, see below. Parameter names may not contain dots (".").

```
miBoolean mi_api_parameter_value(
    miParam_type    type,       /* parameter type */
    void            *value,     /* pointer to value */
    int             *offs,      /* offset in parm blk */
    int             *size)      /* size in parm block */
```

Assign a value to the parameter named with the previous call. The type of the value being assigned and a pointer to the value must be passed. The *type* must agree with the declared type of the parameter, following these rules:

- For all textures miTYPE_TEX must be used, regardless of whether a color, scalar, or vector texture has been declared.

- Instead of miTYPE_SCALAR, miTYPE_INTEGER can be passed. The value will automatically be converted to a miScalar if the parameter has been declared as miTYPE_SCALAR.

- Similarly, a *type* of miTYPE_STRING can be passed for parameters declared as miTYPE_TEX, miTYPE_LIGHT, miTYPE_SHADER, miTYPE_MATERIAL, or miTYPE_GEOMETRY. The value will be interpreted correctly.

- A *type* of miTYPE_INTEGER can be passed for parameters declared as miTYPE_TEX, miTYPE_LIGHT, miTYPE_SHADER, miTYPE_MATERIAL, or miTYPE_GEOMETRY. The value will be interpreted as a numeric tag. This is a deviation from the similarity between .mi syntax and API calls, but simplifies matters for automatic procedural construction of phenomena.

- Values consisting of multiple scalars, such as vectors, colors, and matrices, can be given piecewise, one miTYPE_SCALAR at a time. If fewer than three scalars for a vector, four scalars for a color, or sixteen scalars for a matrix (row-major order) are provided, the remaining scalars are set to zero.

These rules are all consequences of the fact that a .mi2 language parser, when it sees a value, does not have access to the declaration.

```
miBoolean mi_api_parameter_shader(
    char            *name)      /* shader name */
```

Instead of providing a value to a parameter, register another function by name that is called at runtime to calculate the value. This is used to build dynamic shader trees.

```
miBoolean mi_api_parameter_interface(
    char            *name)      /* interface parm name */
```

Instead of providing a value to a parameter, register a link to an interface parameter that provides the value at runtime.

```
miBoolean mi_api_parameter_push(
    miBoolean        is_array)  /* pushing array? */
```

After the call to *mi_api_parameter_name* for a structure or array, before values can be stored, the context must be pushed one level down into the structure's or array's parameter subtree. The *is_array* argument is `miFALSE` for structures and `miTRUE` for arrays. After the push, structure members and array elements can be assigned with regular *mi_api_parameter_value* calls. Every new array member must be preceded with a call to the following function.

```
miBoolean mi_api_new_array_element (void)
```

After the push operation, before a new array value can be assigned, this function must be used to make room for another array element. After the first call to this function, *mi_api_parameter_value* assigns to array element [0], after the next [1] is assigned, and so on. Array elements can only be assigned sequentially. If no values or not enough values are assigned to a parameter, its remaining scalars remain zero.

```
miBoolean mi_api_parameter_pop (void)
```

After a structure or array has been assigned its component values, the parameter subtree of the structure or array must be exited with a pop operation. For example, to assign the scalars 1 and 2 to members a and b of structure s, the call sequence is `name(s), push, name(a), value(1), name(b), value(2),` pop. The order of assignment to a and b is not significant. To assign 3 and 4 to an array a of length 2, the call sequence is `name(a), push, new_element, value(3), new_element, value(4),` pop. Push/pop pairs can be nested.

```
miTag mi_api_function_call_end(
    miTag            oldtag)     /* for incr change */
```

After all parameter values have been assigned, the function definition is completed with this call. The tag of the new function is returned and can now be used where a function is expected during scene definition. Since functions (as opposed to declarations) are not generally named, the standard incremental method cannot be applied; therefore a *tag* argument can be supplied. If *tag* is not the null tag, the existing function identified by *tag* is replaced with the new one such that all references in the scene that referred to the old function now refer to the new one. In this case *tag* is also returned.

```
miTag mi_api_function_append(
    miTag            list,       /* append to this list */
    miTag            func)       /* function to append */
```

Most regular shaders (not output shaders and inheritance shaders) can be given as a list of shaders. In this case mental ray will call all shaders in the list in sequence, with each successive shader operating on the result of the previous. The main application are lens shaders, which are often lists of lens shaders. To append a function *func* to another function or function list *list* this call is used. The first function in the list is the anchor of the list; it can be passed as *list* when appending to the list but it is more efficient to pass the last function added to the list.

```
miBoolean mi_api_function_delete(
    miTag           *list)      /* func list to delete */
```

When a scene element referencing functions is changed incrementally, it is usually desired to delete the old function list before a new one is built with calls to *mi_api_function_append*. This call deletes all functions of the function list, and stores a null tag in the list anchor. The *list* argument is a pointer to the function list tag to permit this call to clear the function list tag itself.

```
miBoolean mi_api_shader_add(
    char            *name,      /* shader name */
    miTag           func_tag)   /* shader function */
```

Normally functions are unnamed. This call can be used to assign a name to a function. The main application are procedural textures, which are nothing but a texture shading function accessible by name (the name can be provided as parameter value to texture parameters of other functions). Named shaders also appear in the .mi2 language as `shader` statements. Note that lights, materials, and other scene elements are more than just shading functions, a named shader can not be used where a material or light is expected.

```
miTag mi_api_function_assign(
    char            *name)      /* name of shader */
```

This call can be used to look up a named shader (was given a name by the preceding call) to obtain its tag. The returned tag can be used like a tag returned by *mi_api_function_call_end*. This is called an "assignment" because the .mi2 language allows assigning an existing named shader wherever a shading definition is called; such assignments are introduced with an equals sign.

```
miBoolean mi_api_shader_call(
    miTag           func_tag,      /* function to call */
    char            *c_inst_name, /* camera instance */
    char            *option_name) /* options element */
```

This function can be used to call a shading function immediately. This call returns after the called function returns. If *func_tag* is a function list, all functions in the list are called in sequence. The functions are provided with a dummy state containing mostly nulls; if a camera instance or options element are passed by name, appropriate camera and options substructures are placed in the state. Either *c_inst_name* or *option_name* may be null pointers.

4.3.11 Phenomenon Definitions

Phenomena are declared after all the subshaders to be used inside the phenomenon have been declared. Inside the phenomenon, subshaders will be defined, complete with shader name and parameters. Parameters may have constant values, like in a regular shader definition, or they may have subshaders assigned to them, or they may have phenomenon interface parameters assigned to them. It is important to understand that the phenomenon *declaration* contains shader *definitions*.

```
miFunction_decl *mi_api_phen_begin(
    miParameter     *outparms, /* one of miTYPE_* */
    char            *name,     /* phenomenon name */
    miParameter     *inparms)  /* parameter list */
```

Begin the declaration of a new phenomenon *name*, along with its result and input parameters that must have been previously built with calls to *mi_api_parameter_decl*, *mi_api_parameter_append*, and *mi_api_parameter_child*.

```
miTag mi_api_phen_end(void)
```

After the declaration returned by the previous function has been set up, this function terminates the phenomenon declaration. If an error occurs, a null tag is returned; otherwise the tag of the new phenomenon element is returned. The type of the returned element is `miSCENE_FUNCDECL`.

4.3.12 Verbatim C Sources

In most cases, compiled C shading functions will be linked to the program as shared libraries. The library can also link existing object files and C source files. This is handled by the LINK module and is outside the scope of the API module. However, API allows verbatim specification of C sources as part of the scene definition with the following three calls. Use of these functions is discouraged except when parsing .mi2 scene files because the overhead is significantly higher than linking shared libraries.

```
miBoolean mi_api_code_verbatim_begin (void)
```

Begin the definition of verbatim code. This call opens a temporary file in `/usr/tmp` with a unique file name that receives the C sources.

```
miBoolean mi_api_code_byte_copy(
    int             length,    /* # of data bytes */
    miUchar         *bytes)    /* C src data array */
```

Append ascii source text to the C source file opened by the preceding call. The *bytes* string is expected to contain *length* characters, not counting a trailing null byte (which is not required). The *bytes* pointer, like any other string passed to an API call, is released using *mi_mem_release*.

```
miBoolean mi_api_code_verbatim_end (void)
```

After the sources have been stored with one or more byte copy calls, this call completes the verbatim source definition. The temporary file is closed, compiled, linked, loaded, and removed.

4.3.13 Scopes

Scopes disambiguate name spaces. The current scope is defined by a string that is prepended to all toplevel element names (objects, materials, lights, functions, declarations, etc) passed to API. Non-toplevel entities such as surfaces, curves, and shader parameters whose lifetime are limited to the enclosing toplevel element are not scoped. The scope string is initially empty. Scopes can be nested. Scopes in the scope string are separated by double colons; the scope string "`a::b::`" is the result of first beginning scope "`a`" and then scope "`b`". If applied to a name "`x`", the resulting name is "`a::b::x`". Since symbol tables contain scoped names, this can be used to distinguish different "`x`".

For example, *mi_api_phen_begin* automatically begins a new scope with the phenomenon name. This causes the phenomenon name and a double colon to be prepended to all shaders defined inside the phenomenon, which allows different phenomena to have subshaders with the same name. If phenomena "`phen1`" and "`phen2`" both have a subshader "`shader`", no conflict arises because their internal names are "`phen1::shader`" and "`phen2::shader`". The scoping functions are available to other modules, for example to allow the shader editor to read a declaration file without causing conflicts with the loaded scene. The name of the declared phenomenon itself, like the name of any other declaration, is global and does not get a scope prepended.

Every context has its own scope string (see LIB module about contexts).

```
miBoolean mi_api_scope_begin(
    char             *name)    /* new scope name */
```

Enter a scope. The given *name* and two colons (in this order) are appended to the scope string.

```
miBoolean mi_api_scope_end(void)
```

Exit a scope. The last name and double colon is stripped off the scope string.

```
char *mi_api_scope_apply(
    char             *name)   /* name to put in scope */
```

Prepend the scope string to *name*, if any. If *name* contains double colons, check the scope part of *name* against the scope, and return a null pointer if the check fails. For example, it is an error for *name* to contain double colons if there is no scope; assuming that the scope is "`a::b::`", the *names* "`x`", "`b::x`", and "`a::b::x`" are all ok and return the same string "`a::b::x`" but "`a::x`" is an error. As usual, *name* must have been allocated using MEM functions. The returned string is allocated with MEM and may be identical to *name*.

The following functions accept `char*` arguments that are passed through *mi_api_scope_apply* automatically by API:

mi_api_delete	*mi_api_delete_tree*	*mi_api_options_begin*
mi_api_camera_begin	*mi_api_render*	*mi_api_light_begin*
mi_api_light_lookup	*mi_api_material_begin*	*mi_api_material_lookup*
mi_api_texture_begin	*mi_api_texture_lookup*	*mi_api_instance_begin*
mi_api_instance_end	*mi_api_instgroup_begin*	*mi_api_instgroup_additem*
mi_api_object_begin	*mi_api_poly_begin*	*mi_api_surface_begin* (material name only)
mi_api_function_assign	*mi_api_function_call*	*mi_api_parameter_shader*
mi_api_shader_add	*mi_api_shader_call*	*mi_api_gui_begin*

4.3.14 Miscellaneous

```
miBoolean mi_api_delete(
    char            *what)      /* element to delete */
```

Delete a single element from the scene database. This function may be used only after all references to the element have been deleted. For example, before deleting an object all instances referencing it must be deleted, or incrementally changed to reference something else, and so on.

```
miBoolean mi_api_delete_tree(
    char            *what)      /* element to delete */
```

Delete a tree anchored at the named element in the scene database. This function takes care of deleting all members of the tree in the proper order such that references to an element are removed before the element itself is deleted, but only within the named tree - multiple instancing from outside is not recognized, and outside references to *what* itself are also not removed.

```
miBoolean mi_api_debug(
    char            *what,      /* what to dump */
    char            *arg)       /* if scene dump, item */
```

This function is useful for debugging code that calls the API module. It is not essential for scene definition. The *what* argument specifies what to check, and the *arg* argument specifies the name of a scene element to be checked, depending on what is being checked. The following *what* strings are supported:

what	*arg*	operation
sym	–	print all symbol tables
sym global	–	print the global (.mi2) symbol table
sym declare	–	print the declaration symbol table
sym options	–	print the .mi1 options symbol table
sym camera	–	print the .mi1 camera symbol table
sym light	–	print the .mi1 light symbol table
sym object	–	print the .mi1 object symbol table
sym instance	–	print the .mi1 instance symbol table
sym group	–	print the .mi1 instance group symbol table
sym material	–	print the .mi1 material symbol table
sym ctexture	–	print the .mi1 color texture symbol table
sym stexture	–	print the .mi1 scalar texture symbol table
sym vtexture	–	print the .mi1 vector texture symbol table
mem summary	–	print per-module MEM memory usage summary
mem dump	–	print all allocated MEM memory blocks
mem check	–	run a consistency check on MEM memory
db statistics	–	print DB database access statistics
db dump	–	print a list of all DB database entries
task statistics	–	print TASK task queue statistics
img verbose	–	future image file accesses print messages
scene check	element	consistency check of a scene element
scene dump	element	recursively print info on scene element
scene alldump	element	recursively print detailed element info

4.4 Geometry Shader Data Structures

This chapter describes the data structures that define a scene in memory. While the scene is constructed using API calls, there is not an API call for all operations that merely write a value into an existing data structure. Instead, the *mi_api_*_begin* calls return a pointer to the data structure just created and expect the caller to fill in simple parameters. This chapter describes these data structures.

This section discusses every element type in detail. There is one subsection for each element type. Each describes

- the element type (as returned by *mi_db_type*),
- the C data type of the contents. Some elements are arrays of this type.
- the extra arguments given to the create and resize functions to preallocate variable-sized sections.
- a brief descriptions of the defaults stored by the create function.
- the declaration of the data type, with description.

This chapter describes the data structures used by mental ray 2.1. The data structures for mental ray 2.0 are similar, but lack a number of fields. These fields are marked "$^{2.1}$".

4.4.1 Instances

Element type:	miSCENE_INSTANCE
Data type:	miInstance
Sizes:	int param_size
Defaults:	all nulls, two identity matrices, parameter size as given by size argument

```
enum miGenMotionType {
        miGM_INHERIT = 0,
        miGM_TRANSFORM,
        miGM_OFF
};

typedef struct miTransform {
        miTag           function;               /* function, may be null tag */
        float           time;                   /* the last evaluation time */
        miMatrix        global_to_local;        /* transformation in world */
        miMatrix        local_to_global;        /* transformation to world */
        miCBoolean      identity;               /* SCENE: matrices are ident.*/
        miCBoolean      spare[3];               /* SCENE: not used */
        int             id;                     /* SCENE: unique transform ID*/
} miTransform;

typedef struct miInstance {
        miTransform     tf;                     /* space transformation */
        miMatrix        motion_transform;       /* motion transformation */
        miTag           item;                   /* instanced item */
        miTag           material;               /* inherited material or list*/
        miTag           parent;                 /* SCENE: leaf inst. parent */
        miTag           boxes;                  /* SCENE: renderable repres. */
        miTag           next;                   /* SCENE: leaf instance list */
        miTag           prev;                   /* SCENE: leaf instance list */
        int             mtl_array_size;         /* if mtl array, array size */
        int             n_boxes;                /* SCENE: # of boxes attached */
        miTag           userdata;               /* optional user data blocks */
        miUint          label;                  /* optional label */
        miTag           geogroup;               /* SCENE: geomshader group */
        miCBoolean      off;                    /* ignore this instance */
        miUint1         gen_motion;             /* motion information */
        miUint1         visible;                /* visible ? */
        miUint1         shadow;                 /* casts shadow? */
        miUint1         trace;                  /* visible as reflection? */
        miUint1         caustic;                /* caustic bitmap */
        miUint1         globillum;              /* globillum bitmap */
```

```
        miCBoolean      temp_material;          /* SCENE: has inherited mtl */
        int             spare[3];               /* not used */
        miTag           param_decl;             /* parameter declaration */
        int             param_size;             /* parameter size in bytes */
        char            param[8];               /* arbitrary-sized parameters*/
} miInstance;
```

A translator must provide: either `tf.function` and `time`, or `global_to_local` and `local_to_global`; also `item` (using *mi_scene_link*), `param_decl`, `param_size`, and `param`.

All fields except the matrices, the material, and the parameters are reserved for Scene and may not be modified by other modules. The tags can be modified indirectly with the link and unlink functions, which take care of reference counts. The instance element has two variable parts; one for inherited shader parameters and one for the relation list. The latter is maintained exclusively by Scene.

tf.function optionally points to a transformation function that computes a matrix from the current time. If present, this function is called during preprocessing with three parameters: a pointer to the result global–to–local matrix, the instance tag, and the time as given in the preprocessing control structure.

tf.time is the time the evaluation function, if present, was last called with. If it matches the current time, the matrices need not be calculated by calling the function again.

tf.global_to_local transforms the parent space to the local space of the instanced subtree. If a transformation functions exists, it writes its result here; if not, the translator must store an appropriate matrix here.

tf.local_to_global is the inverse matrix, set by Scene after the transformation function (if it exists) has returned the `tf.global_to_local` matrix.

tf.identity is `miTRUE` if the transformation matrices in this instance are identity transforms (this saves the renderer unnecessary ray transformations).

tf.id is a unique transformation ID. Scene creates it during preprocessing, trying to assign identical IDs to identical transformations. This is especially important for leaf instances: the renderer does not have to retransform the current ray if the new box has the same transformation (same ID) as the previous.

motion_transform specifies the transformation from parent space to local space for motion blur transforms. If this is a null matrix, the instance transformation `tf` is used.

item is the tag of the element being instanced. Only groups, cameras, lights, objects, functions and boxes can be referenced. If a box is referenced, it is taken as a "trivial object" that does not need tessellation; boxes that *result* from tessellation are not attached here. If a function-list is instanced, actually the geometry shader created scene elements are intended to be instanced.

material is either a material (if *mtl_array_size* is 0) or a material list (if *mtl_array_size* is nonzero) used for material inheritance (as opposed to parameter inheritance). During scene preprocessing, the non-null material tag closest to a geometrical object (lowest in the DAG hierarchy) becomes the default material for any polygon or surface in the object that does not have its own non-null material tag. If the tag references a list (type `miSCENE_TAG`) or materials, it is expected to contain *mtl_array_size* tags, which will be indexed with the polygon or surface label during rendering.

mtl_array_size Specifies the number of tags in the material tag list if nonzero. If the material tag specifies a material directly, it must be zero. This number is used during rendering as a flag that tells mental ray that the material tag references a list, and also how many items there are in the list to prevent array bounds overflows.

boxes is used to point to boxes that resulted from tessellation. They are used in two cases only: object or box instances attach to the cached untransformed boxes (see above for a definition) if enabled; and leaf instances attach to the final renderable representation.

userdata[2.1] allows attaching a user data block (miUserdata) or a chain of user data blocks. Shaders can retrieve the data with *mi_query*.

n_boxes is the number of boxes attached to **boxes**. Keeping this separate avoids having to access boxes to count them.

geogroup is used to point to the group element which contains all the geometry-shader created scene elements for this instance.

off, if true, stops the recursive descent during preprocessing as if the instance and its instanced item didn't exist. This is useful for temporary suspending subtrees without deleting them.

gen_motion specifies the motion blur generation for the instance. Setting this field to `miGM_OFF` switches off motion blur for this instance. Motion blur is always generated when this field is set to `miGM_TRANSFORM`. The parent instance determines whether motion blur is active or not when it is set to `miGM_INHERIT`.

visible, **shadow**, **trace**, **caustic**, and **globillum**[2.1] flags are inherited in the scene DAG. During scene preprocessing, the non-null flag in the DAG instance closest to a geometrical object (lowest in the DAG hierarchy) is put into the leaf instance. Before rendering starts the leaf instance flags are merged with the object flags and stored in internal raylib rendering data structures. In the merging operation these flags are treated as "fuzzy booleans", that is, a zero value means that the flag is ignored (the object flag is taken), 1 disables the flag (even if the object has enabled it) and 2 enables it (even if the object has not set the flag). The *caustic* bitmap has the same bit interpretation as the corresponding field in the `miObject`, but has three more bits defined here. Bit 2, if set, disables generation of caustics cast by this object. Bit 3, if set, disables receiving caustics. Bit 5, if set, enables photons to intersect with this object. In the merging, bit `0` and bit 1 of the leaf instance and object caustic bitmaps are logically combined with an `OR` operation followed by `AND` of the instance caustic bitmap bits 2 and 3, inverted and shifted right two times. Also in the merging, bit 4 of the leaf instance and object caustic bitmaps are logically `ORed` followed by an `AND` with bit 5 of the instance caustic bitmap inverted and shifted right one position. The *globillum*[2.1] bitmap is similar to the *caustic* bitmap.

temp_material is a flag that tells SCENE postprocessing that the material field contains a material that was created during preprocessing, and must be deleted on postprocessing. This happens if the inheritance shader sets one or more of the material fields in its material argument, to implement Catia aspect inheritance.

param_decl points to a parameter declaration that describes the parameters. If parameters exist, this tag must be set by the translator to allow data exchange with other hosts. If it is missing, no data will be swapped regardless of the remote host's byte order. In leaf instances, Scene stores the most recent parent instance's parameter declaration tag here.

param_size is the size of the parameters in bytes. It is taken from the first and only argument of the create and resize calls. In the leaf instance, the inheritance function determines the size.

param is an arbitrary-sized array of parameters stored by the translator. During preprocessing, the DAG is traversed, and the parameters are passed to an inheritance function that is called for every instance found during traversal. The end result is stored in the leaf instance by Scene.

4.4.2 Groups

Element type:	miSCENE_GROUP
Data type:	miGroup
Sizes:	int max_kids, int max_connections
Defaults:	all nulls, max_* as given by size arguments

```
typedef struct miGroup {
        miGeoScalar     merge;          /* merge tolerance */
        miTag           boxes;          /* SCENE: cached shared tesselation */
        int             n_boxes;        /* SCENE: # of boxes attached */
        miBoolean       merge_group;    /* perform merging on members? */
        int             max_kids;       /* number of kids allocated */
        int             no_kids;        /* number of kids actually used */
        int             max_connections;/* number of connections allocated */
        int             no_connections; /* number of connections used */
        miTag           userdata;       /* optional user data blocks */
        miUint          label;          /* optional label */
        int             spare[3];       /* not used */
        miTag           kids[2];        /* kid list (instances) */
} miGroup;

typedef struct {
        miTag           instance[2];    /* the two face type object instances*/
        miGeoIndex      face[2];        /* indices of the two miFace's */
        miGeoIndex      curve[2];       /* indices of the two miCurves*/
        miGeoRange      range[2];
} miConnection;
```

A translator must provide: nothing.
A translator may provide: `merge_group`, `merge`, the connection array.

Groups have two variable-sized sections, one for the list of instances and one for the list of connections. The latter exists only if the group is a merge group. The macro `miGROUP_GET_CONNECTIONS(n)` returns a `miConnection` pointer to the *n*-th connection. Note that instances must be added to groups with *mi_scene_link*, but the connection tags are written directly to the `miConnection`.

boxes is used to point to boxes that resulted from tessellation. They are used in two cases only: object or box instances attach to the cached untransformed boxes (see above for a definition) if enabled; and leaf instances attach to the final renderable representation.

n_boxes is the number of boxes attached to **boxes**. Keeping this separate avoids having to access boxes to count them.

merge_group is `miTRUE` if this group is a merge group. Merge groups are treated like objects; all their subobjects are tessellated as one object. In fact, the Scene module treats merge groups like objects and lets GAP pick apart the group and its subtrees.

merge is the merge epsilon. It is used only in merge groups.

max_kids is the current size of the *kids* array.

no_kids is the number of instances stored in the *kids* array.

max_connections is the current size of the connection array.

no_connections is the number of connections in the connection array.

userdata[2.1] allows attaching a user data block (miUserdata) or a chain of user data blocks. Shaders can retrieve the data with *mi_query*.

label[2.1] a numeric value assigned by applications.

kids is the beginning of the variable section of `miGroup`, consisting of an array of instance tags followed by an optional array of connections.

4.4.3 Cameras

Element type:	miSCENE_CAMERA
Data type:	miCamera
Sizes:	—
Defaults:	as described below

```
typedef struct miCamera {
        miBoolean       orthographic;            /* orthographic rendering? */
```

```
        float           focal;                  /* focal length */
        float           aperture;               /* aperture */
        float           aspect;                 /* aspect ratio of the image */
        miRange         clip;                   /* min/max clipping */
        int             x_resolution;           /* x resolution */
        int             y_resolution;           /* y resolution */
        struct {int xl, yl, xh, yh;}
                        window;                 /* corners of subwindow */
        miTag           volume;                 /* opt. volume shader */
        miTag           environment;            /* opt. environment shader */
        miTag           lens;                   /* opt. lens shader */
        miTag           output;                 /* opt. output shaders/files */
        int             frame;                  /* current frame number */
        float           frame_time;             /* ... as time in seconds */
        int             frame_field;            /* 0=frame, 1/2=field number */
        float           x_offset;               /* x image offset in pixels */
        float           y_offset;               /* y image offset in pixels */
        miTag           userdata;               /* optional user data blocks */
        int             spare[15];              /* not used */
} miCamera;
```

A translator must provide: nothing.
A translator may provide: all fields.

orthographic (default `miFALSE`) switches the camera from the standard pinhole camera to an orthographic camera.

focal (default 1.0) is the focal length of the camera (the distance between the camera and the viewing plane).

aperture (default 1.0) is the width of the viewing plane in 3D space.

aspect (default 1.0) is the height of a pixel 1 unit wide.

clip (default 0.0001, 1000000.0) describes the minimum (hither) and maximum (yon) limits of the scene. Geometry outside these limits will not be rendered.

x_resolution (default 768) is the width of the rendered image in pixels.

y_resolution (default 576) is the height of the rendered image in pixels.

window (default 0, 0, 65535, 65535) describes the lower left and upper right corners of the rendered subwindow. Pixels outside this window will be black. If the upper right pixel exceeds the resolution, it is clipped to the resolution.

volume (default `miNULLTAG`) is the optional atmosphere volume shader.

environment (default `miNULLTAG`) is the optional view environment shader that is called for all (including primary) rays leaving the scene (the active environment shader for secondary rays may be overridden by materials).

lens (default `miNULLTAG`) is the optional first lens shader.

output (default `miNULLTAG`) is the optional first output shader or output file.

frame (default 0) is the frame number of the current render. It is not used by mental ray but is accessible to shaders.

frame_time (default 0.0) is the same as the frame number, but expressed in seconds. It is not used by mental ray.

frame_field (default 0) is the number after the `field` substatement in a `frame` statement. Since frame numbers are integers, the field number must be used to distinguish the first and second field of the frame, if field rendering is in effect. By convention, 0 means that the entire frame is rendered; 1 is the first (odd) and 2 is the second (even) field. It is not used by mental ray.

x_offset (default 0.0) is the x offset of the rendered image from the center of the camera axis in pixel units.

y_offset (default 0.0) is the y offset of the rendered image from the center of the camera axis in pixel units.

userdata[2.1] allows attaching a user data block (miUserdata) or a chain of user data blocks. Shaders can retrieve the data with *mi_query*.

4.4.4 Lights

Element type:	miSCENE_LIGHT
Data type:	miLight
Sizes:	—
Defaults:	as described below

```
enum miLight_type {
        miLIGHT_ORIGIN,
        miLIGHT_DIRECTION,
        miLIGHT_SPOT
};

enum miLight_area {
        miLIGHT_NONE = 0,
        miLIGHT_RECTANGLE,
        miLIGHT_DISC,
        miLIGHT_SPHERE,
        miLIGHT_CYLINDER
};
```

```
typedef struct miLight {
        enum miLight_type type;           /* light type */
        enum miLight_area area;           /* area? */
        miScalar          exponent;       /* global illum. 1/r^(2*exp)*/
        unsigned int      caustic_store_photons;/*caust. photons to store*/
        unsigned int      global_store_photons; /*glob. photons to store */
        miColor           energy;         /* global illum. intensity */
        miTag             shader;         /* light shader */
        miTag             emitter;        /* photon emitter shader */
        miVector          origin;         /* opt. origin */
        miVector          direction;      /* opt. normalized direction */
        float             spread;         /* size of spot? (cos angle) */
        union {
                struct miLight_rectangle    rectangle;
                struct miLight_disc         disc;
                struct miLight_sphere       sphere;
                struct miLight_cylinder     cylinder;
        }               primitive;        /* area primitive */
        short           samples_u;        /* area u samples */
        short           samples_v;        /* area v samples */
        short           low_samples_u;    /* low area u samples */
        short           low_samples_v;    /* low area v samples */
        short           low_level;        /* switch to low at this lvl */
        short           spare1;           /* not used */

        miBoolean       use_shadow_maps;  /* for this light */
        miTag           shadowmap_file;   /* the shadow map file */
        int             shadowmap_resolution; /* resolution */
        float           shadowmap_softness;   /* sample region size */
        int             shadowmap_samples;    /* #samples */
        miBoolean       visible;          /* visible? area lights only */
        miUint          label;            /* light label */
        miTag           userdata;         /* optional user data blocks */
        unsigned int    caustic_emit_photons;/*caust. photons to emit*/
        unsigned int    global_emit_photons; /*glob. photons to emit */
        int             spare[4];         /* not used */
} miLight;

struct miLight_rectangle {
        miVector        edge_u;
        miVector        edge_v;
};

struct miLight_disc {
        miVector        normal;
        miScalar        radius;
};
```

```
struct miLight_sphere {
        miScalar        radius;
};

struct miLight_cylinder {
        miVector        axis;
        miScalar        radius;
};
```

A translator must provide: `type`, `shader`, `origin` and/or `direction` and `spread` depending on `type`, all primitive fields for area light sources.

type (default `miLIGHT_ORIGIN`) distinguishes between point lights (origin only), directional lights (direction only), and spot lights (origin, direction, and spread angle).

area (default `miLIGHT_NONE` describes the type of area light geometry, and is one of `miLIGHT_NONE`, `miLIGHT_RECTANGLE`, `miLIGHT_DISC`, `miLIGHT_SPHERE`, and `miLIGHT_CYLINDER`.

exponent (default 2) controls the falloff of the light at a given distance. An exponent of 2 is physically correct, but other exponents can be chosen to make the light reach farther or less far than it should. An exponent of 1 means that the light energy does not fall off with distance. Exponents other than 2 disturb the energy balance in the scene.

caustic_store_photons is the maximum number of photons from this light source to store in the caustic photon map. If set to zero, the number of photons to emit must be specified, which then controls the number of emitted photons no matter how many are stored. (The zero value is supported in mental ray 2.1.,37 and later, earlier versions require setting it to a very high number.)

caustic_emit_photons is the maximum number of caustic photons to emit from this light source. Emission of caustic photons from a light stops when either caustic_store_photons or caustic_emit_photons has been reached.

global_store_photons[2.1]is the maximum number of photons from this light source to store in the global illumination photon map. Again, a value of zero disables the store limit in mental ray 2.1.37 and later.

global_emit_photons[2.1]is the maximum number of global illumination photons to emit from this light source. Emission of global illumination photons from a light stops when either globillum_store_photons (if nonzero) or globillum_emit_photons has been reached.

shader (default `miNULLTAG`) is the tag of a database element of type `miSCENE_FUNCTION` containing the light shader, which computes illumination by this light at render time.

emitter (default `miNULLTAG`) is the tag of a database element of type `miSCENE_FUNCTION` containing the light photon emitter shader, which emits photons during the global illumination or caustics preprocessing phase.

origin (default 0, 0, 0) is the origin of the light in object space. It is used only if *type* is miLIGHT_ORIGIN or miLIGHT_SPOT.

direction (default 0, 0, 0) is the direction of a directional light. It is used only if *type* is miLIGHT_DIRECTION or miLIGHT_SPOT.

spread is used only by spot lights and it specifies the size of the outer spotlight cone.

primitive contains the size of the area light source if *area* is not miLIGHT_NONE. Depending on area, the width and height of the rectangle are given in *rectangle.edge_u* and *rectangle.edge_v*, or the orientation and radius of the disc are given in *disc.normal* and *disc.radius*, or the radius of the sphere is given in *sphere.radius*, or the axis and radius of the cylinder are given in *cylinder.axis* and *cylinder.radius*. All defaults are 0.

samples_u (default 3) is the number of samples taken in the U direction of the area light source if *area* is not miLIGHT_NONE.

samples_v (default 3) is the number of samples taken in the V direction of the area light source if *area* is not miLIGHT_NONE.

low_samples_u (default 2) is the number of samples taken in the U direction of the area light source if *area* is not miLIGHT_NONE, when the trace depth specified by *low_level* is reached or exceeded.

low_samples_v (default 2) is the number of samples taken in the V direction of the area light source if *area* is not miLIGHT_NONE, when the trace depth specified by *low_level* is reached or exceeded.

low_level (default 3) is the sum of the reflection and refraction trace depth at which area light sampling switches from *samples* to *low_samples*. 0 means that no switching takes place and *samples* are always used.

use_shadow_maps specifies whether shadow maps are used for this light source.

shadowmap_file is the tag of a string containing the filename for the shadowmap. If the tag is null, no file loading and saving will be done. For point lights, six files will be generated, each with an identifying number (1...6) appended to the filename. If the file name contains the # character, it will be expanded to a hexadecimal number identifying the particular instance of this light. This allows different instances of a light to use different files.

shadowmap_resolution is the resolution of the shadow map. For point lights, the individual images will have a lower resolution, so that the total number of pixels rendered will be approximately *shadowmap_resolution* × *shadowmap_resolution*.

shadowmap_softness when non-zero, enables soft shadows. The value given specifies the rectangular size of the region in the shadow map's projection plane in which samples are placed. If this parameter is 0 only one sample will be used, creating sharp shadows. The size is given in internal space units on the shadowmap projection plane.

shadowmap_samples is the number of samples taken from the shadow map. When `shadowmap_softness` is zero, this value is ignored.

visible is `miTRUE` if the light should be seen in the rendering. This only applies to area light sources.

userdata[2.1] allows attaching a user data block (miUserdata) or a chain of user data blocks. Shaders can retrieve the data with *mi_query*.

label[2.1] a numeric value assigned by applications.

4.4.5 Functions

Element type:	miSCENE_FUNCTION
Data type:	miFunction
Sizes:	int param_size
Defaults:	all nulls

```
enum miFunction_type {
        miFUNCTION_C,                   /* regular C/C++ shader */
        miFUNCTION_PHEN,                /* phenomenon interface */
        miFUNCTION_C_REQ,               /* C/C++ shader with reqmnts */
        miFUNCTION_OUTFILE,             /* write an image to a file */
        miFUNCTION_DATA                 /* user data decl, no miFunc */
};

typedef struct miFunction {
        miPointer       user;               /* for shader (init data etc)*/
        miPointer       cached_address;     /* for RC only */
        miPointer       cached_result;      /* array[thread#] of results */
        miPointer       cached_ghost_ptr;   /* if ghost_offs, tag ptrs */
        miPointer       gcache_timestamp;   /* if ghost_offs, eval time */
        miPointer       lightlist;          /* array of lights for shader*/
        miLock          lock;               /* local shader lock */
        enum miFunction_type type;          /* C/C++, phenomenon, or file*/
        miUint          out_typemap;        /* if output, IMG_TYPE bitmap*/
        miUint          out_interpmap;      /* if output, interpolate bm */
        miTag           function_decl;      /* declaration if C or PHEN */
        miTag           next_function;      /* next function call in list*/
        miTag           parameter_indirect; /* get params from this func */
        miTag           interfacephen;      /* parent phen, if any */
        miBoolean       spare2;             /* not used */
        int             parameter_size;     /* size of parameter block */
        int             result_size;        /* size of result struct */
        int             ghost_offs;         /* offset to tag ghost, or 0 */
        int             spare1[2];          /* not used */
        miCBoolean      has_init_shader;    /* init shader exists */
```

```
        miCBoolean      func_init;          /* was function initialized? */
        miCBoolean      inst_init_req;      /* init every instance too? */
        miCBoolean      inst_init;          /* was instance initialized? */
        miCBoolean      no_expl_params;     /* candidate for indirect par*/
        miCBoolean      spare[4];           /* not used */
        miCBoolean      simple;             /* PHEN: can use fast call */
        miUchar         ret_type;           /* PHEN:return type of shader*/
        miUchar         label;              /* sequential # for bitmasks */
        char            parameters[8];      /* parameter block, then */
                                            /* miTag ghost for phenomena */
} miFunction;
```

A translator must provide: `function_decl` (using *mi_scene_link*), `parameter_size` (as *mi_scene_create* argument), `result_size`, `parameters`.
A translator may provide: `next_function`.

Functions are shading functions are pairs of a function identification (the shader name) and a parameter block. They are used for materials, textures, lights, transformations, and many other purposes. Most are called during rendering; some are called during preprocessing or tessellation.

user is not used by mental ray. It is provided so init shaders can access the function and hang local instance data (color tables etc) off this pointer. Previous versions of mental ray required hacks such as adding dummy integers to the shader parameters as a place to store instance data.

cached_address is used to reduce the number of lookups of shader names. After the first lookup, the result of the lookup is cached, and all future lookups first check the address and skip the lookup if it is nonzero. All addresses are stored as a `miPointer` to ensure that they occupy 64 bits in the data structure, regardless of whether the host uses 32-bit or 64-bit pointers.

cached_result is used by *mi_call_shader* and similar functions to cache the result of the last call to this shader. The cache is an array of `result_size` bytes for each thread. This data structure is maintained by *mi_call_shader* and should not be modified by translators. This and the next two fields exist to support phenomena.

cached_ghost_ptr is also created and used exclusively by *mi_call_shader*. It points to an array that has twice the size of the standard tag ghost array (see `parameters` below), and contains one pointer for every tag in that array. It is twice the size because a `miPointer` must be 64 bits wide. The pointer array is used to avoid looking up tags all the time.

gcache_timestamp is also created and used exclusively by *mi_call_shader*. It points to an array that contains one timestamp for every render thread. Whenever a new phenomenon is executed, a global time (per thread) is incremented. If this global time does not agree with the timestamp, `cached_result` is not valid and the shader must be called. If they do agree, the shader has been called before inside the current phenomenon, and the cached result can be used directly.

lightlist is a pointer to an array of light tags. It is used for shaders that have their light list modified according to the global light list.

lock is a lock shared by all instances of a shader. Every shader such as *soft_material* has exactly one local lock that is shared by all concurrent invocations of this shader.

out_typemap is a bitmap that contains the image types needed for the function if it is either an output shader or an output file.

out_interpmap is a bitmap that contains the interpolation flags for each bit in the *out_typemap* bitmap.

function_decl is the declaration of the function, containing both the shader name and a declaration of the parameters it requires. Declaration database elements have type `miSCENE_FUNCTION_DECL`; see below.

next_function references the next function in a chain. Some shader types allow chaining; for example there may be multiple lens shaders anchored in the camera that are called in sequence.

has_init_shader and the other three flags help to determine whether the function and the function instance have been initialized. Except for *func_init* these flags are copies from the declaration (see below) and are here to find out quickly whether it is necessary to access the declaration and do a full init. They are used internally only to cache declaration flags.

parameter_indirect, if nonzero, is the tag of another function that contains the parameters to be used for this function. *parameter_size* and *parameters* are unaffected. This is used for parameterless shadow and photon shaders, which are called with the corresponding material shader's arguments to avoid having to copy the parameters.

interfacephen is the tag of the phenomenon that contains the shader. Presently only used internally to cache the phenomenon tag for lens shaders required by a phenomenon. Should not be used by translators.

parameter_size is the size of the shader parameter area in bytes. Shader parameters are stored at the beginning of the *parameters* array.

result_size is the number of bytes in the result data structure. By default this is 16 (the size of `miColor`, which is the default return type). It *must* be set to match the `result_size` field of the declaration.

ghost_offs is nonzero for phenomenon `miFunctions` and provides an offset into the `parameters` array where the tags begin. This value is either zero or the smallest multiple of 4 equal to or greater than `parameter_size` because tags are integers that must be properly aligned.

ret_type is internally used by the PHEN module for caching the function declaration return type.

label is a number in the range `0` ... 255 that helps distinguishing shaders. A new number is assigned automatically whenever a new function is created, but no attempt is made to keep the numbers unique. This helps the incremental rendering heuristics to decide whether a pixel should be re-rendered.

parameters contains one or two variable-sized data areas: the function parameters, arranged as described in the mental ray User Manual, and the optional tag ghost array. A pointer to the parameter block is passed to the shader whenever it is called. The parameters are expected to be laid out as described by the function declaration.

The tag ghost array is used for phenomenon `miFunctions`. It exists only if `ghost_offs` is nonzero. It has the same layout as the parameter array, such that there is one tag for every parameter at the same offset in the respective array. If the tag for a parameter is nonzero, the tag points to another `miFunction` which must be called (unless its cache is valid, in which case the previous result is re-used; see above) to provide the parameter instead of using the parameter directly. In this case the parameter in the parameter array is the offset into the result returned by the call.

4.4.6 User Data

Element type:	miSCENE_USERDATA
Data type:	miUserdata
Sizes:	int parameter_size
Defaults:	all nulls

```
typedef struct miUserdata {
        miTag           data_decl;              /* parameter declaration */
        miTag           next_data;              /* next data block in list */
        miUint          label;                  /* user-defined label integer*/
        int             parameter_size;         /* size of parameter block */
        short           one;                    /* ==1, for byte order check */
        short           spare1;                 /* not used */
        int             spare2;                 /* not used */
        char            parameters[8];          /* parameter block */
} miUserdata;
```

This element describes a user-definable opaque data block. The API supports setting up these blocks from literal data, from a file, or from shader-like declared parameters. The purpose is carrying user data to shaders that would be too large, contain nonstandard data types, or be repeated in too many places to make storing it as shader parameters feasible. Except in the shader-like parameter case, the data is not byte-swapped by mental ray when transported to another host; this becomes the responsibility of the data recipient.

data_decl is the tag of the declaration of the parameters, if the user data block is defined with parameters. If it was defined with literal data or read from a file, this field is a null tag.

next_data allows chaining of user data blocks, much like shaders can be chained.

parameter_size is the number of bytes stored in this data block, beginning at *parameters*. The rest of the header leading up to the data is not included. Zero is allowed but not useful. mental ray warns if a data block is defined larger than 16 MB.

one is set to 1 when the data block is defined, and when it was defined with parameters and has been imported and byte-swapped. Since literal and file user data blocks are not swapped, the data recipient must assume that non-byte data read from the user data block must be byte-swapped if *one* has the value 0x0100 instead of 1.

parameters contains the user data. Although declared with only eight characters, it is allocated smaller or larger depending on the user data block size such that it holds *parameter_size* bytes.

4.4.7 Function Declarations

Element type:	miSCENE_FUNCTION_DECL
Data type:	miFunction_decl
Sizes:	int decl_size
Defaults:	all nulls, type miFUNCTION_C

```
typedef enum {
        miTYPE_BOOLEAN = 0,                 /* simple types: used for */
        miTYPE_INTEGER,                     /* returns and parameters */
        miTYPE_SCALAR,
        miTYPE_STRING,
        miTYPE_COLOR,
        miTYPE_VECTOR,
        miTYPE_TRANSFORM,
        miTYPE_SHADER,                      /* complex types: used for */
        miTYPE_SCALAR_TEX,                  /* parameters only */
        miTYPE_COLOR_TEX,
        miTYPE_VECTOR_TEX,
        miTYPE_LIGHT,
        miTYPE_STRUCT,
        miTYPE_ARRAY,
        miTYPE_TEX,
        miTYPE_MATERIAL,                    /* phenomenon types */
        miTYPE_GEOMETRY,
        miTYPE_DATA,                        /* free-form user data */
        miNTYPES
} miParam_type;
```

```
typedef struct miPhen_decl {
        int             n_subtags;          /* # of subshader/mtl tags */
        miTag           root;               /* root attachment point */
        miTag           lens;               /* optional lens shaders */
        miTag           output;             /* optional output shaders */
        miTag           volume;             /* optional volume shaders */
        miTag           environment;        /* optional environm. shaders*/
        miTag           geometry;           /* optional geometry shaders */
        miTag           contour_store;      /* opt'l contour store func */
```

```
        miTag           contour_contrast;       /* opt'l contour contrast f. */
        int             lens_seqnr;             /* opt'l sequence number */
        int             output_seqnr;           /* opt'l sequence number */
        int             volume_seqnr;           /* opt'l sequence number */
        int             environment_seqnr;      /* opt'l sequence number */
        /* Fuzzy booleans (0=dont care, 1=false, 2=true) */
        miCBoolean      scanline;               /* need scanline? */
        miCBoolean      trace;                  /* need ray tracing? */
        /* Normal Booleans (these cannot be set explicitly off): */
        miCBoolean      deriv1;                 /* need first derivatives? */
        miCBoolean      deriv2;                 /* need second derivatives? */
        miUchar         mintextures;            /* not used */
        miUchar         minbumps;               /* not used */
        miUchar         minusers;               /* not used */
        miUchar         parallel;               /* parallel output shader */
        char            shadow;                 /* 0, 1, 'l' sort, 's' segm */
        char            face;                   /* 'f'ront, 'b'ack, 'a'll */
        char            render_space;           /* 'c'amera, 'o'bject, 0 any */
        char            spare2;                 /* not used */
} miPhen_decl;


typedef struct miFunction_decl {
        miLock          lock;                   /* local shader lock */
        miPointer       cached_address;         /* for RC only */
        enum miFunction_type type;              /* C function or phenomenon */
        miParam_type    ret_type;               /* return type of shader */
        int             declaration_size;       /* size of declaration */
        int             result_size;            /* size of result struct */
        int             version;                /* shader version from .mi */
        miUint          apply;                  /* what can it be used for? */
        miPhen_decl     phen;                   /* if type==miFUNCTION_PHEN */
        int             spare[2];               /* not used */
        miCBoolean      has_init_shader;        /* init shader exists */
        miCBoolean      has_no_init_shader;     /* checked before, no init sh*/
        miCBoolean      inst_init_req;          /* init every instance too? */
        miCBoolean      func_init;              /* was function initialized? */
        char            name[miNAMESIZE];       /* ascii name */
        char            declaration[4];         /* declaration string */
} miFunction_decl;

#define miDECL_SUBTAG(d,i) (...)
```

A translator must provide: `name`, `result_size`, `declaration`, `version`.
A translator may provide: `type`, `ret_type`.
Provided by *mi_scene_create*: `parameter_size`, `declaration_size`, `parallel`, `apply`.

lock is a lock shared by all instances of a shader. Every shader such as *soft_material* has exactly one local lock that is shared by all concurrent invocations of this shader.

cached_address is used to reduce the number of lookups of shader names. After the first lookup, the result of the lookup is cached, and all future lookups first check the address and skip the lookup if it is nonzero. The address is a `miPointer` because the structure must have the same size regardless of whether pointers are 32 or 64 bits.

type must currently be `miFUNCTION_C`.

ret_type is the return type of the function. For backwards compatibility, undefined return types default to `miTYPE_COLOR`. The type is important for subshaders in shader trees. Only "simple types" are allowed here.

has_init_shader and the other three flags help the renderer to determine whether the function and the function instance have been initialized. *has_no_init_shader* is intended for remembering whether the renderer has already checked whether there is an init shader; if not, no further tests are needed.

name is an ASCII string identifying the shader. This name will be looked up in LINK's symbol table at runtime.

parameter_size helps the translator decide how many bytes to allocate when a new `miFunction` entry is allocated, see above. The parameter size does not include space needed for parameter arrays.

declaration_size is the size of the declaration array in bytes, including the trailing null byte.

result_size is the number of bytes in the result data structure. By default this is 16 (the size of `miColor`, which is the default return type). It *must* be set to match the `result_size` field of the declaration.

version is the declaration version. It can be queried by the shader using *mi_query* and allows the shader to ensure that the declaration and the shader agree. Also, if a shader library contains a function named *shadername*`_version`, it is caled and its returned integer value must match the *version*. It is highly recommended to use this feature.

apply is a bitmap that specifies what the shader can be used for. Each bit stands for a specific type of shader:

miAPPLY_LENS	lens shader in a camera
miAPPLY_MATERIAL	material shader in a material
miAPPLY_LIGHT	light shader
miAPPLY_SHADOW	shadow shader in a material
miAPPLY_ENVIRONMENT	environment shader in a material or camera
miAPPLY_VOLUME	volume shader in a material or camera
miAPPLY_TEXTURE	texture shader
miAPPLY_PHOTON	photon shader in a material
miAPPLY_GEOMETRY	geometry shader
miAPPLY_DISPLACE	displacement shader in a material
miAPPLY_PHOTON_EMITTER	photon emitter shader in a light
miAPPLY_OUTPUT	output shader in a camera

If the apply bitmap is zero (the default), it is not known what the shader can be used for, and all uses are legal. mental ray does not currently enforce non-applicability, this is only a hint.

phen is a substructure containing fields used if the `type` is `miFUNCTION_PHEN`. The `miPhen_decl` substructure is still under development. Note that phenomena keep a list of tags of shaders, materials, lights, and other sub-objects defined in the scope of the phenomenon in a tag list that follows the *declaration* string. Tags in this list can be accessed with the `miDECL_SUBTAG` macro.

declaration describes the parameter layout required by the shader. It is a sequence of ascii characters, each describing a type or structure; the sequence is an abbreviated form of the declaration syntax in the .mi file. The declaration is a list of return and parameter declarations. Each list item begins with an optional `'a'` for array, followed by the type (one of `biscvtSCVlS$` for boolean, integer, scalar, color, vector, transform, scalar texture, color texture, vector texture, light, shader, and string) followed by a double-quoted name. Substructures are defined with {"*name*" followed by the structure name followed by the structure definition followed by }. The declaration has two parts separated by an equals sign; the first part declares the return type and the second part declares the parameters. The first part may have only one field that may not be an array and whose double-quoted name part is omitted, but it may be a structure containing named fields. One null byte terminates the entire declaration.

For example, a shader returning a color *r* and accepting three parameters, a scalar *s*, an array of structures *t* containing two integers *i1* and *i2*, followed by a light array *l* would lead to the following declaration string:

```
c=s"s"a{"t"i"i1"i"i2"}al"l"
```

If the return type were a structure containing a color *c* and a boolean *b*, the declaration changes to:

```
{c"c"b"b"}=s"s"a{"t"i"i1"i"i2"}al"l"
```

4.4.8 Boxes

Element type:	miSCENE_BOX
Data type:	miBox
Sizes:	miVector_list *, miVertex_content *, int nvert, npri, enum miBox_type type, miBoolean moving
Defaults:	all nulls except stored arguments

```
enum miBox_type { miBOX_TRIANGLES, miBOX_ALGEBRAICS };

typedef struct miBox {
      miUint           label;           /* translator: object label */
      miTag            next_box;        /* translator or gap: box list  */
      enum miBox_type  type;            /* type of primitives */
      miBoolean        visible;         /* visible? */
      miBoolean        shadow;          /* casts shadow? */
      miBoolean        trace;           /* visible as reflection? */
      miBoolean        mtl_is_label;    /* triangle mtls are labels */
      miUint1          caustic;         /* bit0=cast, bit1=receive */
      miUint1          globillum;       /* bit0=cast, bit1=receive */
      miCBoolean       spare[6];        /* not used */
      miTag            userdata;        /* optional user data blocks */
      int              spare2[2];       /* not used */
      miVertex_content vert_info;       /* size  content of vertices */
      miVector_list    vect_info;       /* sections of vector array */
      miIndex          no_vertices;     /* number of vertices */
      miIndex          no_primitives;   /* number of primitives */
      miVector         bbox_min;        /* bounding box: low corner */
      miVector         bbox_max;        /* bounding box: high corner */
      miVector         vectors[1];      /* vectors, vertices, primitives */
} miBox;
```

A translator must provide: `vectors`, vertices[1], primitives.
A translator may provide: `label`, `next_box` (using `mi_scene_link`), `visible`, `shadow`, `trace`, `caustic`, `globillum`[2.1], and `mtl_is_label`. Provided by *mi_scene_create*: `type`, `vert_info`, `vect_info`, `no_vertices`, and `no_primitives`

Boxes consists of a `miBox` header, followed by three variable-sized parts: the vector list, the vertex list, and the primitive list. Currently only triangles can be used as a primitive type. All primitives must have the same data type. All primitives in a box were always generated from the same object, no two objects share a box.

label is the label value copied from the object. It is used by shaders only, and can be written to label frame buffers.

[1]The next generation of mental ray will remove the limit of 65536 vectors, vertices, and triangles, and all miIndex types will be replaced with miGeoIndex. miBox will be replaced with miGeoBox. Shaders using miBox will need to be changed.

next_box is used to chain boxes when more than one box results from an object. The maximum size of boxes is limited by the capacity of `miIndex`.

type is either `miBOX_TRIANGLES` and `miBOX__ALGEBRAICS`. Algebraics are not currently supported. Together with *vert_info.motion_offset* (which indicates moving motion-blurred geometry if nonzero), the type determines the data type of the primitives, currently only (`miTriangle`.

visible (default `miTRUE`) makes the triangles visible to primary rays.

shadow (default `miTRUE`) enables shadows cast by the triangles.

trace (default `miTRUE`) makes the triangles visible to second-generation rays.

caustic is a bitmap with three valid bits. Bit 0, if set, enables generation of caustics cast by this object. Bit 1, if set, enables receiving caustics. Bit 4, if set, makes this object invisible to caustic photons.

globillum[2.1] is a bitmap with three valid bits. Bit 0, if set, enables generation of global illumination from this object. Bit 1, if set, enables receiving of global illumination. Bit 4, if set, makes this object invisible to global illumination photons.

mtl_is_label is a flag that informs the renderer that the *material* field in the triangles does not hold a material but an integer label. The renderer must ignore the material in this case and use the inherited material. This flag is set for *tagged* objects in the mi2 language.

userdata[2.1] allows attaching a user data block (miUserdata) or a chain of user data blocks. Shaders can retrieve the data with *mi_query*.

no_vertices is the number of vertices, each of which consists of *vert_info.sizeof_vertex* `miIndex` values.

no_primitives is the number of primitives (triangles or algebraics).

There are two data structures that are used in boxes and several other places to describe the format of vertices and boxes:

```
typedef struct miVertex_content {
        miUchar         sizeof_vertex;  /* size of a vertex
                                           (in the input in miGeoIndex's;
                                            in boxes     in miIndex's) */
        miUchar         normal_offset;  /* when 0, not present */
        miUchar         motion_offset;  /* when 0, not present */
        miUchar         derivs_offset;  /* surf derivs, when 0, not present */
        miUchar         derivs2_offset; /* 2nd derivs, when 0, not present */
        miUchar         texture_offset; /* when 0, not present */
        miUchar         no_textures;    /* number of textures */
        miUchar         bump_offset;    /* when 0, not present */
        miUchar         no_bumps;       /* number of bumps */
```

```
        miUchar         user_offset;        /* when 0, not present */
        miUchar         no_users;           /* number of user vectors */
} miVertex_content;
```

A translator must provide: all fields.
This structure is used in `miBox` to describe which information is stored with each vertex. It is also used to inform the tessellator what information to create vertices with. Vertices always consist of at least one vector reference for the point in space. The normal, the motion vector, the surface derivative pair, the list of textures, the list of bump basis vectors, and the list of user vectors are all optional.

As described in the subsection for boxes below, a vertex is a list of indices into the actual vector table. Each such list begins with the index for the point in space, said to be at offset `0` in the list. The `miVertex_content` structure describes at which offset in the list other vector indices can be found. For example, if there is an index for a normal in the list directly after the index for the point in space, `normal_offset` would be 1. Offset value `0` is reserved for nonexisting items; no item can have offset `0` because the point in space index is stored there.

If some vertices have a certain type type of index and others do not (like some vertices have normals and others do not), the offset in the `miVertex_content` structure is nonzero but the index is set to `miNULL_INDEX` resp. `miNULL_GEOINDEX` in those vertices that do not need it. Using `0` for nonexistent offset members is ok because the first index in a vertex (which has offset `0`) is the point in space, which must always exist. Do not confuse null offsets with null indices, which must use `miNULL_INDEX` resp. `miNULL_GEOINDEX` instead of `0` because the first vector in a polygon vector list can be something other than a point in space. This is inconvenient for the polygon-to-box tessellation code because box vector lists are divided into sections, and the vector list *does* begin with points in space so non-point-in-space indices cannot be `0`, but this rule applies only to boxes. Polygon lists mirror the order in the .mi file, which traditionally does allow index `0` for vectors that are not points in space.

The second recurring structure is the vector list header. Depending on whether the list contains miGeoVectors (in the input) or miVectors (in the boxes) miGeoIndex or miIndex variables are used to reference them.

```
typedef struct miGeoVector_list {
        miGeoIndex      no_vectors;         /* total number of input vectors */
        miGeoIndex      no_points;          /* number of points in space */
        miGeoIndex      no_normals;         /* number of normals */
        miGeoIndex      no_derivs;          /* number of 1st/2nd surface derivs */
        miGeoIndex      no_motions;         /* number of motion vectors */
        miGeoIndex      no_textures;        /* number of texture coordinates */
        miGeoIndex      no_bumps;           /* number of bump basis vectors */
        miGeoIndex      no_users;           /* number of user-defined vectors */
} miGeoVector_list;

typedef struct miVector_list {
        miIndex         no_vectors;         /* total number of box vectors */
```

```
        miIndex         no_points;      /* number of points */
        miIndex         no_normals;     /* number of normals */
        miIndex         no_derivs;      /* number of surf. derivs. */
        miIndex         no_motions;     /* number of motion vectors */
        miIndex         no_textures;    /* number of texture vectors */
        miIndex         no_bumps;       /* number of bump vectors */
        miIndex         no_users;       /* number of user vectors */
} miVector_list;
```

A translator must provide: all fields.

All the vertex indices described by the `miVertex_content` structure are indices into the actual vector list. The vector list itself is partitioned in the seven "sections": one for points in space, one for normals, one for surface derivatives, and so on. This partitioning allows the preprocessing stage to quickly transform a box without traversing the vertex index list; points are transformed in a different way than normals or motion vectors, and some vectors such as user vectors are not transformed at all.

The complete box structure can be summarized as:

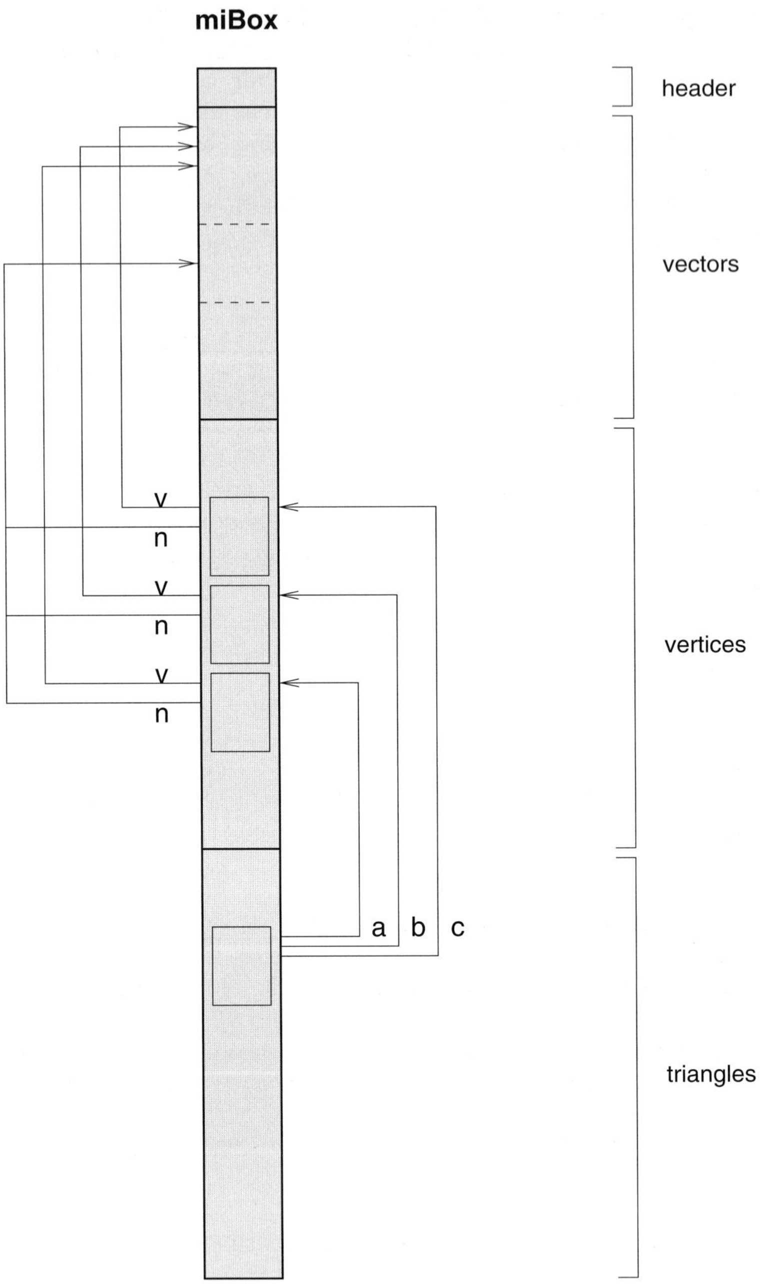

Box Geometry Storage

The header is declared as `miBox` itself. The vector part is a `miVector` array. The vertex part is a `miIndex` array. The primitive part is an array of triangles, which are declared as follows. Fields marked "R:" are reserved for the renderer and should not be used by any other module.

```
enum miTriangle_projection { TRI_XY_P = 0, TRI_YZ_P, TRI_ZX_P,
                             TRI_XY_N = 4, TRI_YZ_N, TRI_ZX_N };

/* gap_flags */
#define miISOLATED_TRI  0x1
#define miIS_STRIP      0x2
#define miSTRIP_BEGIN   0x4
#define miSTRIP_RIGHT   0x8

typedef struct {
        miUchar         proj;           /* R: miTriangle_projection flag */
        miUchar         gap_flags;      /* flags for strip output */
        miIndex         a;              /* vertex index */
        miIndex         b;              /* vertex index */
        miIndex         c;              /* vertex index */
        miTag           material;       /* opt. material */
        miVector        normal;         /* R: normal */
        miScalar        d;              /* R: distance */
} miTriangle;
```

A translator must provide: a, b, c, material.

projection is a flag used by the renderer to cache the best projection plane of the triangle. Possible values are TRI_XY, TRI_XZ, and TRI_YZ. It is declared as a miUchar because declaring it as an enum miTriangle_projection (a 4-byte int) would cause a structure misalignment.

gap_flags store information about triangle strips indicating whether the triangle is not adjacent to its predecessor or successor in the box (miISOLATED_TRI), whether it belongs to a strip or fan (miIS_STRIP), whether it is the first triangle of a fan or strip (miSTRIP_BEGIN), and the type of strip (miSTRIP_RIGHT). gap_flags are computed when the option strips is set.

a, b, c are indices into the vertex list. The first vertex is numbered 0. The indices are multiplied by *vert_info.sizeof_vertex* before the actual array lookup; up to 65536 vertices can be indexed.

material is the tag of a material for this primitive. The referenced database element must have type miSCENE_MATERIAL.

normal is the geometric triangle normal. Normals are calculated and accessed by the renderer only.

4.4.9 Objects

Element type:	miSCENE_OBJECT
Data type:	miObject
Sizes:	—
Defaults:	as described below

```
enum miObject_type {
        miOBJECT_POLYGONS,
        miOBJECT_FACES,
        miOBJECT_BOXES,
        miOBJECT_SPACECURVES,               /* for future use */
        miOBJECT_SUBDIVSURFS,               /* for future use */
        miOBJECT_ALGEBRAICS                 /* for future use */
};

typedef struct miObject {
        miTag               boxes;          /* SCENE: cached shared tess */
        int                 n_boxes;        /* SCENE: # of boxes attached */
        miTag               geogroup;       /* SCENE: geomshader group */
        enum miObject_type  type;           /* which in union to use */
        miBoolean           visible;        /* object visible? */
        miBoolean           shadow;         /* cast a shadow? */
        miBoolean           trace;          /* reflection and refraction? */
        miUint1             caustic;        /* bit0=cast, bit1=receive */
        miUint1             globillum;      /* bit0=cast, bit1=receive */
        miCBoolean          spare_1[2];     /* not used */
        miBoolean           view_dependent; /* miOBJECT_FACES only */
        miBoolean           mtl_is_label;   /* poly/surf mtls are labels */
        miScalar            maxdisplace;    /* max return of displ shader*/
        miBoolean           spare_2[1];     /* not used, for padding */
        miTag               userdata;       /* optional user data blocks */
        miUint              label;          /* optional label */
        miVector            bbox_min;       /* bounding box: low corner */
        miVector            bbox_max;       /* bounding box: high corner */
        miTag               functions;      /* SCENE: material req list */
        unsigned int        n_functions;    /* SCENE: # tags in functions*/
        union {
            miPolygon_list    polygon_list;
            miFace_list       face_list;
            miTag             box_list;
            miSpacecurve_list spacecurve_list;/* for future use */
            miSubdivsurf_list subdivsurf_list;/* for future use */
        }                   geo;            /* geometry */
} miObject;

typedef struct miPolygon_list {
        miGeoIndex          no_polygons;
        miGeoIndex          no_indices;
        miGeoIndex          no_vertices;
        miGeoVector_list    vect_info;      /* contents of vector array */
        miVertex_content    vert_info;      /* vertex size & content */
        miTag               polygons;       /* array of miPolygon */
        miTag               indices;        /* array of miGeoIndex */
        miTag               vertices;       /* see vert_info */
```

```
        miTag                  vectors;           /* array of miGeoVector */
        miApprox               approx;            /* poly approx technique */
} miPolygon_list;

typedef struct miFace_list {
        miGeoIndex      no_faces;
        miGeoIndex      no_surfaces;
        miGeoIndex      no_curves;
        miGeoIndex      no_specpnts;
        miGeoIndex      no_surf_scalars;
        miGeoIndex      no_curve_scalars;
        miTag           faces;                    /* array of miFace */
        miTag           surfaces;                 /* array of miSurface */
        miTag           curves;                   /* array of miCurve */
        miTag           specpnts;                 /* array of miCurve_point */
        miTag           surf_scalars;             /* array of miGeoScalar */
        miTag           curve_scalars;            /* array of miGeoScalar */
        miTag           basis_list;               /* miBasis_list */
} miFace_list;

typedef struct miSpacecurve_list {
        miGeoIndex      no_spacecurves;
        miGeoIndex      no_curves;
        miGeoIndex      no_specpnts;
        miGeoIndex      no_curve_scalars;
        miTag           spacecurves;              /* array of miSpacecurve */
        miTag           curves;                   /* array of miCurve */
        miTag           specpnts;                 /* array of miCurve_point */
        miTag           curve_scalars;            /* array of miGeoScalar */
        miTag           basis_list;               /* miBasis_list */
        miBoolean       pad;                      /* not used */
} miSpacecurve_list;
```

A translator must provide: `type`; all `miPolygon_list` fields for polygonal objects; `no_faces`, `no_surfaces`, `no_surf_scalars`, `faces`, `surfaces`, `surf_scalars`, `basis_list`.

boxes is used to point to boxes that resulted from tessellation. They are used in two cases only: object or box instances attach to the cached untransformed boxes (see above for a definition) if enabled; and leaf instances attach to the final renderable representation.

n_boxes is the number of boxes attached to **boxes**. Keeping this separate avoids having to access boxes to count them.

geogroup is used to point to the group element which contains all the geometry-shader created scene elements for this object.

type (default `miOBJECT_POLYGONS`) specifies the type of the geometry attached to this object. It may be one of miOBJECT_POLYGONS, miOBJECT_FACES, miOBJECT_BOXES, or miOBJECT_ALGEBRAICS. This field determines which member of the union is used. Algebraics are not currently supported.

visible (default miTRUE) makes the object visible to primary rays.

shadow (default miTRUE) enables shadows cast by this object.

trace (default miTRUE) makes the object visible to second-generation rays.

view_dependent (default miFALSE) enables view-dependent tessellation if the object has type miOBJECT_FACES. It should be set to miTRUE iff any of the surfaces in the object references a view-dependent approximation. It should not be changed between preprocessing and postprocessing.

caustic is a bitmap with three valid bits. Bit 0, if set, enables generation of caustics cast by this object. Bit 1, if set, enables receiving caustics. Bit 4, if set, makes this object invisible to caustic photons.

globillum[2.1] is a bitmap with three valid bits. Bit 0, if set, enables generation of global illumination from this object. Bit 1, if set, enables receiving of global illumination by this object. Bit 4, if set, makes this object invisible to global illumination photons.

mtl_is_label is a flag that informs the renderer that the *material* field in the polygons or surfaces does not hold a material but an integer label. The renderer must ignore the material in this case and use the inherited material. This flag is set for *tagged* objects in the mi2 language.

userdata[2.1] allows attaching a user data block (miUserdata) or a chain of user data blocks. Shaders can retrieve the data with *mi_query*.

label is a 32-bit integer that may be used to identify the object in shaders. mental ray does not use it in any way.

functions if this is not a null tag, it points to a list of material tags. This list represents the required materials for the object.

n_functions the number of tags in the *functions* taglist.

geo is a union containing type-specific data. The suffix "_list" indicates that several types store the actual geometry in one or more lists of specific types; these lists are anchored here. The box_list case is a tag of a database element of type miSCENE_BOX. The box data type has been described above. Polygonal geometry is stored in four lists, all anchored in the geo.polygon_list structure.

The following diagram shows the connections between the four lists:

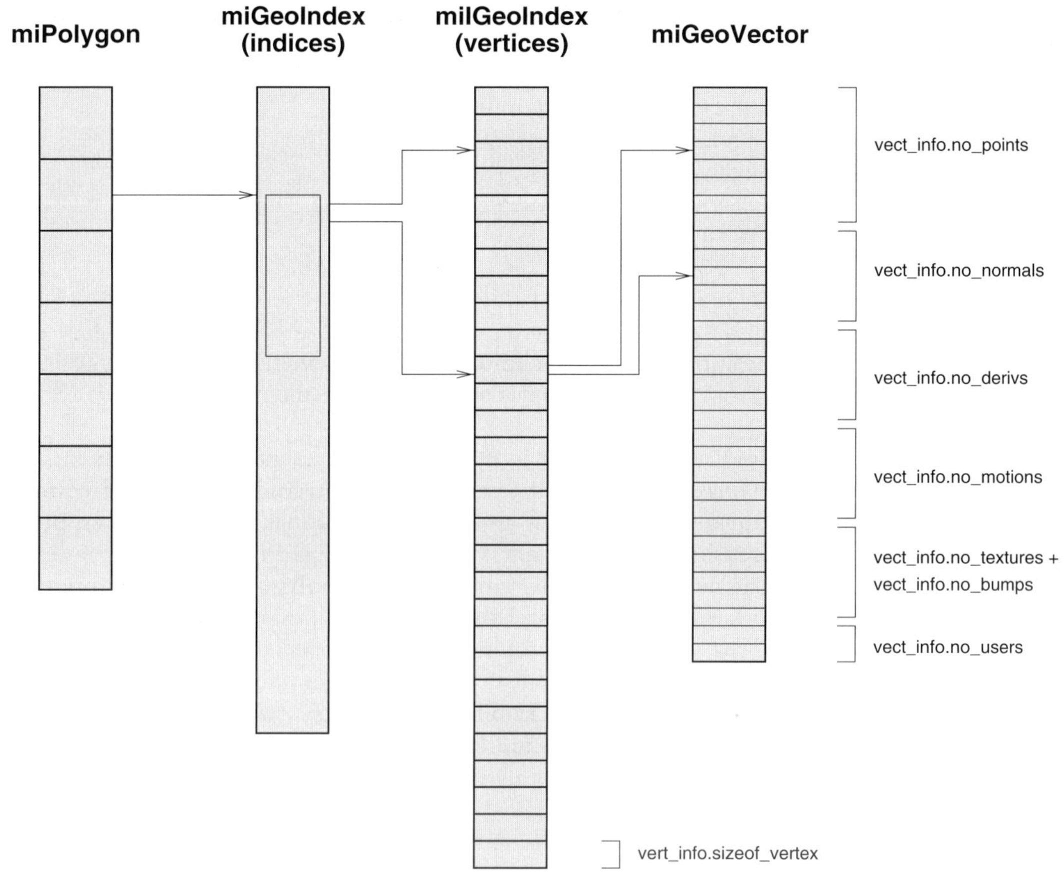

Polygonal Geometry Storage

Arrows indicate indices into the pointed-to data structure. All four grey boxes are separate Scene database element types, refer to the sections for `miSCENE_POLYGON`, `miSCENE_GEOINDEX`, and `miSCENE_GEOVECTOR`, respectively. The data structures are similar to the box data structure, except that the lists are stored in separate database elements, and that an index list is inserted that allows storing polygons with different numbers of vertices in a `miPolygon` data structure that has a constant size. The polygon points to the first vertex index in the index list and gives the number of vertices, as opposed to triangles in boxes that contain the three vertex indices directly.

geo.polygon_list.no_polygons is the number of polygons in the *polygons* list.

geo.polygon_list.no_indices is the number of indices in the *indices* list.

geo.polygon_list.no_vertices is the number of vertices in the *vertices* list. Each vertex consists of *vert_info.sizeof_vertex* indices.

geo.polygon_list.vect_info describes the sections of the vector list. For details, see the section for boxes above.

geo.polygon_list.vert_info describes the layout of the indices in the vertex list. For details, see the section for boxes above.

geo.polygon_list.polygons is the tag of the polygon list.

geo.polygon_list.indices is the tag of the index list.

geo.polygon_list.vertices is the tag of the vertex list.

geo.polygon_list.vectors is the tag of the vector list.

geo.polygon_list.approx is the approximation technique for displacement-mapped polygons. (It does not apply to polygons whose material does not specify displacement maps.)

Surface geometry is more complex. It is stored in up to seven different database elements, all of which are anchored in *geo.face_list*. The term *face* describes one complete visible free-form surface, which is built from one geometry *surface* and multiple optional texture surfaces, bump surfaces, and/or motion surfaces that provide certain types of mappings on the surface. For details on texture surfaces, refer to the mental ray User Manual. Unlike polygons, surfaces store their parameter lists and vectors in large `miGeoScalar` lists. This simplifies storing one, two, three, and four dimensional data in the same list. Trimming, hole, and special curves can optionally be attached to faces; they have their own scalar lists. Both surfaces and curves may reference optional special points. Every surface references two bases, and every curve references one base. Again, all lines in the following diagram indicate indices.

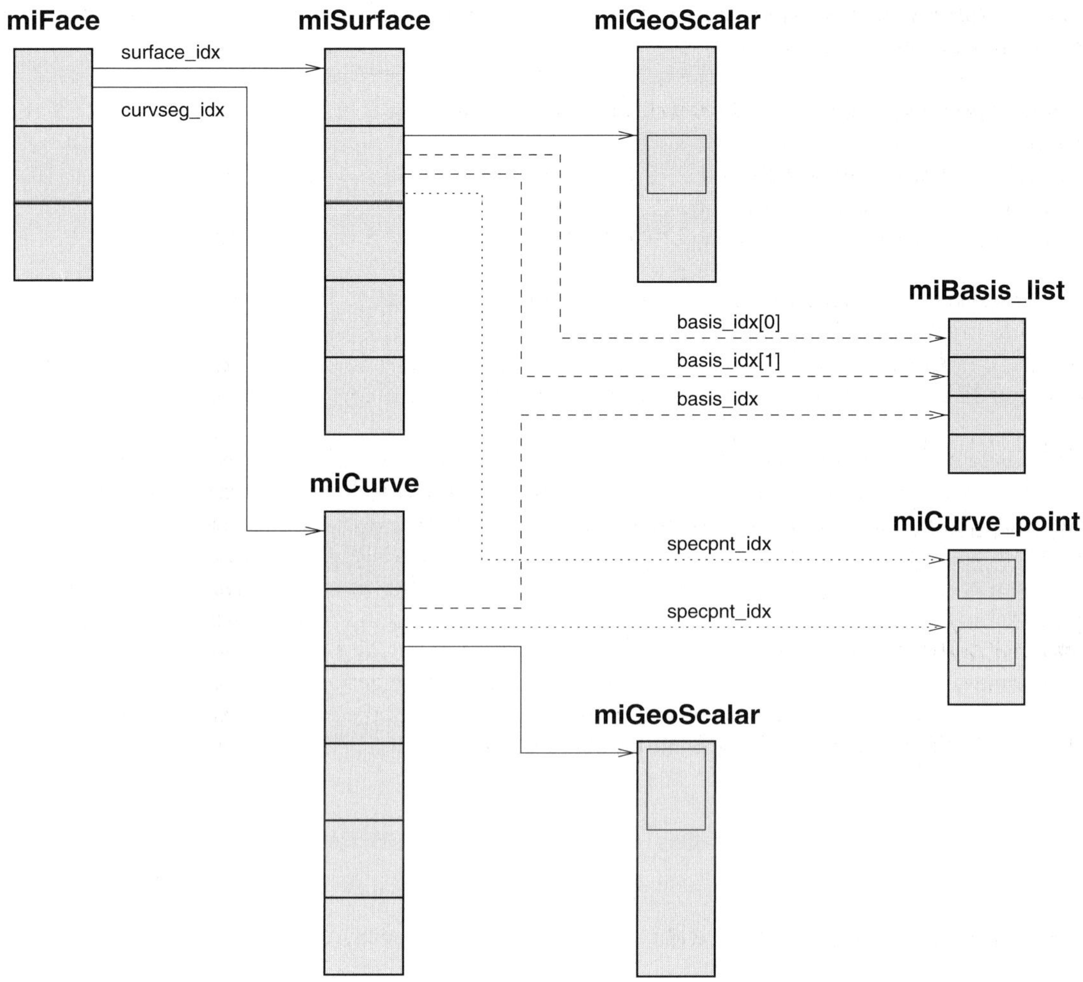

Free-form Surface Geometry Storage

geo.face_list.no_faces is the number of faces in the *geo.face_list.faces* list.

geo.face_list.no_surfaces is the number of surfaces in the *geo.face_list.surfaces* list.

geo.face_list.no_curves is the number of curves in the *geo.face_list.curves* list.

geo.face_list.no_specpnts is the number of special points in the *geo.face_list.specpnts* list.

geo.face_list.no_surf_scalars is the number of surface scalars in the *geo.face_list.surf_scalars* list.

geo.face_list.no_curve_scalars is the number of curve scalars in the *geo.face_list.curve_scalars* list.

geo.face_list.faces is the tag of the list of faces.

geo.face_list.surfaces is the tag of the list of surfaces.

geo.face_list.curves is the tag of the list of curve.

geo.face_list.specpnts is the tag of the list of special points.

geo.face_list.surf_scalars is the tag of the list of surface scalars, which are used for parameter vectors, control points, weights etc. that define all surfaces in this object.

geo.face_list.curve_scalars is the tag of the list of curve scalars, which are used for parameter vectors, control points, weights etc. that define all curves in this object.

geo.face_list.basis_list is the tag of the list of all bases.

An object of type `miOBJECT_SPACECURVE` contains a list of space curves. A single space curve consists of curve segments which are approximated as a single three dimensional curve. The approximation result is stored in a *miLinebox*.

geo.spacecurve_list.no_spacecurves is the number of space curves in the *geo.spacecurve_list.spacecurves* list.

geo.spacecurve_list.no_curves is the number of curves in the *geo.spacecurve_list.curves* list.

geo.spacecurve_list.no_specpnts is the number of special points in the *geo.spacecurve_list.specpnts* list.

geo.spacecurve_list.no_curve_scalars is the number of curve scalars in the *geo.spacecurve_list.curve_scalars* list.

geo.spacecurve_list.spacecurves is the tag of the list of spacecurves.

geo.spacecurve_list.curves is the tag of the list of curves.

geo.spacecurve_list.specpnts is the tag of the list of curve special points.

geo.spacecurve_list.curve_scalars is the tag of the list of curve scalars.

geo.spacecurve_list.basis_list is the tag of the list of all bases used by the curves.

4.4.10 Approximations

Element type:	—
Data type:	miApprox
Sizes:	—
Defaults:	as set by miAPPROX_DEFAULT()

```
enum miApprox_method {
```

```
        miAPPROX_PARAMETRIC,
        miAPPROX_REGULAR,
        miAPPROX_SPATIAL,
        miAPPROX_CURVATURE,
        miAPPROX_LDA,
        miAPPROX_ADJACENCY,           /* only for curves */
        miAPPROX_ALGEBRAIC,           /* only for surfaces */
        miAPPROX_DEFTRIM,             /* only for miFace def_trim_approx */
        miAPPROX_NMETHODS
};

enum miApprox_style {
        miAPPROX_STYLE_NONE,
        miAPPROX_STYLE_GRID,
        miAPPROX_STYLE_TREE,
        miAPPROX_STYLE_DELAUNAY,
        miAPPROX_NSTYLES
};

#define miCNST_UPARAM   0             /* regular/parametric only */
#define miCNST_VPARAM   1
#define miCNST_LENGTH   0             /* curvature/spatial only */
#define miCNST_DISTANCE 1
#define miCNST_ANGLE    2

typedef struct miApprox {
        miGeoScalar          cnst[3];   /* indexed with miUPARAM...miANGLE */
        miCBoolean           spare0[2]; /* not used                        */
        miCBoolean           any;       /* stop if any criterion is met    */
        miCBoolean           view_dep;  /* view dependent ?                */
        enum miApprox_method method;
        enum miApprox_style  style;
        miUshort             subdiv[2]; /* recursive subdivision depth     */
        miGeoIndex           max;       /* maximum number of triangles     */
        miGeoIndex           spare1;    /* not used                        */
} miApprox;
#define miSWAP_SCENE_APPROX "dddiiiss"

#define miAPPROX_MAX_SUBDIV     7
#define miAPPROX_DEFAULT(A)                     \
        (A).style         = miAPPROX_STYLE_TREE;\
        (A).method        = miAPPROX_PARAMETRIC;\
        (A).view_dep      = miFALSE;            \
        (A).cnst[0]       = 1.0;                \
        (A).cnst[1]       = 1.0;                \
        (A).cnst[2]       = 0.0;                \
        (A).subdiv[miMIN] = 0;                  \
        (A).subdiv[miMAX] = 5;
```

A translator may provide: all fields.

The approximation structure is a substructure of **miPolygon_list**, **miCurve**, and **miSurface**. It does not have its own database entry and no associated SCENE functions of its own.

method is the approximation method, and must be one of `miAPPROX_PARAMETRIC`, `miAPPROX_REGULAR`, `miAPPROX_SPATIAL`, `miAPPROX_CURVATURE`, `miAPPROX_LDA`, `miAPPROX_ADJACENCY` (available for curves only), and `miAPPROX_ALGEBRAIC` (available for surfaces only). The default is `miAPPROX_PARAMETRIC`. "LDA" stands for Length, Distance, Angle; this mode combines the spatial and curvature-dependent modes.

style is the approximation style, and must be one of `miAPPROX_NONE`, `miAPPROX_GRID`, `miAPPROX_TREE`, and `miAPPROX_STYLE_MESH`. Tree mode is the default. The API and GAP module will automatically change the style field to grid mode if the method is parametric or regular.

any, if `miTRUE`, makes the tessellation stop if *any* criterion is met, instead of when *all* criteria are met. Close faces are tessellated more finely than distant faces. This mode is not available for the parametric and regular method.

view_dep, if `miTRUE`, turns on view-dependent tessellation. Close faces are tessellated more finely than distant faces. This mode is not available for the parametric and regular method.

cnst[0], **cnst[1]**, and **cnst[2]** specify the approximation precision. They depend on the approximation method. The defaults are 1.0 (which is not ideal for curvature-dependent tessellation). The **cnst** array should be indexed using the `miCNST_*` constants.

technique	cnst[0]	cnst[1]	cnst[2]
parametric	$\frac{\textit{number of U subdivs}}{\textit{degree}}$	$\frac{\textit{number of V subdivs}}{\textit{degree}}$	—
regular	*number of U subdivs*	*number of V subdivs*	—
spatial	edge length limit	—	—
curvature	—	distance tolerance	angle tolerance
lda	edge length limit	distance tolerance	angle tolerance

subdiv[0] and **subdiv[1]** specify the recursion limits. The defaults are 0 and 5, respectively. The maximum value is 7. A subdivision level n means that the curve, triangle, or surface is halved in each parameter direction n times, yielding on the order of 2^n segments. The limits have no effect on Delaunay triangulation.

max is used only for Delaunay triangulation. It specifies the maximum number of triangles to create. The number may be exceeded if the trimming and hole curves have too many vertices.

4.4.11 Polygon Lists

Element type: miSCENE_POLYGON
Data type: miPolygon[ ]
Sizes: int no_polys
Defaults: all nulls

```
typedef struct miPolygon {
        miGeoIndex      no_loops;       /* 1 + (number of holes) */
        miGeoIndex      no_vertices;    /* total number of vertices + headers*/
        miGeoIndex      vertex_idx;     /* into indices list, for sharing */
        miTag           material;       /* surface properties */
        miCBoolean      convex;         /* is polygon convex ? */
        miCBoolean      spare[3];       /* not used */
} miPolygon;
```

A translator must provide: all fields except `spare`.

no_loops is the number of loops of the polygon. Every polygon has exactly one outer boundary loop, plus any number of optional hole loops. Every loop is stored as a pseudo-index called a "header" that doesn't actually refer to the vector list but gives the number of indices to follow, followed by that many indices.

no_vertices is the total number of headers (the number of holes plus 1) plus the total number of vertices for this polygon.

vertex_idx is an index to the first header of the polygon in the index list. *no_vertices* indices beginning at *vertex_idex* define the polygon.

material is the tag of the material of the polygon. It must refer to a database element of type `miSCENE_MATERIAL`.

convex is a flag telling the tessellator that the polygon has no holes and is guaranteed to be convex. This saves time because GAP can use a very simple tessellation algorithm.

4.4.12 Polygon Indices

Element type: miSCENE_GEOINDEX
Data type: miGeoIndex[ ]
Sizes: int no_indices
Defaults: all nulls

Polygon indices are simple `miGeoIndex` arrays. As described above, each polygon indexes a consecutive block of indices that describes one or more loops, each of which begins with a header pseudo-index giving the number of loop indices to follow. Each index indexes into the vertex list, after being multiplied by *vert_info.sizeof_vertex*.

4.4.13 Polygon Vertices

Element type: miSCENE_GEOVERTEX
Data type: miGeoIndex[ ]
Sizes: int no_indices
Defaults: all nulls

The vertex list is an `miGeoIndex` array. It works exactly like the vertex section of boxes; see above. The *vert_info* structure in `miPolygon` determines how many indices make up one vertex, and how it is laid out. Note that the *no_indices* argument of the create and resize functions is the number of indices, not the number of vertices.

4.4.14 Polygon Vectors

Element type: miSCENE_GEOVECTOR
Data type: miGeoVector[ ]
Sizes: int no_vectors
Defaults: all nulls

The vector list is a `miGeoVector` array. It is partitioned into sections as described by the *vect_info* structure in `miPolygon`.

4.4.15 Surfaces: Face List

Element type: miSCENE_FACE
Data type: miFace[ ]
Sizes: int no_faces
Defaults: all nulls except where otherwise noted

```
typedef struct miFace {
        miApprox         def_trim_approx;  /* approx techn. for default trims */
        miGeoRange       range[miUV_DIM];  /* min/max for parameter vals*/
        miGeoIndex       no_curves;        /* total number of curves */
        miGeoIndex       no_surfaces;      /* total # of surfs: 1 geo. + xtras */
        miGeoIndex       surface_idx;      /* surface list index */
        miGeoIndex       curve_idx;        /* index into the 'curves' list*/
        miTag            material;         /* optional: material of the face */
        miVertex_content gap_vert_info;    /* For calculating box sizes */
} miFace;
```

A translator must provide: `range`, `no_surfaces`, `surface_idx`, `material`, `gap_vert_info`.
A translator may provide: `def_trim_approx`, `no_curves`, `curve_idx`.

def_trim_approx is the approximation for default trimming curves. Default trimming curves are automatically created if the face has no explicit trimming curves attached. The default trimming curve follows the edges of the face. The `miAPPROX_DEFTRIM` approximation technique, which is allowed only here, should be used as default to create a default trim curve that does not introduce new vertices.

range[miU] and **range[miV]** specify the minimum and maximum values of the U and V parameter vectors.

no_curves specifies the total number of curves used by this face.

no_surfaces is the total number of surfaces for this face. This is at least 1 for the geometric surface, plus the numbers of texture, bump, and/or motion surfaces.

surface_idx is the index of the first surface in the surface list anchored in the object (see above) that is used for this face. This is the first of *no_surfaces* consecutive surfaces to use.

curve_idx is the index of the first curve in the curve list anchored in the object that is used for this face. This is the first of *no_curves* consecutive curves to use.

material specifies the tag of a material to use for the face.

gap_vert_info describes the layout and size of the vertices to create during tessellation. The boxes created during tessellation will get a copy of this vertex info structure.

4.4.16 Surfaces: Surface List

Element type:	miSCENE_SURFACE
Data type:	miSurface[ ]
Sizes:	int no_surfaces
Defaults:	all nulls, except where otherwise noted

```
typedef struct miSurface {
        miApprox        approx;                 /* approx techn. for surface */
        miApprox        disp_approx;            /* approx for disp. surface */
        miGeoIndex      no_parms[miUV_DIM];     /* no of parameter values */
        miGeoIndex      no_ctls;                /* no of control points */
        miGeoIndex      no_specpnts;            /* no of special points */
        miGeoIndex      scalar_idx;             /* surf_scalar list index */
        miGeoIndex      specpnt_idx;            /* special points list index */
        miGeoIndex      basis_idx[miUV_DIM];    /* index into basis list */
        enum miSurface_type type;
        miUshort        degree[miUV_DIM];       /* from bases, for GAP */
        miUshort        ctl_dim;                /* control pnt dimension */
```

```
    miUshort        spare[3];
} miSurface;
```

A translator must provide: type, approx, disp_approx, ctl_dim, degree, no_parms, no_ctls, scalar_idx, basis_idx.
A translator may provide: no_specpnts, specpnt_idx.

type must be one of the following: miSURFACE_GEOMETRIC, miSURFACE_GEOMOTION, miSURFACE_-TEXTURE, miSURFACE_BUMP, miSURFACE_TEXBUMP_2D, or miSURFACE_TEXBUMP_3D. The 2D variants perform seam rewind correction, the 3D variants do not. All surfaces begin with either miSURFACE_GEOMETRIC or miSURFACE_GEOMOTION, optionally followed by one of the others for each texture space, beginning with space 0 up to a maximum of space 63.

approx is the approximation technique as described above, in the miFace description.

disp_approx is the approximation technique for the displaced surface, if a displacement shader is available.

ctl_dim is the number of scalars per control point:

miSURFACE_GEOMETRIC, non-rational:	3
miSURFACE_GEOMETRIC, rational:	4
miSURFACE_GEOMOTION, non-rational:	6
miSURFACE_GEOMOTION, rational:	7
miSURFACE_TEXTURE_2D	2
miSURFACE_TEXTURE_3D	3
miSURFACE_BUMP:	3
miSURFACE_TEXBUMP_2D, non-rational:	5
miSURFACE_TEXBUMP_2D, rational:	6
miSURFACE_TEXBUMP_3D, non-rational:	5
miSURFACE_TEXBUMP_3D, rational:	6

degree[0] and **degree[1]** contains the degree of the surface in the U and V directions, respectively. This is used by GAP to cache the degree from the surface bases.

no_parms[0] and **no_parms[1]** are the lengths of the U and V parameter vectors, respectively.

no_ctls is the total number of control points for this surface. The number of scalars required in the scalar list is *no_ctls* · *ctl_dim*.

no_specpoints is the number of special points to be included in the tessellation.

scalar_idx is the index of the first scalar in the surface scalar list (also anchored in the object, see above). The scalar list for one surface consists of the U parameter vector, followed by the V parameter vector, followed by the geometric control points (all X first, then all Y, then all Z, then all W, then all motion X, then all motion Y, then all motion Z, if present), followed by the texture and bump control points in the same XYZW order if present.

specpnt_idx is the index of the first special point in the special points list (anchored in the object) to use.

basis_idx[0] and **basis_idx**[1] are indices for the bases in the basis list (anchored in the object) to use, separate for the U and V parameter directions.

4.4.17 Surfaces: Curve Segment List

Element type:	miSCENE_CURVE
Data type:	miCurve
Sizes:	int no_curves
Defaults:	as described below

```
enum miCurve_type {
        miCURVE_TRIM,
        miCURVE_HOLE,
        miCURVE_SPECIAL,
        miCURVE_SPACE
};

typedef struct miCurve {
        enum miCurve_type type;
        miApprox        approx;         /* approx techn. for surface */
        miBoolean       new_loop;       /* F=concatenate to prev, T=begin new */
        miUshort        ctl_dim;        /* control point dimension 2 or 3 */
        miUshort        degree;         /* from basis, for ease in GAP */
        miGeoRange      range;          /* min/max for curve params. */
        miGeoIndex      no_parms;       /* number of curve parameters */
        miGeoIndex      no_ctls;        /* number of control points */
        miGeoIndex      no_specpnts;    /* number of special points */
        miGeoIndex      scalar_idx;     /* index into curve_scalar list */
        miGeoIndex      specpnt_idx;    /* index into special points list */
        miGeoIndex      basis_idx;      /* index into basis list */
} miCurve;
```

A translator must provide: `type`, `approx`, `new_loop`, `ctl_dim`, `degree`, `range`, `no_parms`, `no_ctls`, `scalar_idx`, `basis_idx`.
A translator may provide: `no_specpnts`, `specpnt_idx`.

type specifies what the curve is used for. It must be one of `miCURVE_TRIM`, `miCURVE_HOLE`, `miCURVE_SPECIAL` or `miCURVE_SPACE`. The default is `miCURVE_TRIM`.

approx is the approximation technique as described above, in the `miFace` description.

new_loop is `miTRUE` for every new loop. Loops can be pieced together from multiple consecutive curves. The default is `miTRUE`.

ctl_dim is the control point dimension; 2 for UV curves or 3 for space curves. The default is 2.

degree is the degree of the curve. The default is 3.

range is the range over which the curve is evaluated. The value depends on the parameter list. The defaults are `0.0` and `1.0`.

no_parms is the length of the parameter vectors.

no_ctls is the number of control points for this curve. The number of scalars required in the curve scalar list is $no\_ctls \cdot ctl\_dim$.

no_specpoints is the number of special points to be included in the approximation.

scalar_idx is the index of the first scalar in the curve scalar list (also anchored in the object, see above). The scalar list for one curve consists of the parameter vector, followed by the control points (all X first, then all Y, then all Z, if present).

specpnt_idx is the index of the first special point in the special points list (anchored in the object) to use.

basis_idx is the index of the basis in the basis list (anchored in the object) to use.

4.4.18 Surfaces: Scalar Lists

Element type:	miSCENE_SCALAR
Data type:	miGeoScalar[ ]
Sizes:	int no_scalars
Defaults:	all nulls

Both surfaces and curves store all their geometric data (parameter lists and control points) in unstructured scalar lists. The exact layout and the size of each control point depends on the surface or curve. Surfaces and curves store their scalars in separate scalar lists, but all surfaces in an object share one scalar list, and all curves in the object share the other (which is omitted if there are no curves). Each surface and curve has an index that specifies where in the respective scalar list the scalars for the surface or curve begin. All scalars for a single surface or curve are consecutive. The internal layout of each such curve depends on the surface or curve; see above for details. In general, the parameter vectors come first, followed by the control points in X, Y, Z, W order. All the X are given before the Y, etc.

4.4.19 Surfaces: Curve Point Lists

Element type: miSCENE_CURVPNT
Data type: miCurve_point[ ]
Sizes: int no_points
Defaults: all nulls

```
typedef struct miCurve_point {
        miGeoVector     v;              /* xyz point on surface of curve at t */
        miGeoVector2d   uv;             /* uv value of curve at t */
        miGeoScalar     t;              /* curve parameter value */
        miUshort        flags;          /* GAP: */
        miCBoolean      is_t;           /* is t value present */
        miCBoolean      is_uv;          /* is uv value present */
        miCBoolean      is_v;           /* is xyz value present */
        miCBoolean      spare;          /* not used */
} miCurve_point;
```

A translator must provide: all fields except `spare`.

(Despite the name, curve points may also be referenced as special points by surfaces.)

is_t, **is_uv**, and `is_v`, if `miTRUE`, specify that *t*, *uv*, or *v* are valid, respectively.

t, if enabled by *is_t*, gives the parameter value of the special point.

uv, if enabled by *is_uv*, gives the UV value of the curve at the special point.

v, if enabled by *is_v*, gives the location in space of the special point.

4.4.20 Surfaces: Basis Lists

Element type: miSCENE_BASIS_LIST
Data type: miBasis_list[ ]
Sizes: int no_bases, int no_scalars
Defaults: all nulls

```
enum miBasis_type {
        miBASIS_NONE = 0,               /* for internal use */
        miBASIS_BEZIER,
        miBASIS_BSPLINE,
        miBASIS_CARDINAL,
        miBASIS_MATRIX,
        miBASIS_TAYLOR
```

```
};

typedef struct {
        miGeoIndex      no_bases;
        miGeoIndex      no_scalars;
        miBasis         bases[1];
} miBasis_list;

typedef struct miBasis {
        enum miBasis_type type;
        miGeoIndex      degree;         /* undefined for Cardinal */
        miGeoIndex      stepsize;       /* only for miBASIS_MATRIX */
        miGeoIndex      value_idx;      /* index into the basis scalar list */
} miBasis;
```

A translator must provide: `type`, `degree`; if the type is basis matrix, also `stepsize` and `value_idx`.

no_bases specifies the number of bases in the basis list.

no_scalars specifies the number of scalars that follow the basis list. Scalars are used for basis matrix bases, which require $degree^2$ scalars for a matrix defining the basis. The first scalar in the list has index `0`.

bases is the basis array. It is actually allocated larger.

type is one of `miBASIS_BEZIER`, `miBASIS_BSPLINE`, `miBASIS_CARDINAL`, `miBASIS_MATRIX`, and `miBASIS_TAYLOR`.

degree is the degree of the basis.

stepsize is used for basis matrix bases only. For an explanation, see the description of bases in the mental ray User Manual.

4.4.21 Surfaces: Algebraic Lists

Element type:	miSCENE_ALGEBRAIC
Data type:	miAlgebraic[ ]
Sizes:	—
Defaults:	—

This type is not currently supported.

4.4.22 Space Curves[2.1]

Element type: miSCENE_SPACECURVE
Data type: miSpacecurve[ ]
Sizes: int no_spacecurves
Defaults: all nulls except where otherwise noted

```
typedef struct miSpacecurve {
        miApprox        def_approx;         /* default approximation */
        miGeoIndex      no_curves;          /* total number of curves */
        miGeoIndex      curve_idx;          /* index into the 'curves' list*/
        miBoolean       pad;                /* not used */
        miVertex_content gap_vert_info;     /* For calculating box sizes */
} miSpacecurve;
```

A translator must provide: `no_curves`, `curve_idx`, `gap_vert_info`.
A translator may provide: `def_approx`.

def_approx is the default approximation for curve segments which do not have their own approximation defined.

no_curves specifies the total number of curves used by this space curve.

curve_idx is the index of the first curve in the curve list anchored in the object that is used for this space curve. This is the first of *no_curves* consecutive curves to use.

gap_vert_info describes the layout and size of the vertices to create during tessellation. The boxes created during tessellation will get a copy of this vertex info structure.

4.4.23 Books and Pages

Element type: miSCENE_BOOK
Data type: miBook
Sizes: miGeoIndex line_size, no_lines
Defaults: all nulls except where otherwise noted

```
#define miSCENE_BOOK_MAXSWAP     16

typedef struct miBook {
        miUint          label;          /* type of book                  */
        miGeoIndex      no_pages;       /* number of used pages          */
        miGeoIndex      page_size;      /* number of lines on first page */
        miGeoIndex      line_size;      /* size of elments in bytes      */
        miGeoIndex      next_free_line; /* index of next free line       */
```

```
        char            swap[miSCENE_BOOK_MAXSWAP];
                                         /* string for change of byte order  */
        miTag           next_book;       /* tag for next book                */
        miTag           pages[1];        /* array of page tags               */
} miBook;
```

When a box is created the line size and the swap string must be supplied. The number of lines influences the size of the page. If it is smaller than some threshold a default page size is used.

label is a variable at the disposal of the application using `miBooks`. It is not used by any of the book management functions described below.

no_pages is the number of used memory pages.

page_size is the number of lines on the first page. Consecutive pages grow in geometric progression. The details are implementation dependent and may change in the future.

line_size is the size of the lines in bytes in the current book.

next_free_line is the index of the element of the linked list of free lines.

swap is string of at most `miSCENE_BOOK_MAXSWAP - 1` characters which indicates how the bytes in a line of a book should be swapped when being transferred between machines of different byte order.

next_book is a tag that allows to build chains of books. These may be accessed and enumerated more efficiently than single books.

pages is an array of page tags. It is guaranteed to be big enough to hold all pages that might be allocated to keep the maximum total number of `miMAX_GEOINDEX` lines.

None of the structure elements above except the `label` should be accessed directly. The same applies to the pages the books consist of.

Element type:	miSCENE_PAGE
Data type:	miPage
Sizes:	miGeoIndex page_size, line_size
Defaults:	all nulls except where otherwise noted

```
typedef struct miPage {
        char            swap[miSCENE_BOOK_MAXSWAP];
                                         /* string for change of byte order  */
        miGeoIndex      page_size;       /* number of lines on current page  */
        miGeoIndex      line_size;       /* size of elments in bytes         */
} miPage;
```

When a page is created the page and line sizes and the swap string must be supplied. However, pages should not be created directly but only through the calls to manage books described below.

swap is a string to indicate how lines should be swapped when pages are transferred between machines of different byte order. It has to stored in the pages too, because they are swapped independently of the books.

page_size is the number of lines on the current page.

line_size is the size of the lines on this page in bytes.

Apart from the Scene module calls to create books etc. the calls to manage books are:

```
void *mi_scene_book_get_line(
        miBook              *book,
        miGeoIndex          line_num)
```

Access a line with index line_num of a given book and returns a void pointer to it.

```
void *mi_scene_book_allocate_line(
        miBook              *book,
        miGeoIndex          *line_num)
```

Return a void pointer to a free element in a given book and set the line_num passed by reference. This may be a yet unused line or one that has been previously deleted with a call to mi_scene_book_release_line. If the lines on existing pages are exceeded a new page is allocated.

```
void mi_scene_book_release_line(
        miBook              *book,
        miGeoIndex          line_num)
```

Delete a line from a given book.

```
void mi_scene_book_enumerate(
        miBook              *book,
        void                (*cb_func)(void *,
                                       miGeoIndex,
                                       void *),
        void                *cb_data)
```

Look at each element in a book in turn and if it is in use executes a call-back function. mi_scene_book_enumerate takes three arguments. The first is a pointer to an miBook, the second a pointer to the call-back function, and the third a pointer to optional data that are passed to the call-back when it is called. If either the book or the call-back pointer is NULL nothing is done. Otherwise the book is traversed and for each valid element the function pointed to by the second argument is called. The argument of this call-back function are a pointer to the element in the book, its index and the optional data pointer. An element in a book is valid if it has been allocated by a call to mi_scene_book_allocate_line and not been free-d subsequently by a call to mi_scene_book_release_line. Neither the call-back function nor mi_scene_book_enumerate return a value.

```
miGeoIndex mi_scene_book_free_blk_start(
        miBook                  *book)
```

Return the index of the first line in the completely unused part of a book.

```
miGeoIndex mi_scene_book_no_used_lines(
        miBook                  *book)
```

Return the number of used lines in a book.

```
miGeoIndex mi_scene_book_max_lines(
        miBook                  *book)
```

Return the maximum allocated number of lines in a book.

```
miBoolean mi_scene_book_line_valid(
        miBook                  *book,
        miGeoIndex              line)
```

Return miTRUE if a given line index refers to a used line and miFALSE otherwise.

```
miTag mi_scene_book_attach(
        miTag                   old_book,
        miTag                   new_book,
        miGeoIndex              position)
```

Concatenate chains of books. Insert the new book at the specified position in the chain and returns the tag of the first book in the chain after insertion.

```
miTag mi_scene_book_detach(
        miTag                   book,
        miGeoIndex              position)
```

Split off a component from a chain of books. Return the tag of the first book in the remaining chain.

4.4.24 Subdivision Surfaces

Element type: miSCENE_SUBDIVSURF
Data type: miSurf_subsurf[ ]
Sizes: int nsdsurfs
Defaults: all nulls except where otherwise noted

```
typedef struct miSurf_subsurf {
        miApprox        approx;          /* approximation technique for      */
                                         /*   subdivision surface            */
        miCBoolean      spare[4];
        miGeoIndex      max_subdiv_level;/* maximum level of vertices and    */
                                         /*   faces in the surface           */
        miTag           base_tris;       /* tag for book of base mesh        */
                                         /*   triangles                      */
        miTag           hira_tri_kits;   /* tag for book of hierarchy        */
                                         /*   triangle kits                  */
        miTag           base_quads;      /* tag for book of base mesh        */
                                         /*   quadrangles                    */
        miTag           hira_quad_kits;  /* tag for book of hierarchy        */
                                         /*   quadrangle kits                */
        miSurf_vertex_content vert_info;/* tag for miSurf_vertex_content     */
        miTag           vertices;        /* tag for array of tags for books  */
                                         /*   of vert_info.sizeof_vertex     */
                                         /*   components                     */
} miSurf_subsurf;
```

A translator must provide: approx, max_subdiv_level, a tag for base_tris or base_quads, vert_info and vertices. The default of approx is set by miAPPROX_DEFAULT(). The default of the tt sizeof_vertex field of the miSurf_vertex_content structure is 1.

4.4.25 Materials

Element type: miSCENE_MATERIAL
Data type: miMaterial
Sizes: —
Defaults: all nulls

```
typedef struct miMaterial {
        miBoolean       opaque;                 /* no transparency? */
        miTag           shader;                 /* material shader */
```

```
        miTag           displace;               /* opt. displacement shader */
        miTag           shadow;                 /* opt. shadow shader */
        miTag           volume;                 /* opt. volume shader */
        miTag           environment;            /* opt. environment shader */
        miTag           contour;                /* opt. contour shader */
        miTag           photon;                 /* opt. photon RT shader */
        miTag           photonvol;              /* opt. photon volume shader */
        int             spare[2];               /* not used */
} miMaterial;
```

A translator must provide: `shader`.
A translator may provide: all others.

opaque informs mental ray that the material is always opaque and casts an opaque shadow. This is a hint to mental ray and may not be used by all renderers.

shader is the tag of a material shading function. It must refer to a database element of type `miSCENE_FUNCTION`. This tag may not be `miNULLTAG`.

displace is the tag of an optional displacement shader function.

shadow is the tag of an optional shadow shader function.

volume is the tag of an optional volume shader function.

environment is the tag of an optional environment shader function.

contour is the tag of an optional contour shader function.

photon is the tag of an optional photon shader function.

photonvol is the tag of an optional photon volume shader function.

4.4.26 Rendering Options

Element type:	miSCENE_OPTIONS
Data type:	miOptions
Sizes:	—
Defaults:	as described below

The rendering options were designed to accommodate as wide a range of renderers as possible, from simple wireframe displayers to complex ray tracers. The interpretation of the structure members is left to the renderer. Generally, no renderer will require all provided fields; each renderer may use a different subset. This data structures was named `miRc_options` in earlier versions of raylib; the old name still works.

```
typedef struct miOptions {
        miBoolean       trace;                  /* 2nd generation ray trace? */
        int             scanline;               /* 0=off, 1=on, 'o'=OpenGL */
        miBoolean       motion;                 /* motion blur? : miFALSE */
        miBoolean       shadow_sort;            /* Obsolete! Do not use */
        miBoolean       preview_mode;           /* for future use */
        int             reflection_depth;       /* refl. trace depth : 1 */
        int             refraction_depth;       /* refr. trace depth : 1 */
        int             trace_depth;            /* refl. + refr. depth : 1 */
        int             min_samples;            /* min. sampling level : -2 */
        int             max_samples;            /* max. sampling level : 0 */
        miColor         contrast;               /* sampling contrast: .1 */
        miColor         time_contrast;          /* temporal sampling contrast*/
        miTag           contour_contrast;       /* NULLTAG */
        miTag           contour_store;          /* NULLTAG */
        miBoolean       caustic;                /* enable caustics: miFALSE */
        miBoolean       globillum;              /* enable global il.: miFALSE*/
        int             caustic_accuracy;       /* no. caus. photons in est. */
        float           caustic_radius;         /* maxdist for caus. photons */
        int             globillum_accuracy;     /* no. glob. photons in est. */
        float           globillum_radius;       /* maxdist for glob. photons */
        float           caustic_filter_const;   /* filter const. for caus. */
        float           filter_size_x;          /* filter size in x : 1.0 */
        float           filter_size_y;          /* filter size in y : 1.0 */
        float           jitter;                 /* sample jittering : 0.0 */
        float           shutter;                /* shutter speed for motion:0*/
        int             subdivision;            /* ray class. adjustment : 0 */
        int             subdivision_2d;         /* eye + shadow adjustment:0 */
        int             subdivision_memory;     /* ray class. memory (mb): 6 */
        int             space_max_size;         /* space subdiv. leaf size: 4*/
        int             space_max_depth;        /* space subdiv. depth : 25*/
        float           grid_size;              /* typical # voxels per tri */
        int             no_images;              /* # images : 1 */
        miImg_type      image_types[miRC_MAX_IMAGES]; /* image types */
        miBoolean       write_image[miRC_MAX_IMAGES]; /* write image?*/
        miBoolean       interp_image[miRC_MAX_IMAGES]; /* interpolate image? */
        miTag           shader_tree_image;      /* for previewing */
        miTag           pixel_sample_image;     /* for previewing */
        miCBoolean      use_shadow_maps;        /* use shadow maps ? 0 */
        miCBoolean      rendering_shadow_maps;  /* Shadow map mode? 0 */
        char            recompute_shadow_maps;  /* 'n'o,'y'es (could be Bool)*/
        char            shadow;                 /* shadow casting? */
        char            caustic_filter;         /* filter-type */
        miCBoolean      spare3;
        char            filter;                 /* sample filter type */
        char            acceleration;           /* acceleration: 'b' */
        char            face;                   /* primitive facing */
        char            field;                  /* field rendering? */
        char            smethod;                /* sampling algorithm */
        char            render_space;           /* coordinate space */
        miCBoolean      pixel_preview;          /* pixel selective sampling */
        miCBoolean      task_preview;           /* task selective sampling */
        miCBoolean      visible_lights;         /* any visible area lights? */
```

```
        miCBoolean      shadow_map_motion;      /* motion blurred shadowmaps?*/
        int             task_size;              /* image task size */
        miBoolean       strips;                 /* create triangles in strips*/
        miTag           photonmap_file;         /* photon map file name */
        miBoolean       photonmap_rebuild;      /* photon map rebuild ? */
        int             photon_reflection_depth;/* photon refl. depth */
        int             photon_refraction_depth;/* photon refl. depth */
        int             photon_trace_depth;     /* total photon trace depth */
        int             space_max_mem;          /* maximum bsp memory (mb):0 */
        miPointer       image[miRC_MAX_IMAGES]; /* pointers to frame buffers */
        miCBoolean      no_lens;                /* disable lens shaders */
        miCBoolean      no_volume;              /* disable volume shaders */
        miCBoolean      no_geometry;            /* disable geometry shaders */
        miCBoolean      no_displace;            /* disable displace shaders */
        miUint1         no_output;              /* disable output shaders */
        miCBoolean      no_merge;               /* disable surface merging */
        miUint1         caustic_flag;           /* def. caustic flag for objs*/
        char            diagnostic_mode;        /* miSCENE_DIAG_* flags */
        int             photonvol_accuracy;     /* no. vol. photons in est. */
        float           photonvol_radius;       /* maxdist for vol. photons */
        miUint1         globillum_flag;         /* def. globil. flag for objs*/
        miCBoolean      spare1[9];              /* future disable flags */
        miCBoolean      first_cut;              /* first cookie cut */
        miCBoolean      last_cut;               /* last cookie cut */
        int             cut_windows;            /* cookie cutter cuts: 1 */
        miScalar        cut_expand;             /* tessellate outside frustr.*/
        miTag           userdata;               /* optional user data blocks */
        miApprox        approx;                 /* approximation overrides if*/
        miApprox        approx_displace;        /* style != APPROX_STYLE_NONE*/
        miBoolean       finalgather;            /* fg. for globillum: miFALSE*/
        int             finalgather_rays;       /* no. rays in final gather */
        float           finalgather_maxradius;  /* maxdist for finalgather */
        float           finalgather_minradius;  /* mindist for finalgather */
        float           diag_photon_density;    /* density for diag */
        float           diag_grid_size;         /* gridsize for diag */
        int             spare2[14];             /* not used */
} miOptions;
```

A translator must provide: nothing.
A translator may provide: all fields.

The parameters are described very briefly; for a detailed description refer to the mental ray User Manual.

trace (default `miTRUE`) enables ray tracing.

scanline (default `miTRUE`) enables the first-generation scanline algorithm if applicable to improve speed. `miFALSE` disables scanline rendering, and `'o'` replaces the standard scanline renderer with an OpenGL renderer that used the OpenGL hardware of the system for fast rendering (SGI only).

motion (default `miFALSE`) enables motion blurring.

preview_mode (default `miFALSE`) not currently used.

shadow (default `1`) controls shadow casting. It is one of `0` (no shadows), `1` (normal shadows), `'s'` (shadow segments with separate volume shaders), and `'l'` (shadow intersections sorted from the light source towards the illumination point). **Note:** Version 2.0.8 older versions do not yet support shadow sorting and shadow segments, and use a simple *shadow* boolean and a nonfunctional *shadow_sort* flag. Shadow segments belong to a new set of space probing features introduced in 2.0.4.

filter (default `'b'`) is one of `'b'` (box filter), `'t'` (triangle filter), `'g'` (Gaussian filter), `'m'` (Mitchell filter[2.1]), or `'l'` (Lanczos filter[2.1]).

acceleration (default `'b'`) is one of `'b'` (space subdivision, BSP), `'c'` (ray classification), and `'g'` (grid).

face (default `'a'`) enables backface culling, one of `'f'` (front-facing only), `'b'` (back-facing only), and `'a'` (both).

field (default `0`) enables field rendering, one of `0` (no field rendering), `'e'` (even fields only), and `'o'` (odd fields only).

reflection_depth (default 1) limits the ray tracing depth for reflection rays.

refraction_depth (default 1) limits the ray tracing depth for refraction or transparency rays.

trace_depth (default 1) limits the ray tracing depth for the sum of all rays.

min_samples (default -2) specifies the minimum number of samples in recursive oversampling mode. At least $2^{min\_samples}$ samples will be taken.

max_samples (default `0`) specifies the maximum number of samples in recursive oversampling mode. At most $2^{max\_samples}$ samples will be taken.

contrast (default `0.1 0.1 0.1 0.1`) specifies the contrast limit above which more spatial samples are taken.

time_contrast (default `0.3 0.3 0.3 0.3`) specifies the contrast limit for motion blurring above which more time samples are taken. Because of blurring, this can usually be much higher than the spatial contrast.

contour_contrast (default no shader) specifies a function that computes contrasts in contour rendering mode.

contour_store (default no shader) specifies a function that collects and stores sample information for use by the contour contrast function, in contour rendering mode.

caustic specifies whether caustics should be rendered.

globillum specifies whether global illumination should be rendered. This mode is available only in version 2.1 or later.

caustic_accuracy specifies the number of photons to use when estimating radiance for caustics.

caustic_radius specifies the maximum distance in which photons used in the radiance estimate for caustics are located. If the radius is 0.0 then an estimate based on the scene extent will be used.

global_accuracy specifies the number of photons to use when estimating radiance for global illumination.

global_radius specifies the maximum distance in which photons used in the radiance estimate for global illumination are located. If the radius is 0.0 then an estimate based on the scene extent will be used.

caustic_filter_const is a constant used when filtering caustics radiance estimates.

caustic_filter is the type of filter used: 'b' box filter, 'c' cone filter and 'g' gauss filter.

rendering_caustics is set when caustics are being rendered.

filter_size_x (default 1.0) specifies the width of the filter specified in the `filter` field.

filter_size_y (default 1.0) specifies the height of the filter specified in the `filter` field.

jitter (default 0.0) is the jitter interval. Jittering displaces samples to avoid sampling artifacts.

shutter (default 1.0) is the shutter time of the camera if motion blurring is enabled.

subdivision (default 0) is a correction factor for the number of ray space subdivisions in ray classification acceleration mode.

subdivision_2d (default 0) is a correction factor for the number of shadow ray space subdivisions in ray classification acceleration mode.

subdivision_memory (default 6) specifies how many megabytes the ray classification algorithm should use for acceleration data structures.

space_max_mem (default 0) specifies the maximum memory in megabytes used in the BSP preprocessing. A value of zero indicates that there is no limit on the memory consumption, this is the default. This flag is useful only on multiprocessor machines since the memory consumption increases with the number of rendering threads. When the specified amount of allocated memory is reached, mental ray will prevent threads from being scheduled for preprocessing, thus reducing the memory requirements.

space_max_size (default 4) is the maximum leaf size in BSP mode.

grid_size (default 10.0) specifies the grid size for the grid acceleration method.

space_max_depth (default 24) is the maximum tree depth in BSP mode.

image_types (default `miIMG_TYPE_RGBA`) is an array specifying the image types to be generated during rendering. See the documentation of the IMG module for a list of allowed types.

write_image (default `miTRUE, miTRUE, ...`) specifies for each image whether it is written to a file after rendering completes.

interp_image (default `miTRUE, miFALSE, ...`) specifies for each image whether it is to be interpolated. This means that if fewer than one sample per pixel is taken, the holes are filled in.

shader_tree_image (internal to rc) is an image which remembers which shaders have been used to render each individual pixel. Each pixel contains 32 bits corresponding to 32 different shaders. If shader 31 is used to render a pixel then bit 31 is set in this image for this pixel. If the image uses more than 32 shaders then then the shader number modulo 32 are used to identify the right bit.

pixel_sample_image (internal to rc) is an image in which each pixel set indicates a pixel which should be re-rendered.

no_images (default 1) is the number of valid entries in the three image arrays above.

use_shadow_maps if miTRUE specifies that shadow maps should be used for the light sources which have shadow maps. This is the global on/off control. The default is off.

rendering_shadow_maps is miTRUE when the shadow maps are being rendered. This option is internal to RC and only used to optimize the rendering of shadow maps.

recompute_shadow_maps can be 'y' or 'n'. 'y' means that all shadow maps are recomputed even if they could have been loaded from a file. 'n' means that shadow maps are only computed if they could not be re-used or loaded from a file (shadow maps are recomputed "intelligently" meaning that the shadow map code tries to identify those light sources for which a new shadow map needs to be recomputed. This recomputation currently only applies to light sources for which the position or direction of the emitted light – ie. the transformation matrix – changes in an animation).

pixel_preview is set when pixel previewing should be used. The default is off.

task_preview is set when task previewing should be used. The default is off.

visible_lights is set if there are any area lights with the 'visible' flag. This option is internal to RC and used to optimize rendering.

shadow_map_motion enables motion blurring of shadowmap shadows. The default is on.

task_size (default 0) is the size of the image tasks to be rendered. If it is zero, a heuristic based on the image resolution will be used in RC in order to calculate an appropriate value. task_size can also be specified explicitly.

strips specifies whether the approximated geometry is represented as triangle strips and fans. The default is off.

photonmap_file is a string containing the filename of a file from which a photon map should be loaded (if possible) or otherwise saved to. If this tag is a miNULLTAG then no photon map is loaded or saved.

photonmap_rebuild will, if true, enforce a recomputation of the photon map even if it could have been loaded from a file.

photon_reflection_depth controls the trace depth of reflected photons. The default is 5.

photon_refraction_depth controls the trace depth of refracted photons. The default is 5.

photon_trace_depth controls the combined trace depth of reflected and refracted photons. The default is 5.

image is an array of pointers to frame buffers. It is valid only in output shaders. Use `(miImg_image *)image[n].p` to access.

no_lens, if `miTRUE`, disables all lens shaders. The default is `miFALSE`.

no_volume, if `miTRUE`, disables all volume shaders. The default is `miFALSE`.

no_geometry, if `miTRUE`, disables all geometry shaders. The default is `miFALSE`.

no_displace, if `miTRUE`, disables all displacement shaders. The default is `miFALSE`.

no_output is a bitmap. Bit zero, it set, disables all output shaders. Bit one, if set, disables writing of output image files. The default is zero for both bits.

no_merge, if `miTRUE`, disables all edge merging and adjacency detection. The default is `miFALSE`.

caustic_flag is the default caustic flag for objects. The default value is 3, making all objects caustic generators and caustic receivers.

diagnostic_mode controls alternate rendering modes for diagnostic purposes. It is a bitmap. The only currently supported bit is `miSCENE_DIAG_SAMPLES` which, when set, turns on sample view mode. The default value is zero for all bits.

photonvol_accuracy specifies the number of photons to use when estimating radiance inside participating media.

photonvol_radius specifies the maximum distance in which photons used in the radiance estimate for participating media are located. If the radius is 0.0 then an estimate based on the scene extent will be used.

cut_windows enables rendering every image as $n \times n$ cut windows if set greater than zero. This is available in mental ray 2.0 and 2.1 only.

cut_expand increases the cut window frustum by a factor all around the frustum if greater than zero, to catch invisible outside geometry that becomes visible because it is displaced into the frustum. The default is 0.1. It has an effect only if cut windows are enabled.

globillum_flag[2.1] is the default globillum flag for objects. The default value is 3, making all objects globillum generators and receivers.

approx overrides all base surface approximations in objects, both free-form surfaces and polygonal, if the approximation style is not `miAPPROX_STYLE_NONE`. This style is the default, and all other fields are 0. Use the `miAPPROX_DEFAULT` macro to activate this approximation. See the `miApprox` data structure description above.

approx_displace is the same thing for displacement approximations.

finalgather enables final gathering. The default is off.

finalgather_rays is the number of rays shot in each final gather. The default is 1000.

finalgather_maxradius is the maximum radius in which a final gather result can be used for interpolation or extrapolation. If this radius is 0.0 then an estimate based on the scene extent will be used.

finalgather_minradius indicates that a final gather result must be used for interpolation or extrapolation if it is within this distance. If this radius is 0.0, it will be set to 10% of finalgather-_maxradius.

4.4.27 Images

Element type:	miSCENE_IMAGE
Data type:	miImg_image
Sizes:	—
Defaults:	all nulls

```
typedef struct miImg_image {
        miBoolean       filter;          /* caller wants filtered lookups */
        int             dirsize;         /* valid # of filter levels */
        int             dir[miIMG_DIRSIZE]; /* offs from this to other imgs */
        int             width, height;   /* width and height in pixels */
        int             bits;            /* requested bits per comp, 8/16/32 */
        int             comp;            /* requested components/pixel, 1..4 */
        miBoolean       local;           /* local texture, use image/mmap/path*/
        int             null[3];         /* unused */
        int             c[4];            /* local==miFALSE: */
                                         /*     indexed by miIMG_*; 4*height */
```

```
                                            /*      component indices follow, */
                                            /*      then component scanlines */
        miPointer       image;              /* local==miTRUE: */
        miImg_file      ifp;                /*      describes open file */
        miBoolean       mmapped;            /*      mmapped, not mi_mem_allocated*/
        char            path[4];            /*      local file name to open */
} miImg_image;
```

A translator must provide: nothing.
A translator may provide: nothing.
Provided by *mi_scene_create*: all fields.

Images consist of three sections: the header (type `miImg_image`), a list of scanlines indices, and the actual uncompressed pixel data. There are $height \cdot 4$ scanline indices, one set of *comp* (up to 4) indices for each scanline. They contain indices relative to the first pixel data byte. The pixel data is arranged in one-component scanlines of *width* component values each. All images are scanned bottom-up. For more details, see the documentation of the IMG module.

filter, if nonzero, enables pyramid texture mode.

dirsize and `dir` are used for internal purposes.

width is the number of pixels per scanline.

height is the number of scanlines.

bits is the number of bits per component pixel.

comp is the number of components per pixel.

local, if false, specifies a local image with scanline index list `c` followed by pixel data. If true, the image is local, which means there is no image data but a reference to an image file, which is loaded or mapped at runtime, once on each host. See the IMG documentation for details.

c is the first scanline index block. Only *comp* of the 4 available indices are used. It is unused if `local` is true.

image is used to cache the pointer to the local image. This and the remaining fields are used only if `local` is true.

host is the local host ID. The image pointer is valid only if the host ID matches the local host ID. This guards against network transfers.

ifp is used internally to save information about the open local texture file if memory-mapped.

mmapped is true if the local texture is memory-mapped and needs to be unmapped when the texture is invalidated.

path is the path of the file where each host can find the texture when the image is accessed for the first time.

4.4.28 Strings

Element type:	miSCENE_STRING
Data type:	char[ ]
Sizes:	int no_chars
Defaults:	—

Strings hold standard null-terminated character strings. They are used for the `string` shader parameter type and for shadowmap file names in lights, and for other purposes. The number of characters passed when creating or resizing the string must include the trailing null byte.

4.4.29 Tag Lists

Element type:	miSCENE_TAG
Data type:	miTag[ ]
Sizes:	—
Defaults:	—

Tag lists are not currently used.

Chapter 5

Usage and Command Line Options

When started from a shell command line, mental ray accepts a large number of options. Most of these correspond to similar commands or camera or options statements as described in the Scene Description chapter. The relevant explanations there are repeated in this chapter. When an option is given on the command line, it overrides the corresponding command or statement in the scene file, which in turn overrides the defaults. The defaults for certain options given in the option list below apply only if the corresponding command or statement is not present in the scene file.

For the option description, the same metasymbols as in the Scene Description chapter are used: a bar " | " denotes alternatives, items enclosed in tall square brackets "[ ]" are optional, and the ellipsis "..." denotes omission. Literal text is set in `teletype`, while variable metasymbols are set in *italics*. All other punctuation characters are literals. Strings are quoted with double quotes; this includes all names. The double quotes protect names from interpretation by the shell, they should be entered as shown here.

mental ray is started as

`ray` [*options*] [*scenefile*]

If no scene file is given, the scene is read from standard input. Scene file names should end in `.mi`; if the extension is missing mental ray will read the name as specified, and if this fails, retry with `.mi` added.

5.1 Command Line Options

Options can be abbreviated as long as the given substring is unambiguous. mental ray checks for ambiguities and prints an error message listing the choices. For example, -resolution can be abbreviated as `-res`. For frequently-used options such as `-verbose` and `-filename`, short forms are available. The available options are:

`-acceleration bsp`

Selects the binary space partitioning (BSP) rendering algorithm. This algorithm is often, but not always, the fastest. It is controlled by the `-bsp_size` and `-bsp_depth` options.

`-acceleration grid`

Selects the grid rendering algorithm. It provides faster preprocessing especially on multiprocessor systems. Memory usage is more conservative than with the BSP algorithm. Speed is comparable to BSP but more scene-dependent. It is controlled by the `-grid` option.

`-acceleration raycl`

Selects the ray classification rendering algorithm. This algorithm is recommended for very large scenes. It operates with a constant acceleration memory size, controlled by the `-subdivision_memory` and `-subdivision` options.

`-aperture` *aperture*

The aperture is the width of the viewing plane. The height of the viewing plane is *aperture* divided by *aspect*. Together with the `focal` and `aspect` *viewdefs*, `aperture` defines the lens of the camera.

`-aspect` *aspect*

This is the aspect ratio of the camera. The default is 1.33. In camera space, *aperture* is the width of the viewing plane and *aperture* divided by *aspect* is the height. The viewing plane is divided into pixels as specified by the `resolution` *viewdef*, so the aspect will result in nonsquare pixels if it is not equal to the X resolution divided by the Y resolution. For example, to render a PAL image at a resolution of 720×576 pixels (equivalent to CCIR 601, also called D1), at an image ratio of 3:4 as defined by the PAL standard, pixels are slightly wider than tall, by a factor of $\frac{576}{720} \cdot \frac{4}{3} = 1.0667$. If this number is specified as *aspect*, objects will appear undistorted on a PAL video display (but not on a computer display with square pixels). The NTSC standard has 486 instead of 576 lines.

`-bsp_depth` $depth_{int}$

The maximum number of levels in the BSP tree. This option is used only if binary space partitioning is enabled. Larger tree depths reduce rendering time but increase memory consumption, and also slightly increase preprocessing time. The default is 40.

`-bsp_memory` $memory_{int}$

The maximum memory in megabytes used in the BSP preprocessing. A value of zero indicates that there is no limit on the memory consumption, this is the default. This flag is useful only on multiprocessor machines since the memory consumption increases with the number of rendering threads. When the specified amount of allocated memory is reached, mental ray will prevent threads from being scheduled for preprocessing, thus reducing the memory requirements.

`-bsp_size` $size_{int}$

The maximum number of primitives in a leaf of the BSP tree. This option is used only if binary space partitioning is enabled, it has no effect on the ray classification algorithm. Larger leaf sizes reduce memory consumption but increase rendering time. The default is 10.

`-caustic on|off`

Enable or disable the generation of caustics defined in the scene. The default is `off`. To actually create caustics, lights must have an energy, and materials must have photon shaders.

`-caustic_accuracy` $nphotons_{int}$ [*radius*]

Controls how caustics are estimated from the photon map during rendering. *nphotons* is the maximum number of photons to examine and *radius* the maximum radius to search. if $nphotons = 0$, all photons are examined up to the *radius* limit. $radius = 0.0$ means that a scene-size dependent radius will be used. The defaults are 100 and 0.0.

`-clip` *hither yon*

The *hither* (near) and *yon* (far) planes are planes parallel to the viewing plane that delimit the rendered scene. Points outside the space between the hither and yon planes will not be rendered (this does not apply to the infinite-radius environment maps because they are not geometric objects). The `clip` statement specifies the distance of the hither and yon planes from the camera.

`-code "`*filename*`" ... --`

The named *filename* is interpreted as a C source file, ending with the extension ".c", is compiled and linked into mental ray. The shaders it defines are available in mental ray as shading functions. Multiple file names can be given. The list must be terminated with a double minus sign.

`-colorclip rgb|alpha|raw`[2.1]

This option controls how colors are clipped into a valid range $[0, 1]$ before being written to a non-floating point frame buffer or file. The `rgb` mode is the default. In this mode, RGB is first clipped to $[0, 1]$ and alpha subsequently to $[max(R, G, B), 1]$. In `alpha` mode, alpha is first clipped to $[0, 1]$ and RGB subsequently to $[0, A]$. In `raw` mode, RGB and A are both clipped to $[0, 1]$ independently of each other. In all modes, the RGB components are clipped as specified by the `desaturate` option. The `rgb` and `alpha` modes ensure that the resulting color is a valid premultiplied color. `rgb` should be used if the alpha channel is considered less important than preserving the RGB color and intensity. `alpha` mode is intended for alpha compositing, where the alpha channel is more important than the absolute color value to preserve correct transparencies. `raw` mode should only be used if no layering based on alpha is going to take place. This mode also forces the `premultiply` mode to `on`. It should be used with care because shaders might receive "illegal" colors (colors that cannot be composited in standard ways).

`-contrast` *r g b* [*a*]

The contrast controls supersampling. If neighboring samples differ by more than the color *r, g, b, a*, supersampling is done as specified by the sampling options (see above). Default for *a* is the average of *r*, *g*, and *b*. The recursive supersampling algorithm controlled by `-samples` modifies the contrast based on the recursion level: at sample level 0, the contrast is used directly; at sample level 1, the contrast is doubled (effectively requiring a higher contrast to force another subdivision), and so on. Negative levels divide the contrast, i.e. use a fraction $\frac{1}{2}$, $\frac{1}{4}$, and so on. In general, the contrast is multiplied by 2^{level} at the supersampling level *level*, which is bounded by `-samples`. See the Scene Description chapter for more information on how to optimize performance and quality with contrast values.

`-cut_window` num_{int} [*expand*]

Cut a frame into $num \times num$ sub-frames, each of which is rendered individually. When all are finished, they are combined to the final image. This can greatly reduce memory consumption if the scene is built such that each sub-frame is much less complex than the entire frame, but it may take much longer to run all the extra rendering cycles. If the scene contains few polygons and many free-form surfaces and/or displacement maps, memory usage often goes down by factors of five or ten, while rendering time doubles. Mostly polygonal scenes usually do not benefit from cut windows, and in fact can behave worse. Tessellation caching in animations is disabled in cut window mode.

Before deciding whether geometry outside the cut window frustum should be tessellated, the frustum is enlarged by 10% all around to catch geometry outside the frustum that is displaced into the frustum. This value can be changed with the optional *expand* argument, which is a factor of the cut window size. `0.1` expands the cut window by 10% all around, which increases its area by a factor of 1.44.

This is a temporary feature in version 2.0 and 2.1 of mental ray and not supported in version 2.2 and later.

`-c_compiler "`*filename*`"`

If this option is given, the standard C compiler `"cc"` is replaced with *filename*.

`-c_flags "`*options*`"`

The *options* string replaces the standard options given to the C compiler. The defaults depend on the machine used; for example, the default option string for single-processor SGI IRIX machines is `"-O2"`. The `-c` option is always inserted, as is `-o` if the compiler supports it.

`-c_linker "`*filename*`"`

If this option is given, the standard linker `"ld"` is replaced with *filename*. See the chapter on Writing Shaders for platform-specific information on compiling and linking.

`-desaturate on|off`

If a color is output to a frame buffer that does not have 32-bit (floating-point) precision, and its RGB components are outside the range [0, *max*], mental ray will clip the color to this legal range. If desaturation is turned off, the individual components are simply clipped into range. Otherwise, mental ray tries to maintain the brightness of the color by moving it towards the grayscale axis of the color cube, until the RGB components are in the legal range. *max* is determined by the `colorclip`[2.1] mode. Desaturation is turned off by default.

`-diagnostic grid off|object|world|camera` *size*[2.1]

This diagnostic mode is intended for scene debugging. Unless set to `off`, it draws a colored grid on all objects in the scene that indicate object, world, or camera space coordinates. Steps on the X, Y, and Z axes are shown with red, green, and blue grid lines, respectively. The distance between grid lines is *size* units. This is useful to estimate the size and distances between objects in mental ray, or to visualize object space coordinates. The `off` argument disables the grid. The default is `off`.

`-diagnostic photon off|density|irradiance` *max*[2.1]

When rendering caustics or global illumination, this option disables all material shaders in the scene and produces a false-color rendering of photon density, or the average of the red, green, and blue irradiance components. Photon density is the number of photons per unit surface area. *max* is the density (or irradiance) that is assigned to 100%, or red. The colors are, from 0% to 100%: Blue, cyan, green, yellow, and red. Higher values fade to white. *max* can be given as zero in which case the appropriate maximum is automatically found. This is done after the whole image has been rendered. This mode is useful when tuning the number of photons in a photonmap and setting the various `_accuracy` options, since the density (or irradiance) is estimated using those settings. The default is `off`.

`-diagnostic samples on|off`[2.1] (p. 73)

If set to on, switch to sampling visualization mode and create grayscale images representing sampling densities instead of color images. A black pixel has had no samples, whereas a white pixel has had the maximum amount as specified by the `-samples` option. In addition, a red grid is drawn indicating task boundaries. The default is `off`.

`-displace on|off`

Ignore all displacement shaders if set to `off`. The default is on.

`-dither on|off`

mental ray supports both 8 and 16 bits per color component. In some cases, 8 bits per pixel, as supported by all popular picture file formats, can cause visible banding when the floating-point color values calculated by the material shader are quantized to the 8-bit values used in the picture file. Dithering mitigates the problem by introducing noise into the pixel such that the round-off errors are randomly distributed. Note that this can cause run-length encoded picture files to be larger than without dithering. Dithering is turned off by default.

`-echo` "*filename*" `[ascii] [source] [approx] [norendercommand] [textures] --`

Echo the current scene to the file *filename*. The options specify the format of the echoed file. Allowed options are:

`ascii` uses ascii format for the vectors (default is binary),

`source` prefers source geometry over triangles if available (default),

`approx` prefers triangles over source geometry if available,

`norendercommand` disables the echo of the **render** command,

`textures` includes texture pixel data verbatim.

Note that triangle echos have displacement mapping already applied to the triangles, but the displacement shaders are not removed from the materials so the echoed file will get displaced twice when rendered. The echo option must be terminated with a double minus.

`-face front|back|both`

The *front* side of a geometric object in the scene is defined to be the side its normal vector points away from. By specifying that only front-facing triangles are to be rendered, speed can be improved because fewer triangles need to be tested for a ray. This works well unless there are objects whose back side is seen by refracted or reflected rays – with `face front`, the back side would not be visible. The default is `face both`.

`-file_name "`*filename*`"`

Overrides the file name given by the first file `output` statement in the camera in the scene file. The full file or path name must be given, including extension if desired.

`-file_type "`*format*`"`

Overrides the file format given by the first file `output` statement in the camera in the scene file. File formats include `rgb` for SGI RGBA files, `jpg` for JPEG files, `"pic"` for SOFTIMAGE image files, `"rla"` for Wavefront RLA files, and `"ps"` for PostScript files if contour mode is enabled. For a complete list, see the Output Shaders subsection in the Functionality chapter.

`-filter box|triangle|gauss|mitchell|lanczos` [*width* [*height*]]

The -filter option specifies how multiple samples are to be combined into a single pixel value. The filter defaults to a box filter of width and height 1.0, optimized for speed. This option allows replacing the box filter, or its size (in pixels). If the size of the filter is not specified, default values are used. These are 1.0 for box, 2.0 for triangle, 3.0 for Gauss and 4.0 for Mitchell[2.1]and Lanczos[2.1]. If the height is omitted, it defaults to the width. Other values can be specified: larger filter sizes result in softer images. If the size is too small, artifacts may appear. Filters must be larger than 0.0 but sizes smaller than 1.0 are generally wasteful since they will discard some samples. Filters larger than 1.0 can reduce rendering speed. For further details on filtering, see the description of the `filter` statement in the Scene Description chapter.

`-finalgather on|off`[2.1]

Enables or disables final gathering. It is disabled by default. Final gathering is a rendering technique used for computing indirect illumination with a one-generation raytracing step.

`-finalgather_accuracy` $nrays_{int}$ `[`*maxdist* `[`*mindist*`]]`[2.1]

nrays is the number of rays cast in a final gathering step during rendering. The default is 1000. *maxdist* is the maximum distance within which a final gather result can be reused. The default is scene dependent. *mindist* is the minimum distance within which final gather results must be reused. The default is scene dependent.

`-focal` *distance* `| infinity`

The focal distance is set to *distance*. The focal distance is the distance from the camera to the viewing plane. The viewing plane is the plane in front of the camera that the rendered scene is projected onto; its edges correspond to the edges of the rendered image. However, objects between the camera and the viewing plane will still be rendered; a common approach is to place the viewing plane in the middle of the interesting objects in the scene and then set the aperture such that it is a bit larger than the horizontal extent of the objects in camera space. If `infinity` is used in place of the *distance*, an orthographic view is rendered. An orthographic view turns off perspective, all camera rays are parallel. View-dependent surface tessellation is not possible in orthogonal mode.

`-gamma` *gamma_factor*

Gamma correction can be applied to rendered color pixels to compensate for output devices with a nonlinear color response. All R, G, B, and alpha component values are raised to *gamma_factor*. The default gamma factor is 1.0, which turns gamma correction off.

`-geometry on|off`

Ignore all geometry shaders if set to `off`. The default is `on`.

`-globillum on|off`[2.1]

Enable or disable the computation of global illumination. The default is `off`. To actually compute global illumination, lights must have an energy, and materials must have photon shaders.

`-globillum_accuracy` $nphotons_{int}$ [*radius*][2.1]

Controls how global illumination is estimated from the photon map during rendering. *nphotons* is the maximum number of photons to examine and *radius* the maximum radius to search. if *nphotons* = 0, all photons are examined up to the *radius* limit. *radius* = 0.0 means that a scene-size dependent radius will be used. The defaults are 500 and 0.0.

`-grid_size` *factor*

Adjust the scene-dependent default grid voxel size. The default is 1.0. Larger values increase the number of voxels and shrink each voxel accordingly.

`-help`

Print a summary of all options with their allowed parameters, and terminate.

`-hosts` "*hostname*[:*portnumber*] [*remote parameters*]" ... --

The host list overrides the host list taken from the `.rayhosts` file, if present. One server is started on each host specified. Host names must be given as expected by the local name resolving method (such as `/etc/hosts`) or as a numeric internet address (`nnn.nnn.nnn.nnn`). Machines used as servers must be correctly configured; see the installation notes. The host list must be terminated by a double minus.

`-I` *path*

Overrides the path used to resolve `$include` statements in the .mi scene file. The default path is `/usr/include`. Note that only one `-I` option can be specified. It may contain a colon-separated (Unix only) or semicolon-separated (Unix and NT) list of directory paths that are tried in sequence if a `$include` statement using angle brackets is used in the .mi scene file. Paths introduced with an exclamation point are special; they are applied to quoted `$include` paths too, and substitute the entire directory path. This can be used to force mental ray to use a specified path regardless of the path specified in the `$include` statement, for example because that path points to an obsolete (1.9) version of a declaration file. For example, `-I /a:/b:!/new` tries to find a path `<x/y/z>` first as `/a/x/y/z`, then `/b/x/y/z`, then `/new/z`.

`-imgpipe` fd_{int}

Normally mental ray prints connection information into the output image file that let programs like *imf_disp* connect and display pictures while being rendered. If `-imgpipe` is used, the relevant information is printed to the given file descriptor *fd* instead. This can be used for command lines such as "`ray -imgpipe 1 scene.mi | imf_disp -`". The *imf_disp* program is a viewer provided by mental images that supports image piping.

`-jitter` *jitter*

The jittering factor introduces systematic variations into sample locations. Without jittering, samples are taken at the corners of pixels or subpixels. Jittering displaces the samples by an amount calculated by lighting analysis, limited to *jitter* pixels. This is used to reduce artifacts. Jittering is turned off by default, or by specifying a *jitter* of 0.0. Jittering works best in ray tracing mode. The *jitter* value is always set to 1.0 if jittering is turned on.

`-ld_libs "`*libraries*`"`

The *libraries* string replaces the standard library options given to the linker. The defaults depend on the machine used, typically `"-lm -lc"`. Linker options are highly machine dependent and operating system dependent and cannot be changed.

`-ld_path "`*path1;path2;...*`"`

Supply a list of paths that mental ray searches for dynamic shared objects (DSO) containing shader code. The paths given here precede those that can be given by an environment variable (`MI_LIBRARY_PATH`) and the built-in search path (`/usr/local/mi/lib;.`). `-ld_path` is synonymous with `-L`.

`-lens on|off`

Ignore all lens shaders if set to `off`. The default is on.

`-link "`*filename*`" ... --`

Like the code command, the link command attaches external shaders to mental ray, which can then be used as shading functions. While the code command accepts ".c" files as *filename*, the link command expects either object files ending in ".o", or dynamic shared object (DSO) files ending in ".so". Object files are linked, while DSOs are just attached without any preprocessing. DSOs are the fastest way of attaching an external shader, and require no compilers or development options, which are sometimes sold separately by system vendors. On Windows NT, `.so` extensions are automatically converted to `.dll` for cross-platform compatibility.[1] However, not all systems support DSOs; see "Dynamic Linking of Shaders". The file name list must be terminated with a double minus sign.

`-merge on|off`
: Ignore all merge epsilons and all connections in the scene.

`-message` *module class_list* `... --`
: Enable or disable individual message classes, per module. The module names are printed at the beginning of every message printed by mental ray; `all` can be used to modify the message classes of all modules. The *class_list* is a comma-separated list of classes to print. Supported message classes are `phase`, `progress`, `vprogress`, `time`, `scene`, `memory`, `render`, `vrender`, `resources`, `network`, `files`, and `debug`. The special words `default`, `all`, and `none` are also supported. A class can be inverted by prepending an exclamation point. For example, to print less verbose RC progress messages and make all modules report every file accessed, specify

```
-message rc default,!vprogress all default,files --
```

`-o "`*filename*`"`
: This is an abbreviation for `-file_name`.

`-offset` *x y*[2.1]
: Specifies an offset for the rendered image. The default is 0.0 for both values, which means that the image will be centered on the camera's Z axis. Positive values translate the image up and to the right. The *offset* is measured in pixel units.

`-output on|off`
: Ignore all output shaders if set to `off`. The default is on. File output statements are not affected.

`-photonmap_file "`*filename*`"`
: Use *filename* for the photon map, in all frames. If the photon map file does not exist, it is created and saved. If it exists, it is loaded and used. For multiple frames it is only created for the first frame and then loaded for the remaining frames.

[1] For system and development software requirements, see the Release and Installation Notes.

`-photonvol_accuracy` *nphotons*$_{int}$ [*radius*]

Controls how global illumination[2.1] or caustics in participating media are estimated from the photon map during rendering. *nphotons* is the maximum number of photons to examine and *radius* the maximum radius to search. if *nphotons* = 0, all photons are examined up to the *radius* limit. *radius* = 0.0 means that a scene-size dependent radius will be used. The defaults are 30 and 0.0.

`-photon_depth` *reflect*$_{int}$ [*refract*$_{int}$ [*sum*$_{int}$]]

`photon_depth` is similar to `trace_depth` except that it applies to photons. *reflect* thus limits the number of recursive reflection photons. If it is set to 0, no photons will be reflected; if it is set to 1, one level is allowed but a photon cannot be reflected again, and so on. Similarly, *refract* controls the maximum depth of refracted photons. Additionally, it is possible to limit the sum of reflected and refracted photon levels with *sum*. Note that custom shaders may override these values. The default value is 5 5 5.

`-premultiply on|off`

Premultiplication means that colors are stored with alpha multiplied to R, G, and B. For example, white at 10% opacity is not stored as (1, 1, 1, 0.1) but as (0.1, 0.1, 0.1, 0.1). This is the standard method in computer graphics to represent colors; mental ray always uses it internally and in all shaders. One implication is that R, G, and B can never exceed A. mental ray normally enforces this when storing color values into frame buffers. The `-premultiply off` option instructs mental ray to always store colors *unpremultiplied* into frame buffers and files. It does this by undoing the internally applied premultiplication. (mental ray internally always works with premultiplied colors to present a uniform interface to shaders; since this is done with floating-point values there is no precision penalty.) This option is ignored if the `-colorclip raw`[2.1] mode is in effect.

`-raycl_memory` *memory*$_{int}$

This option sets the amount of memory to be used by the ray space subdivision algorithm for acceleration data structures to *memory* megabytes on each CPU. It has no effect if the BSP algorithm is used. mental ray allows presetting the amount of rendering acceleration memory independently of scene complexity without sacrificing speed. The default is set to 6 megabytes, which is sufficient for most scenes. Even for extremely large scenes, little can be gained from memory sizes greater than 12 megabytes. Note that this option does not affect the amount of memory used for the scene description, which depends on the complexity of the geometry in the current frame.

`-raycl_subdivision` *subdiv*$_{int}$ *subdiv_2d*$_{int}$

mental ray uses a ray tracing algorithm that subdivides the space of all rays. The optimal subdivision is determined automatically by a built-in scene analysis. The `-subdivision` option can be used to modify the result of this analysis; arguments of 0 leave the calculated subdivision unchanged, positive numbers increase and negative numbers reduce the subdivision. *subdiv* controls general subdivision; *subdiv_2d* controls primary (eye) and shadow rays. This option has no effect if the BSP algorithm is used.

`-render` $begin_{int}$ [end_{int} [inc_{int}]]
: Render only frames *begin* through *end*[2]. If *end* is omitted, *begin* and all following frames are rendered. If *inc* is given, only every *inc*-th frame is rendered. Frame 1 is considered the first `render` statement in the scene file; camera frame specifiers are not considered. For example, `4 8 2` will skip the first three frames, then render frame 4, 6, and 8, and omit the rest. It is not an error if the scene file has fewer frames than requested.

`-resolution` x_{int} y_{int}
: Specifies the width and height of the output image in pixels.

`-samplelock on|off`
: Whether to let the sampling of area light sources, motion blur, and depht-of-field be static or depend on the frame number. The default is on, meaning static sampling.

`-samples` min_{int} max_{int}
: This option determines the minimum and maximum sample rate. Each pixel is sampled at least $2^{2 \cdot min}$ times in each direction. If *min* is 0, each pixel is sampled at least once. Positive values increase the minimum sample rate; negative numbers reduce the sample rate to less than one initial sample per pixel (infrasampling). *min* has default -2, which means that at least one sample per 4×4 pixels is taken. If *min* is chosen too small, small features may be lost if all samples happen to miss it (if it is found just once in any pixel of a task, mental ray will analyze the feature and render it correctly). If a `filter` camera statement is used to set a filter other than `box 1 1`, *min* must be set to -1 or greater (mental ray 2.1) or 1 or greater (mental ray 2.0).

The *max* value sets the maximum sample rate. If neighboring samples find a difference in contrast exceeding the contrast limit, the area that contains the contrast is subdivided until the maximum recursion depth specified by *max* is reached. At most $2^{2 \cdot max}$ samples per pixel are taken. If a filter camera statement or option is used to set a filter other than `box 1 1`, *max* must be set to 0 or greater (mental ray 2.1) or 1 or greater (mental ray 2.0).

`-scanline on|off|opengl`
: This statement controls the scanline rendering algorithm. By default,

[2]The -render option was introduced in mental ray 2.1.36.

mental ray uses the scanline algorithm to compute rays traveling in a straight line from the camera, such as primary rays. In most cases this gives better performance than pure ray tracing. Turning scanline off forces mental ray to rely entirely on ray tracing. This will generally slow down rendering but in some cases, for example when the `task size` is very small, the overhead of initializing the scanline algorithm may outweigh its benefit and turning it off can result in a speed improvement.

`-scanline opengl`[2.1]mode will cause mental ray to use OpenGL hardware if available to further accelerate rendering. OpenGL is not used to compute actual colors but only projection and intersection information, so the full mental ray shader feature set remains available. However, there may be a precision loss. Since OpenGL rendering is typically extremely fast compared to network transfer times, only the client host uses its OpenGL hardware. The results are broadcast to server hosts if present. Server hosts never use their OpenGL hardware. Also see `-task_size` below.

OpenGL rendering makes certain demands on the OpenGL hardware present. If a 24 bit frame buffer with a Z buffer is not present, OpenGL rendering may fail. OpenGL may also fail or become slow if the image to be rendered is larger than the workstation display. The *max* parameter to the `-samples` option should not be higher than `0`, or image artifacts may appear. During rendering with OpenGL, a window may briefly appear containing seemingly random colors. On Unix workstations, mental ray will need access to the X server and OpenGL hardware for OpenGL rendering to work. This is usually achieved through the use of the `DISPLAY` environment variable. See your workstation manuals for details. Finally, OpenGL rendering does not work with motion blurring. If, for any reason, OpenGL rendering is not possible on the client host, mental ray falls back on regular scanline rendering.

`-shadow off`

All shadowing is disabled.

`-shadow on`

This flag enables simple shadowing. Shadow shaders determine how much light from a light source passes through a shadow-casting object between the light source and an illuminated point on some other object. In `shadow on` mode (the default), shadows are computed. Shadow shaders are called in random order.

`-shadow sort`

This flag also turns on shadowing, but alters the way shadow shaders are called. The shadow-casting objects are sorted such that the shadow shader of the object closest to the illuminated point is called first and the one closest to the light is called last (unless the sequence terminates early because light is completely blocked).

`-shadow segments`

Like with `shadow sort`, the shadow shaders are called in a sorted fashion. Shadows are computed by tracing the segments between the illumination point, the occluding objects and the light source and applying volume shaders to these segments (shadow segments). This slows down rendering, but is required if volume effects should cast shadows (as for certain complex shaders such as fur shaders).

`-shadowmap [on][off][opengl][only][rebuild][reuse][motion][nomotion]--`

This option can be used to control shadow maps: The allowed options are:

`on` activates use of shadow maps.

`off` disables use of shadow maps. This is the default.

`only` causes only shadow maps to be rendered, without rendering a color image. By default the color image is rendered also.

`rebuild` causes all shadow maps to be recomputed, even if they are found in memory or on disk. By default `reuse` is in effect, meaning that shadowmaps are computed only if they are not found in memory or on disk.

`reuse` causes shadowmaps to be reused. First, internal memory is searched for shadowmaps from a previous frame. If they are not found, a search is made on disk in the current directory, according to the filenames specified in the .mi file if given. If neither is found, the shadowmaps are recomputed.

`motion` activates motion blurred shadow maps. This is the default.

`nomotion` disables motion blurred shadow maps. This improves rendering speed.

`opengl`[2.1]causes mental ray to try to use OpenGL acceleration when rendering shadow maps. The same limitations apply as mentioned with the `-scanline opengl` option. Additionally, because of the difference of the rendering algorithm, shadow maps rendered with this option contain slightly different information from those generated with the regular algorithm, and the resulting shadows may look different. In particular, soft areas of shadows tend to be smaller and some areas may incorrectly be determined to be not in shadow due to the lower precision of OpenGL acceleration. When OpenGL rendering of shadow maps is enabled, only the client host will participate, since the computation cost of the map is so small that the network transfer time would be prohibitive.

`-shutter` *shutter*

This option specifies the shutter open time. A *shutter* value of 0.0 turns motion blurring off, values greater than 0.0 turn motion blurring on. The *shutter* value scales the motion vectors attached to object vertices; if *shutter* is 1.0, each vertex moves the distance given by its motion vector, and is blurred in the image over this distance. Values less than 1.0 reduce this path.

`-task_size` $task\_size_{int}$

This option specifies the size of the image tasks during rendering. Smaller task sizes are convenient for previewing, but also increase the overall rendering time. This option can also be used in order to optimize load balancing for parallel rendering. Note that very small task sizes can cause the scanline algorithm to perform poorly and in such cases it may be desirable to turn it off. See `-scanline` above. If the `task_size` is not specified, an appropriate default value is used.

`-threads` $nthreads_{int}$

Normally, mental ray starts one thread for each CPU in the system. In a single-processor host, the default is always 1. This option changes the number of threads. There is normally no advantage in increasing the number of threads, but it may be lowered to reserve CPUs for other users, to avoid monopolizing a multi-processor machine. Note that Convex machines do not make the number of CPUs in the system available to user programs, so `-threads` should always be used.

`-time_contrast` *r g b* [*a*]

The time contrast controls temporal supersampling for motion blurred scenes. It works similar to the spatial contrast parameter explained above: If neighboring samples in time differ by more than the color *r*, *g*, *b*, *a*, supersampling is done. Default for *a* is the average of *r*, *g*, and *b*; the default for *r*, *g*, and *b* is 0.2. Using values for `-time_contrast` that are higher than `-contrast` can speed up motion blur rendering at the price of more grainy images without degrading the quality of spatial antialiasing.

`-trace on|off`

Normally, mental ray will use a combination of a scanline algorithm and ray tracing to calculate samples of the scene. If `-trace off` is specified, ray tracing is disabled, and mental ray will rely exclusively on the scanline algorithm. Since the scanline algorithm can only compute straight rays from the pinhole camera, reflection rays cannot be cast and refraction rays are computed like transparent rays, which do not allow control over the ray direction based on the index of refraction of the material. Lens shaders cannot alter ray origin and direction. However, reflections onto environment maps do work. Motion blurring and shadows are also affected if ray tracing is turned off. Ray tracing is turned on by default.

`-trace_depth` *reflect*$_{int}$ [*refract*$_{int}$ [*sum*$_{int}$]]

reflect limits the number of recursive reflection rays. If it is set to 0, no reflection rays will be cast; if it is set to 1, one level is allowed but a reflection ray can not be reflected again, and so on. Similarly, *refract* controls the maximum depth of refraction and transparency rays (which implement transparency with and without index of refraction). Additionally, it is possible to limit the sum of reflection and refraction rays with *sum*. For example, if `3 3 4` is given, an eye ray may be reflected 3 times, or refracted 3 times, or reflected twice and then refracted twice, or any other combination that sums up to at most 4. Shaders may override this setting. The default is 1 1 1.

`-v on|off|`*level*$_{int}$

An abbreviation for `-verbose`.

`-verbose on|off|`*level*$_{int}$

This command controls verbose messages. There are seven levels: fatal errors (0), errors (1), warnings (2), progress reports (3), informational messages (4), debugging messages (5), and verbose debugging messages (6). All message categories numerically less than *level* are printed. Verbose `off` is equivalent to level 2 (fatal errors and errors); verbose on is equivalent to level 5 (everything except debugging messages).

`-view_samples on|off`[2.1]

Toggles the sample view mode. When on, the rgb image will be replaced with an image that shows where samples were collected during rendering. This is useful for tuning the `-samples` and `-contrast` parameters and identifying troublesome areas in the image. A pixel's intensity reflects the number of samples collected within the pixel and on its lower and left edges. It is normalized to the maximum number of samples per pixel. In addition, task boundaries are shown as red in the image.

`-volume on|off`

Ignore all volume shaders if set to `off`. The default is on.

`-window` *x_low*$_{int}$ *y_low*$_{int}$ *x_high*$_{int}$ *y_high*$_{int}$

Only the sub-rectangle of the image specified by the four bounds will be rendered. All pixels that fall outside the rectangle will be left black.

`-xcolor ["`*control*`"]`

Print colored messages. Error messages, for example, are printed in red, which makes them stand out much better in verbose reports. The control string allows customization; it consists of seven characters describing the severity level (fatal, error, warning, info, progress, debug, and vdebug). Each character is one of k (black), r (red), g (green), y (yellow), b (blue), m (magenta), c (cyan), w (white), or a dot (no color).

5.2 Startup File

When mental ray starts up, it automatically checks the following list of startup files:

Unix:

```
.rayrc
$HOME/.rayrc
$MI_ROOT/rayrc
/usr/local/mi/rayrc
```

Windows NT:

```
rayrc
%MI_ROOT%\rayrc
%SystemDrive%\rayrc
%SystemDrive%\Program Files\mental images\rayrc
```

If the startup file is found, it is read and parsed like a regular .mi scene file. After one such file was read, the search is terminated without searching in the remaining locations. `HOME`, `MI_ROOT`, and `SystemDrive` are environment variables.

The purpose of the startup file is portable initialization. For example, it may contain `link` statements that load commonly used shader libraries, or `$include` statement to load shader declarations (after the corresponding `link` statement). One important point is that different systems with different directory structures can be handled with different local startup files, such that paths built into scene files that could cause incompatibilities are no longer necessary. On Windows NT systems, for example, paths and library names are generally different than on Unix systems, and startup files can be used to hide the differences.

Remote rendering servers on other hosts also read the startup file, but they ignore all `link` and `code` statements. (It is not a good idea to put `code` statements into a startup file because running the compiler can make mental ray startup time unacceptable.) This is done to make sure that the shader library list on the server is consistent with the shader library list on the client host.

Although startup files support the full .mi language, they should only be used for initialization and not to preload geometry or other scene database elements because this could cause conflicts with scenes that are loaded later. In particular, `render` statements may not be used in a startup file; mental ray will abort parsing the startup file at a `render` statement.

5.3 Stack Size

On highly parallel Unix machines, it is recommended to set the stack size with the following shell command before starting 32-bit versions of mental ray:

```
limit  stacksize  8192
```

The default may be 64 MB or higher, which means that the virtual memory limit is reached with 8 or 16 CPUs (depending on the machine type) because the 32-bit address space is shared by all CPUs. If virtual memory runs out, the kernel may be forced to kill mental ray threads, which may freeze execution. A stack size of 8192 (KB) is generous, 4096 is usually sufficient also. Every thread needs one stack. For systems with a large number of processors, such as 64 or 128, the virtual memory limit can be avoided altogether by using the 64-bit version of mental ray.

When a 32-bit Unix version of mental ray sees a stack size greater than 16 MB, it limits the stack size to 16 MB for all threads except the first one (which is already running), and prints a warning.

The problem does not arise on Windows NT because PCs only have small numbers of processors. mental ray always chooses a stack size of 4 MB on NT because there is no way to set it from a shell. Windows NT is not a 64-bit operating system.

Note that one should not plan on using more than a quarter of available virtual memory on stacks because the executable, heap storage, and normal and memory-mapped textures must also fit into virtual memory.

Chapter 6

Upgrading from mental ray 1.9 to 2.x

With mental ray 2.x a new generation of mental ray has become available. Its internal design greatly differs from mental ray 1.9; it incorporates many new features like networking based on a global shared database, incremental changes support, Phenomena, new rendering techniques for caustics and contour rendering, an improved approach to parallelization, and enhanced extensibility. At the same time, obsolete features such as nonrecursive sampling have been removed.

For the mental ray 1.9 user, this means that the transition from mental ray 1.9 to 2.x requires some attention. mental ray 2.x has been designed for maximum compatibility with mental ray 1.9, so in general no additional work will be required by the user to render existing scenes that do not use contour rendering or custom shaders. However, the mental ray installation procedure is slightly different, and shader writers need to make adjustments to the shader sources. This chapter summarizes all changes required when switching from version 1.9 to 2.x.

mental ray 2.x also introduces a number of new features. Some of them improve on 1.9 features and are recommended for future shader designs; these are also listed in this chapter. However, this is not a complete list of improvements in mental ray 2.x.

6.1 Rendering Algorithms

If incompatible options are given to mental ray, some of them are overridden to return to a consistent state. In mental ray 1.9.9.20 and higher, including mental ray 2.x, the strategy was changed: instead of re-enabling ray tracing if any other feature such as lenses are used and ray tracing was explicitly turned off, the newer versions do not turn ray tracing back on but change the operation of the feature normally requiring ray tracing. The following features are affected:

- If ray tracing is turned off, lens shaders cannot modify the ray origin and direction. Lens shaders are still useful in this mode because they can modify the color returned by the eye ray, or decide to not sample points in certain directions.

- A new algorithm was introduced in mental ray 2.x that supports fast motion blur in scanline mode. Turning ray tracing off no longer disables motion blurring.
- Similarly, shadow maps were introduced that support shadows in scanline mode. Only opaque shadows are supported in this mode; transparent and transparency-mapped shadows still require ray tracing. Shadow maps do support motion-blurred shadows.

6.2 Scene Description Language

mental ray 2.x supports a new generation of the mental images scene description language, called `.mi2`. The language version supported by mental ray 1.9, called `.mi1`, is still available for backwards compatibility. New translator designs should always use `.mi2` because only `.mi2` supports instancing, inheritance, incremental changes, and many other features. Here are some rules for using `.mi2`:

- Use object space coordinates instead of camera coordinates.
- Use options, cameras, instances and groups instead of frames and views.
- Use incremental changes wherever possible.
- Do not use the following statements: `red`, `green`, `blue`, `white`, `recursive`, `adaptive`, `memory`.
- Double-quote names to avoid clashes with new keywords.
- Contour rendering has been rewritten completely. The new algorithms offer much higher flexibility, programmability, and features such as colored contours, varying line widths and styles, parallelism, and contour generation concurrently with color image generation, and compositing. The contour modes of mental ray 1.9 are no longer supported, any `.mi1` scene file containing contour features must be modified.
- Use `contour contrast`, `contour store`, `contour output`, and contour shaders.
- Do not use: `contour line width`, `contour depth`, and `paper transform`.

6.3 Shader Writing

- Even if none of the following points apply, shaders must be recompiled with the `shader.h` file that comes with mental ray 2.x. It is not possible to use the same shader object or library file for both mental ray 1.9 and 2.x. A shader compiled with the wrong `shader.h` file will not be able to access state variables correctly. `shader.h` contains `#define RAY2` to allow shader sources to make sure that the correct file is included.
- The `shader.h` file that comes with mental ray 2.x is fully ANSI-compliant. Old-style K&R compilers cannot be used any longer.

- Always put `min version 2.0` into all shader declaration `$include` files used by mental ray 2.x but not by mental ray 1.9. Add `max version 1.99` for shader declaration files used by mental ray 1.9 but not 2.x.

- All shaders that accept arrays as parameters must be modified. mental ray 1.9 required that arrays are given as `*array` in the parameter `struct`, with `array` being the name of the array. This must be changed to `array[1]` for mental ray 2.x shaders. The `i_array` and `n_array` integers remain unchanged. This change has been announced in the mental ray 1.9 User's Manual, [RAY1 97]; see the discussion there

- Shaders using the *mi_trace_light* function should be rewritten to use *mi_sample_light*. The new function has been available in mental ray 1.9 for upward compatibility but was functionally identical to *mi_trace_light*; in mental ray 2.x it was reimplemented to allow correct behavior in cases where the illuminated surface is close to an area light source. In these cases, only *mi_sample_light* correctly increases the size of the highlight.

- A tag to a light instance is now accessible through $state \rightarrow light\_instance$. In 1.9 it was $state \rightarrow instance$, but this field is now reserved for other purposes.

- The $state \rightarrow contour$ field is not available in 2.x. If a shader wants to test whether there is contours or not, test if ($state \rightarrow options \rightarrow contour\_contrast! = 0$) and ($state \rightarrow options \rightarrow contour\_store! = 0$) instead.

- Do not use $state \rightarrow shadow\_sort$. This variable is still available for backwards compatibility reasons, but may be dropped in future versions of mental ray. Instead, check whether the $state \rightarrow shadow$ variable has the character value `'l'` (lower-case L).

- Shadow shaders and material shaders used as shadow shaders should be written to support shadow segment mode. If this mode is enabled, $state \rightarrow shadow\_sort$ has the character value `'s'`.

- In both mental ray 1.9 and 2.x, *tags* are used to identify scene components such as instances and shaders. A tag is an opaque data type that is not normally used directly, but can be converted to a pointer using the *mi_db_access* function. In mental ray 1.9, the tag value happens to be bit-wise identical to the pointer; this is not the case in mental ray 2.x. Also, mental ray 1.9 does not fail if there is not a *mi_db_unpin* call for every *mi_db_access* call; mental ray 2.x may fail with a pin overflow error. Both of these effects are a problem only for shaders that do not comply with the mental ray shader interface as specified in the 1.9 User's Manual.

- The *mi_db_access* function was a dummy function in mental ray 1.9, but is implemented in mental ray 2.x. It does not accept a null tag as argument, but mental ray 1.9 does not check this. mental ray 2.x does, and fails with a fatal error in this case.

- Shaders that use the (undocumented) transformation fields in the state ($state \rightarrow world\_transform$, $state \rightarrow inv\_world\_transform$, $state \rightarrow object\_transform$ and $state \rightarrow inv\_object\_transform$) have to be rewritten. mental ray version 2.x provides the *mi_query* function that can be called with the *miQ_TRANS_CAMERA_TO_WORLD*, *miQ_TRANS_OBJECT_TO_WORLD* and similar codes in order to provide the appropriate transformations. Note that *mi_query* returns a pointer to the matrix, not the matrix itself, to reduce data copying. See the description of the *mi_query* function.

- Shaders that access opaque data structures by "knowing" that the n-th integer or pointer in undocumented structures contain a certain value will no longer work. All internal data structures have changed. Features not documented in the User's Manual are not portable. Use *mi_query* to access internal data.

- Many shaders use an init shader to set up private data that is later used during shading. In mental ray 1.9 it was common to declare dummy parameters to have a place to store the pointer to the private data. This was dangerous because of alignment problems on systems with 64-bit pointers and is not recommended. mental ray 2.x supports a user pointer for storing the private data pointer; it can be obtained with *mi_query*'s `miQ_FUNC_USERPTR` mode.

- Exit shaders now have *state* as parameter. This was not the case with 1.9 exit shaders. Failing to add this parameter can cause severe problems.

- A number of image access functions are renamed for more consistent use of function names. Every call to these functions must be replaced with the renamed functions as they are defined in shader.h. These functions were available but undocumented in mental ray 1.9.

- *get_no_procs* is no longer available. Use *mi_par_nthreads* instead. Note that some versions of mental ray 1.9 misspelled this function *mi_par_nthread.*

- Some effects require a large number of scene modifications to install various types of shaders, dummy geometry, and rendering options, resulting in lengthy procedures for integrating the effect. mental ray 2.x supports a new feature called *phenomena* that automate the integration and installation of procedural geometry.

Appendix A

Scene File Grammar

This appendix contains the formal syntax of the mental images .mi scene description format. The grammar is in *yacc* format; *yacc* is a Unix compiler generator. Nonterminals that begin with `T_` are typed values:

`T_SYMBOL` is an unquoted string consisting of zero or more letters, numbers, and underscores and does not begin with a number.

`T_INTEGER` is a nonempty sequence of numerical digits.

`T_FLOAT` is a nonempty sequence of digits, followed by a period, followed by a nonempty sequence of digits.

`T_STRING` is a sequence of arbitrary printable characters enclosed in double quotes. Nonprintables such as newlines are not allowed. Backslash and double quote characters that should be part of the string must be prefixed with a backslash.

`T_BYTE_STRING` is a sequence of hexadecimal bytes, each consisting of two characters in the range `0..9` or `a..f`. Line breaks are allowed between bytes. Other characters are not allowed.

`T_VECTOR` is a backquote followed by 12 bytes followed by a backquote. The 12 bytes are the binary image of three floats, not swapped.

This appendix is intended to aid translator writers, and to describe the relationship between the .mi scene description language and the API available to geometry shader writers. This is the complete mental ray grammar including parts that are not part of the shader interface (such as initiating rendering). Refer to the mental ray integration guide for a description of these functions.

Note that the grammars used by mental ray 1.9 and mental ray 2.0 are arranged in a slightly different way, but functionally the 2.0 grammar is a fully compatible superset of the 1.9 grammar with added features such as instancing.

```
%start start

%union {
        miBoolean        boolean;
        char            *symbol;
        char            *string;
        struct          {
                int      len;
                miUchar *bytes;
        }                byte_string;
        int              integer;
        double           floating;
        float            floatoctet[8];
        miMatrix         matrix;
        miVector         vector;
        miGeoVector      geovector;
        miTransform     *transform;
        miParameter     *para_type;
        miDlist         *dlist;
        miTag            tag;
}

%token <symbol>         T_SYMBOL
%token <integer>        T_INTEGER
%token <floating>       T_FLOAT
%token <string>         T_STRING
%token <byte_string>    T_BYTE_STRING
%token <vector>         T_VECTOR

%token ACCELERATION ACCURACY ADAPTIVE ALL ALPHA ANGLE ANY APERTURE APPLY
%token APPROXIMATE ARRAY ASPECT
%token BACK BASIS BEZIER BLUE BOOLEAN BOTH BOX BSP BSPLINE BUFFER BUMP
%token CALL CAMERA CARDINAL CAUSTIC CLASSIFICATION CLIP CODE COLOR COLORCLIP
%token CONE CONIC CONNECT CONSTANT CONTOUR CONTRAST CONTROL CORNER CP
%token CREASE CURVATURE CURVE CUSP CYLINDER
%token D DART DATA DEBUG_ DECLARE DELAUNAY DELETE_ DENSITY DEPTH DERIVATIVE
%token DESATURATE DIAGNOSTIC DIRECTION DISC DISPLACE DISTANCE DITHER
%token ECHO EMITTER END ENVIRONMENT EVEN ENERGY EXPONENT
%token FACE FALSE_ FAN FIELD FILE_ FILTER FINALGATHER FOCAL FRAME FRONT
%token GAMMA GAUSS GEOMETRY GLOBILLUM GRADING GREEN GRID GROUP GUI
%token HIDE HOLE
%token IMP IMPLICIT INCREMENTAL INFINITY_ INHERITANCE INSTANCE INSTGROUP
%token INTEGER INTERFACE_ IRRADIANCE
%token JITTER
%token LANCZOS LENGTH LENS LIGHT LINK LOCAL
%token M MAPSTO MATERIAL MATRIX MAX_ MEMORY MERGE MI MIN_ MITCHELL MIXED MOTION
%token N NOCONTOUR NULL_
%token OBJECT ODD OFF OFFSET ON OPAQUE_ OPENGL OPTIONS ORIGIN OUTPUT
%token P PARALLEL_ PARAMETRIC PHENOMENON PHOTON PHOTONMAP PHOTONS PHOTONVOL
%token PREMULTIPLY PRIORITY
```

```
%token Q QUALITY
%token RATIONAL RAY RAYCL RAW REBUILD RECTANGLE RECURSIVE RED REGISTRY REGULAR
%token RENDER RESOLUTION RGB_ ROOT
%token SAMPLELOCK SAMPLES SCALAR SCANLINE SEGMENTS SET SHADOW SHADOWMAP SHUTTER
%token SIZE SOFTNESS SORT SPACE SPATIAL SPDL SPECIAL SPHERE SPREAD STORE STRING
%token STRIP STRUCT SUBDIVISION SHADER SMART SURFACE SYSTEM
%token T TAG TAGGED TASK TAYLOR TEXTURE TIME TRACE TRANSFORM TREE TRIANGLE TRIM
%token TRUE_
%token U V VALUE VECTOR VERBOSE VERSION VIEW VISIBLE VOLUME
%token W WHITE WIDTH WINDOW WORLD

%type <floating>                floating
%type <boolean>                 boolean
%type <string>                  symbol
%type <string>                  opt_symbol
%type <matrix>                  transform
%type <integer>                 tex_flags
%type <integer>                 tex_flag
%type <integer>                 tex_type
%type <integer>                 simple_type
%type <string>                  inst_item
%type <tag>                     inst_func
%type <tag>                     inst_params
%type <integer>                 filter_type
%type <integer>                 c_filter_type
%type <tag>                     function
%type <tag>                     function_list
%type <tag>                     tex_func_list
%type <tag>                     phen_root
%type <string>                  mtl_or_label
%type <para_type>               shret_type
%type <para_type>               shret_type_nosh
%type <para_type>               shret_decl_seq
%type <para_type>               shret_decl
%type <para_type>               parm_decl_list
%type <para_type>               parm_decl_seq
%type <para_type>               parm_decl
%type <boolean>                 rational
%type <dlist>                   basis_matrix
%type <floating>                merge_option
%type <vector>                  vector
%type <geovector>               geovector
%type <dlist>                   para_list
%type <boolean>                 opt_volume_flag
%type <boolean>                 opt_vector_flag
%type <boolean>                 opt_incremental
%type <integer>                 apply
%type <integer>                 apply_list
%type <floatoctet>              out_parms
%type <integer>                 colorclip_mode

%%
```

```
start           :
                        { functag = 0;
                          mi_api_incremental(is_incremental = miFALSE);
                          mi_reset_time();
                          if (mi_get_subverbosity(miM_MI) & miMSG_PHASE)
                                mi_progress("begin mi scene file parsing"); }
                  command_list
                        { if (mi_get_subverbosity(miM_MI) & miMSG_PHASE)
                                mi_progress("end of scene file, parsing ends");
                        }
                |
                        { mi_info("end of scene file"); }
                ;


/*------------------------------------------------------------------------
 * primitive types
 *----------------------------------------------------------------------*/

boolean         : ON
                        { $$ = miTRUE; }
                | OFF
                        { $$ = miFALSE; }
                | TRUE_
                        { $$ = miTRUE; }
                | FALSE_
                        { $$ = miFALSE; }
                ;

floating        : T_FLOAT       { $$ = $1; }
                | T_INTEGER     { $$ = $1; }
                ;

vector          : floating floating floating
                        { $$.x = $1; $$.y = $2; $$.z = $3; }
                | T_VECTOR
                        { $$ = $1; }
                ;

geovector       : floating floating floating
                        { $$.x = $1; $$.y = $2; $$.z = $3; }
                | T_VECTOR
                        { $$.z = $1.z; $$.y = $1.y; $$.x = $1.x; }
                ;

transform       : TRANSFORM     floating floating floating floating
                                floating floating floating floating
                                floating floating floating floating
                                floating floating floating floating
                        { $$[0] = $2;  $$[1] = $3;  $$[2] = $4;  $$[3] = $5;
                          $$[4] = $6;  $$[5] = $7;  $$[6] = $8;  $$[7] = $9;
                          $$[8] = $10; $$[9] = $11; $$[10]= $12; $$[11]= $13;
                          $$[12]= $14; $$[13]= $15; $$[14]= $16; $$[15]= $17; }
```

```
                  ;

symbol          : T_SYMBOL
                        { $$ = $1; }
                | T_STRING
                        { $$ = $1; }
                ;

opt_symbol      :
                        { $$ = 0; }
                | symbol
                        { $$ = $1; }
                ;

colorclip_mode  :  RGB_
                        { $$ = miIMG_COLORCLIP_RGB; }
                |  ALPHA
                        { $$ = miIMG_COLORCLIP_ALPHA; }
                |  RAW
                        { $$ = miIMG_COLORCLIP_RAW; }
                ;


/*-----------------------------------------------------------------------------
 * top-level commands
 *---------------------------------------------------------------------------*/

command_list    :       { mi_api_incremental(is_incremental = miFALSE); }
                  command
                | command_list
                        { mi_api_incremental(is_incremental = miFALSE); }
                  command
                ;

command         : frame
                | debug
                | set
                | call
                | version
                | incr_command
                | INCREMENTAL
                        { mi_api_incremental(is_incremental = miTRUE); }
                  incr_command
                | DELETE_ symbol
                        { mi_api_delete($2); }
                | RENDER symbol symbol symbol
                        { mi_timing("mi scene file parsing");
                          mi_reset_time();
                          mi_api_render($2, $3, $4,
                                         mi_mem_strdup(ctx->inheritance_func));
                          if (mi_get_subverbosity(miM_MI) & miMSG_PHASE)
                                mi_progress("resume mi scene file parsing");
                          yyreturn MIYYRENDER;
```

```
                  }
                | VERBOSE boolean
                  { if (!ctx->mi_force_verbose)
                          mi_set_verbosity($2? miERR_ALL & ~miERR_DEBUG
                                                         & ~miERR_VDEBUG
                                             : miERR_FATAL|miERR_ERROR);}
                | VERBOSE T_INTEGER
                  { if (!ctx->mi_force_verbose)
                          mi_set_verbosity((1 << $2) - 1); }
                | ECHO T_STRING
                  { mi_info("%s", $2);
                    mi_mem_release($2); }
                | SYSTEM T_STRING
                  { if ((system($2) >> 8) & 0xff)
                    mi_api_warning("system \"%s\" failed", $2);
                    mi_mem_release($2); }
                | MEMORY T_INTEGER
                  { mi_api_warning("memory view parameter ignored"); }
                | CODE T_STRING
                  { mi_link_file_add($2, miTRUE, miFALSE, miFALSE); }
                | CODE
                  { mi_api_code_verbatim_begin(); }
                  code_bytes_list
                  { mi_api_code_verbatim_end(); }
                | LINK T_STRING
                  { mi_link_file_add($2, miFALSE, miFALSE, miFALSE); }
                | DECLARE function_decl
                | DECLARE phenomenon_decl
                | DECLARE data_decl
                | REGISTRY symbol
                  { mi_api_registry_begin($2); }
                  reg_body END REGISTRY
                  { mi_api_registry_end(); }
                ;

reg_body        :
                | reg_item reg_body
                ;

reg_item        : VALUE symbol
                  { mi_api_registry_add(mi_mem_strdup("value"), $2); }
                | LINK symbol
                  { mi_api_registry_add(mi_mem_strdup("link"), $2); }
                | CODE symbol
                  { mi_api_registry_add(mi_mem_strdup("code"), $2); }
                | MI symbol
                  { mi_api_registry_add(mi_mem_strdup("mi"), $2); }
                | SPDL symbol
                  { mi_api_registry_add(mi_mem_strdup("spdl"), $2); }
                | ECHO symbol
                  { mi_api_registry_add(mi_mem_strdup("echo"), $2); }
                | SYSTEM symbol
                  { mi_api_registry_add(mi_mem_strdup("system"), $2); }
```

```
                | symbol symbol
                      { mi_api_registry_add($1, $2); }
                ;

incr_command    : options
                | camera
                | texture
                | material
                | light
                | instance
                | instgroup
                | object
                | userdata
                | gui
                | SHADER symbol function_list
                      { mi_api_shader_add($2, $3); }
                ;

code_bytes_list : T_BYTE_STRING
                      { mi_api_code_byte_copy($1.len, $1.bytes); }
                | code_bytes_list T_BYTE_STRING
                      { mi_api_code_byte_copy($2.len, $2.bytes); }
                ;

set             : SET symbol
                      { mi_api_variable_set($2, 0); }
                | SET symbol symbol
                      { mi_api_variable_set($2, $3); }
                ;

call            : CALL function_list
                      { mi_api_shader_call($2, 0, 0); }
                | CALL function_list ',' symbol symbol
                      { mi_api_shader_call($2, $4, $5); }
                ;

debug           : DEBUG_ symbol opt_symbol
                      { mi_api_debug($2, $3); }
                ;

version         : VERSION T_STRING
                      { mi_api_version_check($2, 0);
                        ctx->mi_did_check_version = miTRUE; }
                | MIN_ VERSION T_STRING
                      { mi_api_version_check($3, 0);
                        ctx->mi_did_check_version = miTRUE; }
                | MAX_ VERSION T_STRING
                      { mi_api_version_check($3, 1);
                        ctx->mi_did_check_version = miTRUE; }
                ;


/*****************************************************************************
```

```
 *************************    mi1 compatibility    ***************************
 ****************************************************************************/

/*----------------------------------------------------------------------------
 * frame
 *---------------------------------------------------------------------------*/

frame           :
                        { mi_api_frame_begin(&camera, &options); }
                  frame_number
                  initial_frame_cmd_list
                  view
                  frame_command_list
                  END FRAME
                        { mi_timing("mi scene file parsing");
                          mi_reset_time();
                          mi_api_frame_end();
                          if (mi_get_subverbosity(miM_MI) & miMSG_PHASE)
                                mi_progress("resume mi scene file parsing");
                          yyreturn MIYYENDFRAME;
                        }
                ;

initial_frame_cmd_list
                :
                | initial_frame_cmd_list initial_frame_cmd
                ;

initial_frame_cmd
                : texture
                | light
                | material
                ;

frame_command_list
                :
                | frame_command_list frame_command
                ;

frame_command
                : texture
                | light
                | material
                | object
                | call
                | debug
                | version
                | gui
                ;


/*----------------------------------------------------------------------------
 * view
```

```
 *-------------------------------------------------------------------------*/

view            : VIEW
                  view_list
                  END VIEW
                ;

view_list       :
                | view_list view_item
                ;

view_item       : camview_item
                | optview_item
                | MIN_ SAMPLES T_INTEGER
                        { options->min_samples = $3; }
                | MAX_ SAMPLES T_INTEGER
                        { options->max_samples = $3; }
                | SAMPLES T_INTEGER
                        { mi_api_warning(
                                "\"samples\" view parameter ignored"); }
                | RECURSIVE boolean
                        { if (!$2)
                                mi_api_warning("\"recursive off\" ignored"); }
                | ADAPTIVE boolean
                        { mi_api_warning("\"adaptive\" statement ignored"); }
                | ACCELERATION RAY CLASSIFICATION
                        { options->acceleration = 'c'; }
                | ACCELERATION SPATIAL SUBDIVISION
                        { options->acceleration = 'b'; }
                | ACCELERATION GRID
                        { options->acceleration = 'g'; }
                | SUBDIVISION MEMORY T_INTEGER
                        { options->subdivision_memory = $3; }
                | SUBDIVISION T_INTEGER T_INTEGER
                        { options->subdivision    = $2;
                          options->subdivision_2d = $3; }
                | MAX_ SIZE T_INTEGER
                        { options->space_max_size = $3; }
                | MAX_ DEPTH T_INTEGER
                        { options->space_max_depth = $3; }
                | SHADOW SORT boolean
                        { if ($3) options->shadow = 'l'; }
                | SHADOW SEGMENTS boolean
                        { if ($3) options->shadow = 's'; }
                | transform
                        { mi_api_view_transform($1); }
                | RED floating floating
                | GREEN floating floating
                | BLUE floating floating
                | WHITE floating floating
                ;
```

```
/*****************************************************************************
 *************************    new mi2 features    ****************************
 *****************************************************************************/

/*---------------------------------------------------------------------------
 * options
 *---------------------------------------------------------------------------*/

options         : OPTIONS symbol
                        { options = mi_api_options_begin($2); }
                  option_list END OPTIONS
                        { mi_api_options_end(); }
                ;

option_list     :
                | option_list option_item
                ;

option_item     : optview_item
                |       { curr_datatag = &options->userdata; }
                  data
                | ACCELERATION RAYCL
                        { options->acceleration = 'c'; }
                | ACCELERATION BSP
                        { options->acceleration = 'b'; }
                | ACCELERATION GRID
                        { options->acceleration = 'g'; }
                | DIAGNOSTIC SAMPLES boolean
                        { miBIT_SWITCH(options->diagnostic_mode,
                                miSCENE_DIAG_SAMPLES,$3);}
                | DIAGNOSTIC PHOTON OFF
                        { miBIT_SWITCH(options->diagnostic_mode,
                                miSCENE_DIAG_PHOTON, miFALSE);}
                | DIAGNOSTIC PHOTON DENSITY floating
                        { miBIT_SWITCH(options->diagnostic_mode,
                                miSCENE_DIAG_PHOTON, miFALSE);
                          miBIT_SWITCH(options->diagnostic_mode,
                                miSCENE_DIAG_PHOTON_D, miTRUE);
                          options->diag_photon_density = $4;}
                | DIAGNOSTIC PHOTON IRRADIANCE floating
                        { miBIT_SWITCH(options->diagnostic_mode,
                                miSCENE_DIAG_PHOTON, miFALSE);
                          miBIT_SWITCH(options->diagnostic_mode,
                                miSCENE_DIAG_PHOTON_I, miTRUE);
                          options->diag_photon_density = $4;}
                | DIAGNOSTIC GRID OFF
                        { miBIT_SWITCH(options->diagnostic_mode,
                                miSCENE_DIAG_GRID, miFALSE);}
                | DIAGNOSTIC GRID OBJECT floating
                        { options->diag_grid_size = $4;
                          miBIT_SWITCH(options->diagnostic_mode,
                                miSCENE_DIAG_GRID, miFALSE);
                          miBIT_SWITCH(options->diagnostic_mode,
```

```
                                  miSCENE_DIAG_GRID_O, $4 != 0.0);}
                   | DIAGNOSTIC GRID WORLD floating
                           { options->diag_grid_size = $4;
                             miBIT_SWITCH(options->diagnostic_mode,
                                  miSCENE_DIAG_GRID, miFALSE);
                             miBIT_SWITCH(options->diagnostic_mode,
                                  miSCENE_DIAG_GRID_W, $4 != 0.0);}
                   | DIAGNOSTIC GRID CAMERA floating
                           { options->diag_grid_size = $4;
                             miBIT_SWITCH(options->diagnostic_mode,
                                  miSCENE_DIAG_GRID, miFALSE);
                             miBIT_SWITCH(options->diagnostic_mode,
                                  miSCENE_DIAG_GRID_C, $4 != 0.0);}
                   | SAMPLES T_INTEGER
                           { options->min_samples = $2-2;
                             options->max_samples = $2;}
                   | SAMPLES T_INTEGER T_INTEGER
                           { options->min_samples = $2;
                             options->max_samples = $3;}
                   | SHADOW SORT
                           { options->shadow = 'l'; }
                   | SHADOW SEGMENTS
                           { options->shadow = 's'; }
                   ;

optview_item       : SHADOW OFF
                           { options->shadow = 0; }
                   | SHADOW ON
                           { options->shadow = 1; }
                   | TRACE boolean
                           { options->trace = $2; }
                   | SCANLINE boolean
                           { options->scanline = $2; }
                   | SCANLINE OPENGL
                           { options->scanline = 'o'; }
                   | LENS boolean
                           { options->no_lens = !$2; }
                   | VOLUME boolean
                           { options->no_volume = !$2; }
                   | GEOMETRY boolean
                           { options->no_geometry = !$2; }
                   | DISPLACE boolean
                           { options->no_displace = !$2; }
                   | OUTPUT boolean
                           { options->no_output = !$2; }
                   | MERGE boolean
                           { options->no_merge = !$2; }
                   | FILTER filter_type
                           { options->filter        = $2;
                             options->filter_size_x =
                             options->filter_size_y = 0.0; }
                   | FILTER filter_type floating
                           { options->filter        = $2;
```

```
            options->filter_size_x =
            options->filter_size_y = $3; }
    | FILTER filter_type floating floating
          { options->filter        = $2;
            options->filter_size_x = $3;
            options->filter_size_y = $4; }
    | FACE FRONT
          { options->face = 'f'; }
    | FACE BACK
          { options->face = 'b'; }
    | FACE BOTH
          { options->face = 'a'; }
    | FIELD OFF
          { options->field = 0; }
    | FIELD EVEN
          { options->field = 'e'; }
    | FIELD ODD
          { options->field = 'o'; }
    | SAMPLELOCK boolean
          { options->samplelock = $2; }
    | PHOTON TRACE DEPTH T_INTEGER
          { options->photon_reflection_depth = $4;
            options->photon_refraction_depth = $4;
            options->photon_trace_depth      = $4 + $4; }
    | PHOTON TRACE DEPTH T_INTEGER T_INTEGER
          { options->photon_reflection_depth = $4;
            options->photon_refraction_depth = $5;
            options->photon_trace_depth      = $4 + $5; }
    | PHOTON TRACE DEPTH T_INTEGER T_INTEGER T_INTEGER
          { options->photon_reflection_depth = $4;
            options->photon_refraction_depth = $5;
            options->photon_trace_depth      = $6; }
    | TRACE DEPTH T_INTEGER
          { options->reflection_depth = $3;
            options->refraction_depth = $3;
            options->trace_depth      = $3 + $3; }
    | TRACE DEPTH T_INTEGER T_INTEGER
          { options->reflection_depth = $3;
            options->refraction_depth = $4;
            options->trace_depth      = $3 + $4; }
    | TRACE DEPTH T_INTEGER T_INTEGER T_INTEGER
          { options->reflection_depth = $3;
            options->refraction_depth = $4;
            options->trace_depth      = $5; }
    | CONTRAST floating floating floating
          { options->contrast.r = $2;
            options->contrast.g = $3;
            options->contrast.b = $4;
            options->contrast.a = ($2 + $3 + $4)/3; }
    | CONTRAST floating floating floating floating
          { options->contrast.r = $2;
            options->contrast.g = $3;
            options->contrast.b = $4;
```

```
            options->contrast.a = $5; }
    | TIME CONTRAST floating floating floating
            { options->time_contrast.r = $3;
              options->time_contrast.g = $4;
              options->time_contrast.b = $5;
              options->time_contrast.a = ($3 + $4 + $5)/3; }
    | TIME CONTRAST floating floating floating floating
            { options->time_contrast.r = $3;
              options->time_contrast.g = $4;
              options->time_contrast.b = $5;
              options->time_contrast.a = $6; }
    | CONTOUR STORE function
            { options->contour_store = $3; }
    | CONTOUR CONTRAST function
            { options->contour_contrast = $3; }
    | JITTER floating
            { options->jitter = $2; }
    | SHUTTER floating
            { options->shutter = $2;
              options->motion  = options->shutter > 0; }
    | TASK SIZE T_INTEGER
            { options->task_size = $3; }
    | RAYCL SUBDIVISION T_INTEGER T_INTEGER
            { options->subdivision    = $3;
              options->subdivision_2d = $4; }
    | RAYCL MEMORY T_INTEGER
            { options->subdivision_memory = $3; }
    | BSP SIZE T_INTEGER
            { options->space_max_size = $3; }
    | BSP DEPTH T_INTEGER
            { options->space_max_depth = $3; }
    | BSP MEMORY T_INTEGER
            { options->space_max_mem = $3; }
    | GRID SIZE floating
            { options->grid_size = $3; }
    | DESATURATE boolean
            { miImg_mode_val val;
              val.b = $2;
              mi_img_mode(miIMG_MODE_DESATURATE,val); }
    | DITHER boolean
            { miImg_mode_val val;
              val.b = $2;
              mi_img_mode(miIMG_MODE_DITHER,val); }
    | PREMULTIPLY boolean
            { miImg_mode_val val;
              val.b = !($2);
              mi_img_mode(miIMG_MODE_NOPREMULT,val); }
    | COLORCLIP colorclip_mode
            { miImg_mode_val val;
              val.i = $2;
              mi_img_mode(miIMG_MODE_COLORCLIP,val); }
    | GAMMA floating
            { miImg_mode_val val;
```

```
            val.d = $2;
            mi_img_mode(miIMG_MODE_GAMMA,val); }
    | OBJECT SPACE
            { options->render_space = 'o'; }
    | CAMERA SPACE
            { options->render_space = 'c'; }
    | MIXED SPACE
            { options->render_space = 'm'; }
    | WORLD SPACE
            { mi_api_warning(
                    "world space statement ignored"); } /*<<<*/
    | INHERITANCE symbol
            { if (ctx->inheritance_func)
                    mi_mem_release(ctx->inheritance_func);
              ctx->inheritance_func = $2;
              if (!(options->inh_funcdecl = mi_api_decl_lookup(
                                            mi_mem_strdup($2))))
                    mi_api_nerror(421, "undeclared inheritance "
                                           "shader \"%s\"", $2);
            }
    | SHADOWMAP MOTION boolean
            { options->shadow_map_motion = $3; }
    | SHADOWMAP REBUILD boolean
            { options->recompute_shadow_maps = (($3)?'y':'n'); }
    | SHADOWMAP boolean
            { options->use_shadow_maps = $2; }
    | SHADOWMAP OPENGL
            { options->use_shadow_maps = 'o'; }
    | CAUSTIC boolean
            { options->caustic = $2; }
    | CAUSTIC T_INTEGER
            { options->caustic_flag = $2; }
    | CAUSTIC ACCURACY T_INTEGER
            { options->caustic_accuracy = $3; }
    | CAUSTIC ACCURACY T_INTEGER floating
            { options->caustic_accuracy = $3;
              options->caustic_radius = $4; }
    | CAUSTIC FILTER c_filter_type
            { options->caustic_filter = $3;
              options->caustic_filter_const = 1.1; }
    | CAUSTIC FILTER c_filter_type floating
            { options->caustic_filter = $3;
              options->caustic_filter_const = $4; }
    | GLOBILLUM boolean
            { options->globillum = $2; }
    | GLOBILLUM T_INTEGER
            { options->globillum_flag = $2; }
    | GLOBILLUM ACCURACY T_INTEGER
            { options->globillum_accuracy = $3; }
    | GLOBILLUM ACCURACY T_INTEGER floating
            { options->globillum_accuracy = $3;
              options->globillum_radius = $4; }
    | FINALGATHER boolean
```

```
                      { options->finalgather = $2; }
                | FINALGATHER ACCURACY T_INTEGER
                      { options->finalgather_rays = $3; }
                | FINALGATHER ACCURACY T_INTEGER floating
                      { options->finalgather_rays = $3;
                        options->finalgather_maxradius = $4;
                        options->finalgather_minradius = 0.0; }
                | FINALGATHER ACCURACY T_INTEGER floating floating
                      { options->finalgather_rays = $3;
                        options->finalgather_maxradius = $4;
                        options->finalgather_minradius = $5; }
                | PHOTONVOL ACCURACY T_INTEGER
                      { options->photonvol_accuracy = $3; }
                | PHOTONVOL ACCURACY T_INTEGER floating
                      { options->photonvol_accuracy = $3;
                        options->photonvol_radius = $4; }
                | PHOTONMAP FILE_ T_STRING
                      { mi_scene_delete(options->photonmap_file);
                        strcpy((char *)mi_scene_create(
                                      &options->photonmap_file,
                                      miSCENE_STRING, strlen($3)+1), $3);
                        mi_db_unpin(options->photonmap_file);
                        mi_mem_release($3); }
                | PHOTONMAP REBUILD boolean
                      { options->photonmap_rebuild = $3; }
                | APPROXIMATE opt_displace
                | FRAME BUFFER T_INTEGER opt_symbol
                      { mi_api_framebuffer(options, $3, $4); }
                ;

filter_type     : BOX
                      { $$ = 'b'; }
                | TRIANGLE
                      { $$ = 't'; }
                | GAUSS
                      { $$ = 'g'; }
                | MITCHELL
                      { $$ = 'm'; }
                | LANCZOS
                      { $$ = 'l'; }
                ;

c_filter_type   : BOX
                      { $$ = 'b'; }
                | CONE
                      { $$ = 'c'; }
                | GAUSS
                      { $$ = 'g'; }
                ;

opt_displace    :     { miAPPROX_DEFAULT(approx); }
                  s_approx_tech ALL
                      { memcpy(&options->approx, &approx, sizeof(miApprox));}
```

```
                | { miAPPROX_DEFAULT(approx); }
                  DISPLACE s_approx_tech ALL
                        { memcpy(&options->approx_displace, &approx,
                                                    sizeof(miApprox)); }
                ;


/*-----------------------------------------------------------------------
 * camera
 *-----------------------------------------------------------------------*/

camera          : CAMERA symbol
                        { camera = mi_api_camera_begin($2);
                          have_l = have_o = have_v = have_e = 0; }
                  camera_list END CAMERA
                        { mi_api_camera_end(); }
                ;

camera_list     :
                | camera_list camera_item
                ;

camera_item     : camview_item
                | frame_number
                | FIELD T_INTEGER
                        { camera->frame_field = $2; }
                ;

camview_item    : OUTPUT
                        { mi_api_function_delete(&camera->output); }
                | OUTPUT T_STRING T_STRING
                        { if (!have_o++)
                                mi_api_function_delete(&camera->output);
                          camera->output = mi_api_function_append(
                                camera->output,
                                mi_api_output_file_def(0, 0, $2, $3)); }
                | OUTPUT T_STRING out_parms T_STRING
                        { miTag ftag;
                          if (!have_o++)
                                mi_api_function_delete(&camera->output);
                          camera->output = mi_api_function_append(
                                camera->output,
                                ftag = mi_api_output_file_def(0, 0, $2, $4));
                          mi_api_output_file_parameter(ftag, 0, $3); }
                | OUTPUT T_STRING T_STRING T_STRING
                        { if (!have_o++)
                                mi_api_function_delete(&camera->output);
                          mi_api_output_type_identify(&tbm, &ibm, $2);
                          camera->output = mi_api_function_append(
                                camera->output,
                                mi_api_output_file_def(tbm, ibm, $3, $4));}
                | OUTPUT T_STRING T_STRING out_parms T_STRING
                        { miTag ftag;
```

```
            if (!have_o++)
                mi_api_function_delete(&camera->output);
            mi_api_output_type_identify(&tbm, &ibm, $2);
            camera->output = mi_api_function_append(
                camera->output,
                ftag = mi_api_output_file_def(tbm, ibm,$3,$5));
            mi_api_output_file_parameter(ftag, 0, $4); }
    | OUTPUT T_STRING function
          { if (!have_o++)
                mi_api_function_delete(&camera->output);
            mi_api_output_type_identify(&tbm, &ibm, $2);
            camera->output = mi_api_function_append(
                camera->output,
                mi_api_output_function_def(tbm, ibm, $3)); }
    | VOLUME
          { mi_api_function_delete(&camera->volume); }
    | VOLUME function_list
          { if (!have_v++)
                mi_api_function_delete(&camera->volume);
            camera->volume = mi_api_function_append(
                                camera->volume, $2); }
    | ENVIRONMENT
          { mi_api_function_delete(&camera->environment); }
    | ENVIRONMENT function_list
          { if (!have_e++)
                mi_api_function_delete(&camera->environment);
            camera->environment = mi_api_function_append(
                                camera->environment, $2); }
    | LENS
          { mi_api_function_delete(&camera->lens); }
    | LENS function_list
          { if (!have_l++)
                mi_api_function_delete(&camera->lens);
            camera->lens = mi_api_function_append(
                                camera->lens, $2); }
    | FOCAL floating
          { camera->focal = $2;
            camera->orthographic = miFALSE; }
    | FOCAL INFINITY_
          { camera->focal = 1;
            camera->orthographic = miTRUE; }
    | APERTURE floating
          { camera->aperture = $2; }
    | ASPECT floating
          { camera->aspect = $2; }
    | RESOLUTION T_INTEGER T_INTEGER
          { camera->x_resolution = $2;
            camera->y_resolution = $3; }
    | OFFSET floating floating
          { camera->x_offset = $2;
            camera->y_offset = $3; }
    | WINDOW T_INTEGER T_INTEGER T_INTEGER T_INTEGER
          { camera->window.xl = $2;
```

```
                        camera->window.yl = $3;
                        camera->window.xh = $4;
                        camera->window.yh = $5; }
                | CLIP floating floating
                      { camera->clip.min = $2;
                        camera->clip.max = $3; }
                |     { curr_datatag = &camera->userdata; }
                  data
                ;

out_parms       : QUALITY T_INTEGER
                      { $$[0] = (float) $2; }
                ;

frame_number    : FRAME T_INTEGER
                      { camera->frame       = $2;
                        camera->frame_time  = 0;
                        camera->frame_field = 0; }
                | FRAME T_INTEGER floating
                      { camera->frame       = $2;
                        camera->frame_time  = $3;
                        camera->frame_field = 0; }
                ;


/*-----------------------------------------------------------------------------
 * instance
 *---------------------------------------------------------------------------*/

instance        : INSTANCE symbol
                      { curr_inst = mi_api_instance_begin($2);
                        if (!curr_inst) curr_inst = &dummy_inst; }
                  inst_item inst_func
                  inst_flags
                  inst_params
                      { mi_api_instance_end($4, $5, $7); }
                  END INSTANCE
                ;

inst_item       :
                      { $$ = 0; }
                | symbol
                      { $$ = $1; }
                ;

inst_func       :
                      { $$ = miNULLTAG; }
                | GEOMETRY function_list
                      { $$ = $2; }
                ;

inst_flags      :
                | inst_flag inst_flags
```

```
                ;

inst_flag       : VISIBLE boolean
                        { curr_inst->visible = $2 ? 2 : 1; }
                | SHADOW boolean
                        { curr_inst->shadow = $2 ? 2 : 1; }
                | TRACE boolean
                        { curr_inst->trace = $2 ? 2 : 1; }
                | CAUSTIC
                        { curr_inst->caustic &= 0x30;
                          curr_inst->caustic |= 0x03; }
                | CAUSTIC boolean
                        { curr_inst->caustic &= 0x0f;
                          curr_inst->caustic |= $2 ? 0x20 : 0x10; }
                | CAUSTIC T_INTEGER
                        { curr_inst->caustic &= 0x30;
                          curr_inst->caustic |= ($2 & 0x0f); }
                | GLOBILLUM
                        { curr_inst->globillum &= 0x30;
                          curr_inst->globillum |= 0x03; }
                | GLOBILLUM boolean
                        { curr_inst->globillum &= 0x0f;
                          curr_inst->globillum |= $2 ? 0x20 : 0x10; }
                | GLOBILLUM T_INTEGER
                        { curr_inst->globillum &= 0x30;
                          curr_inst->globillum |= ($2 & 0x0f); }
                | HIDE boolean
                        { curr_inst->off = $2; }
                | TRANSFORM
                        { curr_inst->tf.function = miNULLTAG;
                          mi_matrix_ident(curr_inst->tf.global_to_local); }
                | TRANSFORM function
                        { curr_inst->tf.function = $2;
                          mi_matrix_ident(curr_inst->tf.global_to_local); }
                | transform
                        { curr_inst->tf.function = miNULLTAG;
                          mi_matrix_copy(
                                curr_inst->tf.global_to_local, $1);
                          if (!mi_matrix_invert(curr_inst->tf.local_to_global,
                                               curr_inst->tf.global_to_local)){
                                mi_api_warning("singular matrix, using "
                                                                "identity");
                                mi_matrix_ident(curr_inst->tf.global_to_local);
                                mi_matrix_ident(curr_inst->tf.local_to_global);
                        }}
                | MOTION OFF
                        { mi_matrix_null(curr_inst->motion_transform);
                          curr_inst->gen_motion = miGM_OFF; }
                | MOTION TRANSFORM
                        { mi_matrix_null(curr_inst->motion_transform);
                          curr_inst->gen_motion = miGM_INHERIT; }
                | MOTION transform
                        { mi_matrix_copy(curr_inst->motion_transform, $2);
```

```
                        curr_inst->gen_motion = miGM_TRANSFORM; }
                | MATERIAL
                        { curr_inst->material = miNULLTAG;
                          curr_inst->mtl_array_size = 0; }
                  inst_mtl
                | TAG T_INTEGER
                        { curr_inst->label = $2; }
                |       { curr_datatag = &curr_inst->userdata; }
                  data
                ;

inst_params     :
                        { $$ = (miTag)-1; }
                | '(' ')'
                        { $$ = miNULLTAG; }
                | '('
                        { if (!ctx->inheritance_func)
                                mi_api_error(
                                        "no inheritance function in options");
                          else {
                                mi_api_function_call(mi_mem_strdup(
                                        ctx->inheritance_func));
                          }
                        }
                  parameter_seq comma_rparen
                        { $$ = mi_api_function_call_end(0); }
                ;

comma_rparen    : ')'
                | ',' ')'
                ;

inst_mtl        :
                | symbol
                        { curr_inst->material = mi_api_material_lookup($1); }
                | '['
                        { taglist = mi_api_dlist_create(miDLIST_TAG); }
                  inst_mtl_array ']'
                        { curr_inst->mtl_array_size = taglist->nb;
                          curr_inst->material = mi_api_taglist(taglist); }
                ;

inst_mtl_array  : symbol
                        { mi_api_dlist_add(taglist,
                                (void *)(miIntptr)mi_api_material_lookup($1));}
                  inst_mtl_next
                ;

inst_mtl_next   :
                | ','
                | ',' inst_mtl_array
                ;
```

```
/*---------------------------------------------------------------------------
 * instgroup
 *---------------------------------------------------------------------------*/

instgroup       : INSTGROUP symbol
                        { curr_group = mi_api_instgroup_begin($2);
                          mi_api_instgroup_clear(); }
                  group_flags
                  group_list END INSTGROUP
                        { mi_api_instgroup_end(); }
                ;

group_flags     :
                | group_flag group_flags
                ;

group_flag      : MERGE floating
                        { curr_group->merge = $2;
                          curr_group->merge_group = $2 >= miMERGE_MIN; }
                | TAG T_INTEGER
                        { curr_group->label = $2; }
                |       { curr_datatag = &curr_group->userdata; }
                  data
                ;

group_list      :
                | symbol
                        { mi_api_instgroup_additem($1); }
                  group_list
                ;

/*****************************************************************************
 *************************     either     ***********************************
 ****************************************************************************/

/*---------------------------------------------------------------------------
 * function declaration
 *---------------------------------------------------------------------------*/

function_decl   : shret_type_nosh T_STRING parm_decl_list
                        { mi_api_funcdecl_begin($1, $2, $3);
                          mi_api_funcdecl_end(); }
                | SHADER shret_type T_STRING parm_decl_list
                        { if (!(curr_decl = mi_api_funcdecl_begin($2, $3, $4)))
                                curr_decl = &dummy_decl; }
                  declare_req_seq END DECLARE
                        { mi_api_funcdecl_end(); }
                ;

shret_type      : shret_type_nosh
                        { $$ = $1; }
```

```
                | SHADER
                        { $$ = mi_api_parameter_decl(miTYPE_SHADER, 0, 0); }
                ;

shret_type_nosh :
                        { $$ = mi_api_parameter_decl(miTYPE_COLOR, 0, 0); }
                | simple_type
                        { $$ = mi_api_parameter_decl($1, 0, 0); }
                | STRUCT '{' shret_decl_seq '}'
                        { miParameter *parm =
                                mi_api_parameter_decl(miTYPE_STRUCT, 0, 0);
                          mi_api_parameter_child(parm, $3);
                          $$ = parm; }
                ;

shret_decl_seq  : shret_decl_seq ',' shret_decl
                        { $$ = mi_api_parameter_append($1, $3); }
                | shret_decl
                        { $$ = $1; }
                ;

shret_decl      : simple_type symbol
                        { $$ = mi_api_parameter_decl($1, $2, 0); }
                | SHADER symbol
                        { $$ = mi_api_parameter_decl(miTYPE_SHADER, $2, 0); }
                | DATA symbol
                        { $$ = mi_api_parameter_decl(miTYPE_DATA,   $2, 0); }
                ;

parm_decl_list  : '(' parm_decl_seq ')'
                        { $$ = $2; }
                | '(' parm_decl_seq ',' ')'
                        { $$ = $2; }
                | '(' ')'
                        { $$ = 0; }
                ;

parm_decl_seq   : parm_decl_seq ',' parm_decl
                        { $$ = mi_api_parameter_append($1, $3); }
                | parm_decl
                        { $$ = $1; }
                ;

parm_decl       : simple_type symbol
                        { $$ = mi_api_parameter_decl($1, $2, 0); }
                | SHADER symbol
                        { $$ = mi_api_parameter_decl(miTYPE_SHADER, $2, 0); }
                | DATA symbol
                        { $$ = mi_api_parameter_decl(miTYPE_DATA,   $2, 0); }
                | STRUCT symbol '{' parm_decl_seq '}'
                        { miParameter *parm =
                                mi_api_parameter_decl(miTYPE_STRUCT, $2, 0);
                          mi_api_parameter_child(parm, $4);
```

```
                          $$ = parm; }
                | ARRAY parm_decl
                        { miParameter *parm =
                                mi_api_parameter_decl(miTYPE_ARRAY, 0, 0);
                          mi_api_parameter_child(parm, $2);
                          $$ = parm; }
                ;

simple_type     : BOOLEAN
                        { $$ = miTYPE_BOOLEAN; }
                | INTEGER
                        { $$ = miTYPE_INTEGER; }
                | SCALAR
                        { $$ = miTYPE_SCALAR; }
                | STRING
                        { $$ = miTYPE_STRING; }
                | COLOR
                        { $$ = miTYPE_COLOR; }
                | VECTOR
                        { $$ = miTYPE_VECTOR; }
                | TRANSFORM
                        { $$ = miTYPE_TRANSFORM; }
                | SCALAR TEXTURE
                        { $$ = miTYPE_SCALAR_TEX; }
                | VECTOR TEXTURE
                        { $$ = miTYPE_VECTOR_TEX; }
                | COLOR TEXTURE
                        { $$ = miTYPE_COLOR_TEX; }
                | LIGHT
                        { $$ = miTYPE_LIGHT; }
                | MATERIAL
                        { $$ = miTYPE_MATERIAL; }
                | GEOMETRY
                        { $$ = miTYPE_GEOMETRY; }
                ;

declare_req_seq :
                | declare_req declare_req_seq
                ;

declare_req     : gui
                | SCANLINE OFF
                        { curr_decl->phen.scanline = 1; }
                | SCANLINE ON
                        { curr_decl->phen.scanline = 2; }
                | TRACE OFF
                        { curr_decl->phen.trace = 1; }
                | TRACE ON
                        { curr_decl->phen.trace = 2; }
                | SHADOW OFF
                        { curr_decl->phen.shadow = 1; }
                | SHADOW ON
                        { curr_decl->phen.shadow = 2; }
```

```
              | SHADOW SORT
                     { curr_decl->phen.shadow = 'l'; }
              | SHADOW SEGMENTS
                     { curr_decl->phen.shadow = 's'; }
              | FACE FRONT
                     { curr_decl->phen.face = 'f'; }
              | FACE BACK
                     { curr_decl->phen.face = 'b'; }
              | FACE BOTH
                     { curr_decl->phen.face = 'a'; }
              | TEXTURE T_INTEGER
                     { curr_decl->phen.mintextures = $2; }
              | BUMP T_INTEGER
                     { curr_decl->phen.minbumps = $2; }
              | DERIVATIVE
                     { curr_decl->phen.deriv1 =
                       curr_decl->phen.deriv2 = 0; }
              | DERIVATIVE T_INTEGER
                     { if ($2 == 1)
                             curr_decl->phen.deriv1 = miTRUE;
                       else if ($2 == 2)
                             curr_decl->phen.deriv2 = miTRUE;
                       else
                             mi_api_error("derivative not 1 or 2"); }
              | DERIVATIVE T_INTEGER T_INTEGER
                     { if ($2 == 1 || $3 == 1)
                             curr_decl->phen.deriv1 = miTRUE;
                       else if ($2 == 2 || $3 == 2)
                             curr_decl->phen.deriv2 = miTRUE;
                       if ($2 != 1 && $2 != 2 || $3 != 1 && $3 != 2)
                             mi_api_error("derivative not 1 or 2"); }
              | OBJECT SPACE
                     { curr_decl->phen.render_space = 'o'; }
              | CAMERA SPACE
                     { curr_decl->phen.render_space = 'c'; }
              | MIXED SPACE
                     { curr_decl->phen.render_space = 'm'; }
              | WORLD SPACE
                     { mi_api_warning("world space statement ignored"); }
              | PARALLEL_
                     { curr_decl->phen.parallel = miTRUE; }
              | VERSION T_INTEGER
                     { curr_decl->version = $2; }
              | APPLY apply_list
                     { curr_decl->apply = $2; }
              ;

apply_list    : apply                  { $$ = $1; }
              | apply ',' apply_list   { $$ = $1 | $3; }
              ;

apply         : LENS                   { $$ = miAPPLY_LENS;          }
              | MATERIAL               { $$ = miAPPLY_MATERIAL;      }
```

```
                | LIGHT                   { $$ = miAPPLY_LIGHT;           }
                | SHADOW                  { $$ = miAPPLY_SHADOW;          }
                | ENVIRONMENT             { $$ = miAPPLY_ENVIRONMENT;     }
                | VOLUME                  { $$ = miAPPLY_VOLUME;          }
                | TEXTURE                 { $$ = miAPPLY_TEXTURE;         }
                | PHOTON                  { $$ = miAPPLY_PHOTON;          }
                | GEOMETRY                { $$ = miAPPLY_GEOMETRY;        }
                | DISPLACE                { $$ = miAPPLY_DISPLACE;        }
                | EMITTER                 { $$ = miAPPLY_PHOTON_EMITTER;  }
                | OUTPUT                  { $$ = miAPPLY_OUTPUT;          }
                ;


/*-----------------------------------------------------------------------
 * function instance
 *-----------------------------------------------------------------------*/

function_list   :
                        { funclist = miNULLTAG; }
                  func_list
                        { $$ = funclist; }
                ;

func_list       : function
                        { funclist = $1; }
                | func_list function
                        { funclist = mi_api_function_append(funclist, $2); }
                ;

function        : T_STRING
                        { mi_api_function_call($1); }
                  parameter_list
                        { $$ = mi_api_function_call_end(functag); functag = 0;}
                | '=' symbol
                        { $$ = mi_api_function_assign($2); }
                | '=' opt_incremental SHADER symbol function
                        { mi_api_shader_add($4, $5); $$ = $5;
                          mi_api_incremental(is_incremental); }
                ;

opt_incremental :
                        { mi_api_incremental(miFALSE); }
                | INCREMENTAL
                        { mi_api_incremental(miTRUE); }
                ;

parameter_list  : '(' ')'
                | '(' parameter_seq ')'
                | '(' parameter_seq ',' ')'
                ;

parameter_seq   : parameter
                | parameter_seq ',' parameter
```

```
                ;

parameter       : symbol
                        { mi_api_parameter_name($1); }
                  value_list
                ;

value_list      : value
                | value_list value
                ;

value           : NULL_
                | boolean
                        { int value = $1;
                          mi_api_parameter_value(miTYPE_BOOLEAN, &value,0,0); }
                | T_INTEGER
                        { int value = $1;
                          mi_api_parameter_value(miTYPE_INTEGER, &value,0,0); }
                | T_FLOAT
                        { float value = $1;
                          mi_api_parameter_value(miTYPE_SCALAR,  &value,0,0); }
                | symbol
                        { mi_api_parameter_value(miTYPE_STRING,  $1, 0, 0); }
                | '=' symbol
                        { mi_api_parameter_shader($2); }
                | '=' INTERFACE_ symbol
                        { mi_api_parameter_interface($3); }
                | '{'
                        { mi_api_parameter_push(miFALSE); }
                  parameter_seq '}'
                        { mi_api_parameter_pop(); }
                | '['
                        { mi_api_parameter_push(miTRUE); }
                  array_value_seq ']'
                        { mi_api_parameter_pop(); }
                | '[' ']'
                ;

array_value_seq :       { mi_api_new_array_element(); }
                  value_list
                  array_value_cont
                ;

array_value_cont:
                | ','
                        { mi_api_new_array_element(); }
                  value_list array_value_cont
                ;


/*-----------------------------------------------------------------------------
 * user data
 *----------------------------------------------------------------------------*/
```

```
userdata        : DATA symbol data_label T_INTEGER
                        { curr_data = mi_api_data_begin($2, 0,
                                                  (void *)(miIntptr)$4);
                          curr_data->label = label; }
                  '[' data_bytes_list ']'
                        { mi_api_data_end(); }
                | DATA symbol data_label symbol
                        { curr_data = mi_api_data_begin($2, 1,
                                                  (void *)(miIntptr)$4);
                          curr_data->label = label;
                          mi_api_data_end(); }
                | DATA symbol data_label symbol '('
                        { mi_api_function_call($4); }
                  parameter_seq comma_rparen
                        { tag = mi_api_function_call_end(0);
                          curr_data = mi_api_data_begin($2, 2,
                                                  (void *)(miIntptr)tag);
                          curr_data->label = label;
                          mi_api_data_end(); }
                ;

data_label      :
                        { label = 0; }
                | TAG T_INTEGER
                        { label = $2; }

data_bytes_list :
                | tex_bytes_list T_BYTE_STRING
                        { mi_api_data_byte_copy($2.len, $2.bytes); }
                ;

data_decl       : DATA T_STRING parm_decl_list
                        { if (curr_decl = mi_api_funcdecl_begin(0, $2, $3))
                                curr_decl->type = miFUNCTION_DATA; }
                  data_decl_req END DECLARE
                        { if (curr_decl) mi_api_funcdecl_end(); }
                ;

data_decl_req   : gui
                | VERSION T_INTEGER
                        { if (curr_decl) curr_decl->version = $2; }
                | APPLY apply_list
                        { if (curr_decl) curr_decl->apply = $2; }
                ;

data            : DATA symbol
                        { *curr_datatag = mi_api_data_append(*curr_datatag,
                                        mi_api_data_lookup($2)); }
                | DATA NULL_
                        { *curr_datatag = 0; }
                ;
```

```
/*------------------------------------------------------------------------
 * phenomenon declaration
 *-----------------------------------------------------------------------*/

phenomenon_decl : PHENOMENON shret_type T_STRING parm_decl_list
                        { curr_decl = mi_api_phen_begin($2, $3, $4);
                          if (!curr_decl) curr_decl = &dummy_decl; }
                  phen_body_list
                  END DECLARE
                        { mi_api_phen_end(); }
                ;

phen_body_list  :
                | phen_body phen_body_list
                ;

phen_body       : SHADER symbol function_list
                        { mi_api_shader_add($2, $3); }
                | material
                | light
                | instance
                | declare_req
                | ROOT phen_root
                        { if (curr_decl->phen.root)
                                mi_api_error("multiple roots not allowed");
                          else
                                curr_decl->phen.root = $2; }
                | OUTPUT T_STRING T_STRING
                        { curr_decl->phen.output = mi_api_function_append(
                                curr_decl->phen.output,
                                mi_api_output_file_def(0, 0, $2, $3)); }
                | OUTPUT T_STRING T_STRING T_STRING
                        { mi_api_output_type_identify(&tbm, &ibm, $2);
                          curr_decl->phen.output = mi_api_function_append(
                                curr_decl->phen.output,
                                mi_api_output_file_def(tbm, ibm, $3, $4));}
                | OUTPUT T_STRING function
                        { mi_api_output_type_identify(&tbm, &ibm, $2);
                          curr_decl->phen.output = mi_api_function_append(
                                curr_decl->phen.output,
                                mi_api_output_function_def(tbm, ibm, $3)); }
                | LENS function_list
                        { curr_decl->phen.lens = mi_api_function_append(
                                                curr_decl->phen.lens, $2); }
                | VOLUME function_list
                        { curr_decl->phen.volume = mi_api_function_append(
                                                curr_decl->phen.volume, $2); }
                | ENVIRONMENT function_list
                        { curr_decl->phen.environment = mi_api_function_append(
                                        curr_decl->phen.environment, $2); }
                | GEOMETRY function_list
                        { curr_decl->phen.geometry = mi_api_function_append(
```

```
                                        curr_decl->phen.geometry, $2);}
                | CONTOUR STORE function
                        { curr_decl->phen.contour_store = $3; }
                | CONTOUR CONTRAST function
                        { curr_decl->phen.contour_contrast = $3; }
                | OUTPUT PRIORITY T_INTEGER
                        { curr_decl->phen.output_seqnr = $3; }
                | LENS PRIORITY T_INTEGER
                        { curr_decl->phen.lens_seqnr = $3; }
                | VOLUME PRIORITY T_INTEGER
                        { curr_decl->phen.volume_seqnr = $3; }
                ;

phen_root       : MATERIAL symbol
                        { if (*curr_decl->declaration != 'm') {
                                mi_api_error("not a material phenomenon");
                                $$ = 0;
                          } else
                                $$ = mi_api_material_lookup($2); }
                | LIGHT symbol
                        { if (*curr_decl->declaration != 'l') {
                                mi_api_error("not a light phenomenon");
                                $$ = 0;
                          } else
                                $$ = mi_api_light_lookup($2); }
                | function_list
                        { $$ = 0;
                          if (*curr_decl->declaration == 'm')
                                mi_api_error("must use ``root material''");
                          else if (*curr_decl->declaration == 'l')
                                mi_api_error("must use ``root light''");
                          else
                                $$ = mi_api_function_append(
                                        curr_decl->phen.root, $1); }
                ;


/*-----------------------------------------------------------------------
 * texture
 *----------------------------------------------------------------------*/

texture         :       { pyramid_filter = 0.; }
                  tex_flags tex_type TEXTURE symbol
                        { functag = mi_api_texture_begin($5, $3, $2); }
                  tex_data
                        { if (pyramid_filter > 0. && functag)
                              if (mi_db_type(functag) == miSCENE_IMAGE) {
                                 mi_img_pyramid_set_filter((miImg_image *)
                                         mi_scene_edit(functag),pyramid_filter);
                                 mi_scene_edit_end(functag);
                              } else
                                 mi_api_nwarning(401, "cannot filter shaders");
                          functag = 0; }
```

```
                ;

tex_flags       :
                        { $$ = 0; }
                | tex_flag tex_flags
                        { $$ = $1 | $2; }
                ;

tex_flag        : LOCAL
                        { $$ = 1; }
                | FILTER
                        { pyramid_filter = 1.; $$ = 2; }
                | FILTER floating
                        { pyramid_filter = $2;
                          $$ = (pyramid_filter > 0.) ? 2 : 0; }
                ;

tex_type        : COLOR
                        { $$ = 0; }
                | SCALAR
                        { $$ = 1; }
                | VECTOR
                        { $$ = 2; }
                ;

tex_data        : '[' T_INTEGER T_INTEGER ']'
                        { mi_api_texture_array_def_begin($2, $3, 1); }
                  tex_bytes_list
                        { functag = mi_api_texture_array_def_end(); }
                | '[' T_INTEGER T_INTEGER T_INTEGER ']'
                        { mi_api_texture_array_def_begin($2, $3, $4); }
                  tex_bytes_list
                        { functag = mi_api_texture_array_def_end(); }
                | tex_func_list
                        { functag = mi_api_texture_function_def($1); }
                | T_STRING
                        { functag = mi_api_texture_file_def($1); }
                ;

tex_func_list   : function
                        { $$ = $1; }
                | function tex_func_list
                        { $$ = mi_api_function_append($1, $2); }
                ;

tex_bytes_list  :
                | tex_bytes_list T_BYTE_STRING
                        { mi_api_texture_byte_copy($2.len, $2.bytes); }
                ;


/*-----------------------------------------------------------------------
 * light
```

```
*-----------------------------------------------------------------------*/

light           : LIGHT symbol
                        { curr_light = mi_api_light_begin($2);
                          light_map = 0; }
                  light_ops
                  END LIGHT
                        { switch(light_map & 6) {
                            case 2: curr_light->type = miLIGHT_ORIGIN;    break;
                            case 4: curr_light->type = miLIGHT_DIRECTION;break;
                            case 6: curr_light->type = miLIGHT_SPOT;      break;
                          }
                          mi_api_light_end(); }
                ;

light_ops       :
                | light_op light_ops
                ;

light_op        : function
                        { if (!(light_map & 1))
                                mi_api_function_delete(&curr_light->shader);
                          light_map |= 1;
                          curr_light->shader = mi_api_function_append(
                                                 curr_light->shader, $1); }
                | EMITTER function
                        { if (!(light_map & 8))
                                mi_api_function_delete(&curr_light->emitter);
                          light_map |= 8;
                          curr_light->emitter = mi_api_function_append(
                                                 curr_light->emitter, $2); }
                | SHADOWMAP
                        { curr_light->use_shadow_maps = miTRUE; }
                | SHADOWMAP boolean
                        { curr_light->use_shadow_maps = $2; }
                | ORIGIN vector
                        { curr_light->origin = $2;
                          light_map |= 2; }
                | DIRECTION vector
                        { curr_light->direction = $2;
                          mi_vector_normalize(&curr_light->direction);
                          light_map |= 4; }
                | ENERGY floating floating floating
                        { curr_light->energy.r = $2;
                          curr_light->energy.g = $3;
                          curr_light->energy.b = $4; }
                | EXPONENT floating
                        { curr_light->exponent = $2; }
                | CAUSTIC PHOTONS T_INTEGER
                        { curr_light->caustic_store_photons = $3;
                          curr_light->caustic_emit_photons = 0; }
                | CAUSTIC PHOTONS T_INTEGER T_INTEGER
                        { curr_light->caustic_store_photons = $3;
```

```
          curr_light->caustic_emit_photons = $4; }
| GLOBILLUM PHOTONS T_INTEGER
        { curr_light->global_store_photons = $3;
          curr_light->global_emit_photons = 0; }
| GLOBILLUM PHOTONS T_INTEGER T_INTEGER
        { curr_light->global_store_photons = $3;
          curr_light->global_emit_photons = $4; }
| RECTANGLE vector vector light_samples
        { curr_light->area = miLIGHT_RECTANGLE;
          curr_light->primitive.rectangle.edge_u = $2;
          curr_light->primitive.rectangle.edge_v = $3; }
| DISC vector floating light_samples
        { curr_light->area = miLIGHT_DISC;
          curr_light->primitive.disc.normal      = $2;
          curr_light->primitive.disc.radius      = $3; }
| SPHERE floating light_samples
        { curr_light->area = miLIGHT_SPHERE;
          curr_light->primitive.sphere.radius    = $2; }
| CYLINDER vector floating light_samples
        { curr_light->area = miLIGHT_CYLINDER;
          curr_light->primitive.cylinder.axis    = $2;
          curr_light->primitive.cylinder.radius  = $3; }
| RECTANGLE
        { curr_light->area = miLIGHT_NONE; }
| DISC
        { curr_light->area = miLIGHT_NONE; }
| SPHERE
        { curr_light->area = miLIGHT_NONE; }
| CYLINDER
        { curr_light->area = miLIGHT_NONE; }
| SPREAD floating
        { curr_light->spread = $2; }
| SHADOWMAP RESOLUTION T_INTEGER
        { curr_light->shadowmap_resolution = $3; }
| SHADOWMAP SOFTNESS floating
        { curr_light->shadowmap_softness = $3; }
| SHADOWMAP SAMPLES T_INTEGER
        { curr_light->shadowmap_samples = $3; }
| SHADOWMAP FILE_ T_STRING
        { mi_scene_delete(curr_light->shadowmap_file);
          strcpy((char *)mi_scene_create(
                        &curr_light->shadowmap_file,
                        miSCENE_STRING, strlen($3)+1), $3);
          mi_db_unpin(curr_light->shadowmap_file);
          mi_mem_release($3); }
| VISIBLE
        { curr_light->visible = miTRUE; }
| VISIBLE boolean
        { curr_light->visible = $2; }
| TAG T_INTEGER
        { curr_light->label = $2; }
|
        { curr_datatag = &curr_light->userdata; }
  data
```

```
                ;

light_samples   :
                | T_INTEGER T_INTEGER
                        { curr_light->samples_u     = $1;
                          curr_light->samples_v     = $2; }
                | T_INTEGER T_INTEGER T_INTEGER
                        { curr_light->samples_u     = $1;
                          curr_light->samples_v     = $2;
                          curr_light->low_level     = $3; }
                | T_INTEGER T_INTEGER T_INTEGER T_INTEGER T_INTEGER
                        { curr_light->samples_u     = $1;
                          curr_light->samples_v     = $2;
                          curr_light->low_level     = $3;
                          curr_light->low_samples_u = $4;
                          curr_light->low_samples_v = $5; }
                ;


/*-----------------------------------------------------------------------------
 * material
 *----------------------------------------------------------------------------*/

material        : MATERIAL symbol
                        { curr_mtl = mi_api_material_begin($2);
                          have_d = have_s = have_v =
                          have_e = have_c = have_p = have_pv = 0; }
                  mtl_flags
                  function_list
                        { curr_mtl->shader = $5; }
                  mtl_args
                  END MATERIAL
                        { mi_api_material_end(); }
                ;

mtl_flags       :
                | mtl_flag mtl_flags
                ;

mtl_flag        : NOCONTOUR
                        { mi_api_warning(
                                "obsolete \"nocontour\" flag ignored"); }
                | OPAQUE_
                        { curr_mtl->opaque = miTRUE; }
                ;

mtl_args        :
                | mtl_arg mtl_args
                ;

mtl_arg         : DISPLACE
                        { mi_api_function_delete(&curr_mtl->displace); }
                | DISPLACE function_list
```

```
                    { if (!have_d++)
                            mi_api_function_delete(&curr_mtl->displace);
                      curr_mtl->displace = $2; }
                | SHADOW
                    { mi_api_function_delete(&curr_mtl->shadow); }
                | SHADOW function_list
                    { if (!have_s++)
                            mi_api_function_delete(&curr_mtl->shadow);
                      curr_mtl->shadow = $2; }
                | VOLUME
                    { mi_api_function_delete(&curr_mtl->volume); }
                | VOLUME function_list
                    { if (!have_v++)
                            mi_api_function_delete(&curr_mtl->volume);
                      curr_mtl->volume = $2; }
                | ENVIRONMENT
                    { mi_api_function_delete(&curr_mtl->environment); }
                | ENVIRONMENT function_list
                    { if (!have_e++)
                            mi_api_function_delete(&curr_mtl->environment);
                      curr_mtl->environment = $2; }
                | CONTOUR
                    { mi_api_function_delete(&curr_mtl->contour); }
                | CONTOUR function_list
                    { if (!have_c++)
                            mi_api_function_delete(&curr_mtl->contour);
                      curr_mtl->contour = $2; }
                | PHOTON
                    { mi_api_function_delete(&curr_mtl->photon); }
                | PHOTON function_list
                    { if (!have_p++)
                            mi_api_function_delete(&curr_mtl->photon);
                      curr_mtl->photon = $2; }
                | PHOTONVOL
                    { mi_api_function_delete(&curr_mtl->photonvol); }
                | PHOTONVOL function_list
                    { if (!have_pv++)
                          mi_api_function_delete(&curr_mtl->photonvol);
                      curr_mtl->photonvol = $2; }
                ;


/*------------------------------------------------------------------------------
 * object
 *----------------------------------------------------------------------------*/

object          : OBJECT opt_symbol
                    { curr_obj = mi_api_object_begin($2); }
                  obj_flags
                  bases_and_groups
                  END OBJECT
                    { mi_api_object_end(); }
                ;
```

```
obj_flags       :
                | obj_flag obj_flags
                ;

obj_flag        : VISIBLE
                        { curr_obj->visible = miTRUE; }
                | VISIBLE boolean
                        { curr_obj->shadow = $2; }
                | SHADOW
                        { curr_obj->shadow = miTRUE; }
                | SHADOW boolean
                        { curr_obj->shadow = $2; }
                | TRACE
                        { curr_obj->trace = miTRUE; }
                | TRACE boolean
                        { curr_obj->trace = $2; }
                | TAGGED
                        { curr_obj->mtl_is_label = miTRUE; }
                | TAGGED boolean
                        { curr_obj->mtl_is_label = $2; }
                | CAUSTIC
                        { curr_obj->caustic |= 3; }
                | CAUSTIC boolean
                        { curr_obj->caustic &= 0x03;
                          if (!$2)
                                  curr_obj->caustic |= 0x10; }
                | CAUSTIC T_INTEGER
                        { curr_obj->caustic &= 0x10;
                          curr_obj->caustic |= ($2 & 0x03); }
                | GLOBILLUM
                        { curr_obj->globillum |= 3; }
                | GLOBILLUM boolean
                        { curr_obj->globillum &= 0x03;
                          if (!$2)
                                  curr_obj->globillum |= 0x10; }
                | GLOBILLUM T_INTEGER
                        { curr_obj->globillum &= 0x10;
                          curr_obj->globillum |= ($2 & 0x03); }
                | TAG T_INTEGER
                        { curr_obj->label = $2; }
                |       { curr_datatag = &curr_obj->userdata; }
                  data
                | transform
                        { mi_api_object_matrix($1); }
                | MAX_ DISPLACE floating
                        { curr_obj->maxdisplace = $3; }
                ;

bases_and_groups:
                | basis bases_and_groups
                | group bases_and_groups
                ;
```

```
basis           : BASIS symbol rational MATRIX T_INTEGER T_INTEGER basis_matrix
                        { mi_api_basis_add($2, $3, miBASIS_MATRIX, $5,$6,$7); }
                | BASIS symbol rational BEZIER T_INTEGER
                        { mi_api_basis_add($2, $3, miBASIS_BEZIER, $5, 0, 0); }
                | BASIS symbol rational TAYLOR T_INTEGER
                        { mi_api_basis_add($2, $3, miBASIS_TAYLOR, $5, 0, 0); }
                | BASIS symbol rational BSPLINE T_INTEGER
                        { mi_api_basis_add($2, $3, miBASIS_BSPLINE, $5, 0, 0);}
                | BASIS symbol rational CARDINAL
                        { mi_api_basis_add($2, $3, miBASIS_CARDINAL, 0, 0, 0);}
                ;

rational        :
                        { $$ = miFALSE; }
                | RATIONAL
                        { $$ = miTRUE; }
                ;

basis_matrix    :       { $$ = mi_api_dlist_create(miDLIST_GEOSCALAR); }
                | basis_matrix floating
                        { miGeoScalar s=$2; mi_api_dlist_add($1, &s); $$=$1; }
                ;

group           : GROUP opt_symbol merge_option
                        { mi_api_object_group_begin($3);
                          mi_mem_release($2); }
                  vector_list
                  vertex_list
                  geometry_list
                  END GROUP
                        { mi_api_object_group_end(); }
                ;

merge_option    :
                        { $$ = 0.0; }
                | MERGE floating
                        { $$ = $2; }
                ;

vector_list     :
                | vector_list geovector
                        { mi_api_geovector_xyz_add(&$2); }
                ;

vertex_list     :
                | vertex_list vertex
                ;

vertex          : V T_INTEGER
                        { mi_api_vertex_add($2); }
                  n_vector
                  d_vector
```

```
                  t_vector_list
                  m_vector
                  u_vector_list
                  vertex_flag
                ;

n_vector        :
                | N T_INTEGER
                        { mi_api_vertex_normal_add($2); }
                ;

d_vector        :
                | D T_INTEGER T_INTEGER
                        { mi_api_vertex_deriv_add($2, $3); }
                | D T_INTEGER T_INTEGER T_INTEGER
                        { mi_api_vertex_deriv2_add($2, $3, $4); }
                | D T_INTEGER T_INTEGER T_INTEGER T_INTEGER T_INTEGER
                        { mi_api_vertex_deriv_add($2, $3);
                          mi_api_vertex_deriv2_add($4, $5, $6); }
                ;

m_vector        :
                | M T_INTEGER
                        { mi_api_vertex_motion_add($2); }
                ;

t_vector_list   :
                | t_vector_list T T_INTEGER
                        { mi_api_vertex_tex_add($3, -1, -1); }
                | t_vector_list T T_INTEGER T_INTEGER T_INTEGER
                        { mi_api_vertex_tex_add($3, $4, $5); }
                ;

u_vector_list   :
                | u_vector_list U T_INTEGER
                        { mi_api_vertex_user_add($3); }
                ;

vertex_flag     :
                | CUSP
                        { mi_api_vertex_flags_add(miAPI_V_CUSP, 1); }
                | CUSP floating
                        { mi_api_vertex_flags_add(miAPI_V_CUSP, $2); }
                | CONIC
                        { mi_api_vertex_flags_add(miAPI_V_CONIC, 1); }
                | CONIC floating
                        { mi_api_vertex_flags_add(miAPI_V_CONIC, $2); }
                | CORNER
                        { mi_api_vertex_flags_add(miAPI_V_CORNER, 0); }
                | DART
                        { mi_api_vertex_flags_add(miAPI_V_DART, 0); }
                ;
```

```
geometry_list   :
                | geometry_list geometry
                ;

geometry        : polygon
                | curve
                | spacecurve
                | surface
                | subdivsurf
                | connection
                | approximation
        /*      | implicit_patch        */
                ;

/* polygons */

polygon         : CP opt_symbol
                        { mi_api_poly_begin(1, $2); }
                  poly_indices
                        { mi_api_poly_end(); }
                | P opt_symbol
                        { mi_api_poly_begin(0, $2); }
                  poly_indices
                        { mi_api_poly_end(); }
                | STRIP opt_symbol
                        { mi_api_poly_begin(2, $2); }
                  strip_indices
                        { mi_api_poly_end(); }
                | FAN opt_symbol
                        { mi_api_poly_begin(3, $2); }
                  strip_indices
                        { mi_api_poly_end(); }
                ;

poly_indices    :
                | T_INTEGER
                        { mi_api_poly_index_add($1); }
                  poly_indices
                | HOLE
                        { mi_api_poly_hole_add(); }
                  poly_indices
                ;

strip_indices   :
                | T_INTEGER
                        { mi_api_poly_index_add($1); }
                  strip_indices
                ;

h_vertex_ref_seq: h_vertex_ref
                | h_vertex_ref_seq h_vertex_ref
```

```
                ;

h_vertex_ref    : T_INTEGER
                        { mi_api_vertex_ref_add($1, (double)1.0); }
                | T_INTEGER T_FLOAT
                        { mi_api_vertex_ref_add($1, $2); }
                | T_INTEGER W floating
                        { mi_api_vertex_ref_add($1, $3); }
                ;


para_list       : T_FLOAT
                        { miDlist *dlp =mi_api_dlist_create(miDLIST_GEOSCALAR);
                          miGeoScalar s = $1;    /* $1 is a double */
                          mi_api_dlist_add(dlp, &s);
                          $$ = dlp; }
                | para_list T_FLOAT
                        { miGeoScalar s = $2;    /* $2 is a double */
                          mi_api_dlist_add($1, &s);
                          $$ = $1; }
                ;


/* curves and space curves */

curve           : CURVE symbol rational symbol
                        { mi_api_curve_begin($2, $4, $3); }
                  para_list h_vertex_ref_seq curve_spec
                        { mi_api_curve_end($6); }
                ;

curve_spec      :
                | SPECIAL curve_special_list
                ;

curve_special_list
                : curve_special
                | curve_special_list curve_special
                ;

curve_special   : T_INTEGER
                        { mi_api_curve_specpnt($1, -1); }
                | T_INTEGER MAPSTO T_INTEGER
                        { mi_api_curve_specpnt($1, $3); }
                ;

spacecurve      : SPACE CURVE symbol
                        { mi_api_spacecurve_begin($3); }
                  spcurve_list
                        { mi_api_spacecurve_end(); }
                ;

spcurve_list    : symbol floating floating
```

```
                        { miGeoRange r;
                          r.min = $2;
                          r.max = $3;
                          mi_api_spacecurve_curveseg(miTRUE, $1, &r); }
                | spcurve_list symbol floating floating
                        { miGeoRange r;
                          r.min = $3;
                          r.max = $4;
                          mi_api_spacecurve_curveseg(miFALSE, $2, &r); }
                ;


/* free-form surfaces */

surface         : SURFACE symbol mtl_or_label
                        { mi_api_surface_begin($2, $3); }
                  rational symbol floating floating para_list
                        { mi_api_surface_params(miU, $6, $7, $8, $9, $5); }
                  rational symbol floating floating para_list
                        { mi_api_surface_params(miV, $12, $13, $14, $15, $11);}
                  h_vertex_ref_seq
                  tex_surf_list
                  surf_spec_list
                        { mi_api_surface_end(); }
                ;

mtl_or_label    : symbol
                        { $$ = $1; }
                | T_INTEGER
                        { $$ = (char *)(miIntptr)$1; }
                ;

tex_surf_list   :
                | tex_surf_list tex_surf
                ;

tex_surf        : opt_volume_flag opt_vector_flag TEXTURE
                  rational symbol para_list
                  rational symbol para_list
                        { mi_api_surface_texture_begin(
                                        $1, $2, $5, $6, $4, $8, $9, $7); }
                  h_vertex_ref_seq

                | DERIVATIVE
                        { mi_api_surface_derivative(1); }
                | DERIVATIVE T_INTEGER
                        { mi_api_surface_derivative($2); }
                | DERIVATIVE T_INTEGER T_INTEGER
                        { mi_api_surface_derivative($2);
                          mi_api_surface_derivative($3); }
                ;

opt_volume_flag :
```

```
                        { $$ = miFALSE; }
                | VOLUME
                        { $$ = miTRUE; }
                ;

opt_vector_flag :
                        { $$ = miFALSE; }
                | VECTOR
                        { $$ = miTRUE; }
                ;


surf_spec_list  :
                | surf_spec_list surf_spec
                ;

surf_spec       : TRIM trim_spec_list
                | HOLE hole_spec_list
                | SPECIAL
                        { newloop = miTRUE; }
                  special_spec_list
                ;

trim_spec_list  : symbol floating floating
                        { miGeoRange r;
                          r.min = $2;
                          r.max = $3;
                          mi_api_surface_curveseg(miTRUE, miCURVE_TRIM,$1,&r);}
                | trim_spec_list symbol floating floating
                        { miGeoRange r;
                          r.min = $3;
                          r.max = $4;
                          mi_api_surface_curveseg(miFALSE,miCURVE_TRIM,$2,&r);}
                ;

hole_spec_list  : symbol floating floating
                        { miGeoRange r;
                          r.min = $2;
                          r.max = $3;
                          mi_api_surface_curveseg(miTRUE,miCURVE_HOLE,$1,&r); }
                | hole_spec_list symbol floating floating
                        { miGeoRange r;
                          r.min = $3;
                          r.max = $4;
                          mi_api_surface_curveseg(miFALSE,miCURVE_HOLE,$2,&r);}
                ;

special_spec_list
                : special_spec
                | special_spec_list special_spec
                ;

special_spec    : T_INTEGER
```

```
                          { mi_api_surface_specpnt($1, -1); }
                | T_INTEGER MAPSTO T_INTEGER
                          { mi_api_surface_specpnt($1, $3); }
                | symbol floating floating
                          { miGeoRange r;
                            r.min = $2;
                            r.max = $3;
                            mi_api_surface_curveseg(newloop,
                                                    miCURVE_SPECIAL, $1, &r);
                            newloop = miFALSE; }
                ;

connection      : CONNECT
                  symbol symbol floating floating
                  symbol symbol floating floating
                          { miGeoRange c1, c2;
                            c1.min = $4;
                            c1.max = $5;
                            c2.min = $8;
                            c2.max = $9;
                            mi_api_object_group_connection($2,$3,&c1,$6,$7,&c2);}
                ;


/* subdivision surfaces */

subdivsurf      : SUBDIVISION SURFACE symbol
                          { mi_api_subdivsurf_begin($3); }
                  sds_base_polys END SUBDIVISION SURFACE
                          { mi_api_subdivsurf_end(); }
                ;

sds_base_polys  :
                | sds_base_poly sds_base_polys
                ;

sds_base_poly   : P opt_symbol
                          { mi_api_subdivsurf_poly(3);
                            mi_api_subdivsurf_mtl($2); }
                  sds_indices sds_flags sds_subdiv_base
                | Q opt_symbol
                          { mi_api_subdivsurf_poly(4);
                            mi_api_subdivsurf_mtl($2); }
                  sds_indices sds_flags sds_subdiv_base
                ;

sds_subdiv_base :
                | '{'
                          { mi_api_subdivsurf_push();
                            mi_api_subdivsurf_kit(); }
                  sds_materials sds_indices sds_flags sds_subdiv_subs '}'
                          { mi_api_subdivsurf_pop(); }
                ;
```

```
sds_subdiv_subs :
                | '{'
                        { mi_api_subdivsurf_push(); }
                  sds_sub_polys '}'
                        { mi_api_subdivsurf_pop(); }
                ;

sds_sub_polys   : sds_sub_poly
                | sds_sub_poly ',' sds_sub_polys
                ;

sds_sub_poly    :
                        { mi_api_subdivsurf_kit(); }
                |
                        { mi_api_subdivsurf_kit(); }
                  sds_materials sds_indices sds_flags sds_subdiv_subs
                ;

sds_materials   :
                | symbol
                        { mi_api_subdivsurf_mtl($1); }
                  sds_materials
                ;

sds_indices     : T_INTEGER
                        { mi_api_subdivsurf_index($1); }
                | T_INTEGER
                        { mi_api_subdivsurf_index($1); }
                  sds_indices
                ;

sds_flags       :
                | CREASE floating
                        { mi_api_subdivsurf_flags(miAPI_E_CREASE, $2); }
                  sds_creaseflags
                ;

sds_creaseflags :
                | floating
                        { mi_api_subdivsurf_flags(miAPI_E_CREASE, $1); }
                  sds_creaseflags;
                ;


/*---------------------------------------------------------------------------
 * approximations (in objects and options)
 *---------------------------------------------------------------------------*/

approximation   :       { miAPPROX_DEFAULT(approx); }
                  approx_body
                ;
```

```
approx_body      : APPROXIMATE SURFACE  s_approx_tech s_approx_names
                 | APPROXIMATE SUBDIVISION SURFACE
                                      c_approx_tech sds_approx_names
                 | APPROXIMATE DISPLACE s_approx_tech d_approx_names
                 | APPROXIMATE CURVE    c_approx_tech c_approx_names
                 | APPROXIMATE SPACE CURVE
                                      c_approx_tech spc_approx_names
                 | APPROXIMATE TRIM     c_approx_tech t_approx_names
                 | APPROXIMATE          s_approx_tech
                        { mi_api_poly_approx(&approx); }
                 ;

s_approx_tech    : s_approx_params
                        { approx.subdiv[miMIN]  = 0;
                          approx.subdiv[miMAX]  = 5;
                          approx.max            = miHUGE_INT; }
                 | s_approx_params T_INTEGER T_INTEGER
                        { approx.subdiv[miMIN]  = $2;
                          approx.subdiv[miMAX]  = $3;
                          approx.max            = miHUGE_INT; }
                 | s_approx_params MAX_ T_INTEGER
                        { approx.subdiv[miMIN]  = 0;
                          approx.subdiv[miMAX]  = 5;
                          approx.max            = $3; }
                 | s_approx_params T_INTEGER T_INTEGER MAX_ T_INTEGER
                        { approx.subdiv[miMIN]  = $2;
                          approx.subdiv[miMAX]  = $3;
                          approx.max            = $5; }
                 ;

c_approx_tech    : c_approx_params
                        { approx.subdiv[miMIN]  = 0;
                          approx.subdiv[miMAX]  = 5; }
                 | c_approx_params T_INTEGER T_INTEGER
                        { approx.subdiv[miMIN]  = $2;
                          approx.subdiv[miMAX]  = $3; }
                 ;

s_approx_params  : s_approx_param
                 | s_approx_param s_approx_params
                 ;

c_approx_params  : c_approx_param
                 | c_approx_param c_approx_params
                 ;

s_approx_param   : x_approx_param
                 | PARAMETRIC floating floating
                        { approx.method                 = miAPPROX_PARAMETRIC;
                          approx.cnst[miCNST_UPARAM]    = $2;
                          approx.cnst[miCNST_VPARAM]    = $3; }
                 | REGULAR PARAMETRIC floating floating
                        { approx.method                 = miAPPROX_REGULAR;
```

```
                        approx.cnst[miCNST_UPARAM]     = $3;
                        approx.cnst[miCNST_VPARAM]     = $4; }
                | IMPLICIT
                      { approx.method                  = miAPPROX_ALGEBRAIC; }
                ;

c_approx_param  : x_approx_param
                | PARAMETRIC floating
                      { approx.method                  = miAPPROX_PARAMETRIC;
                        approx.cnst[miCNST_UPARAM]     = $2;
                        approx.cnst[miCNST_VPARAM]     = 1.0; }
                | REGULAR PARAMETRIC floating
                      { approx.method                  = miAPPROX_REGULAR;
                        approx.cnst[miCNST_UPARAM]     = $3;
                        approx.cnst[miCNST_VPARAM]     = 1.0; }
                ;

x_approx_param  : VIEW
                      { approx.view_dep         = miTRUE; }
                | ANY
                      { approx.any              = miTRUE; }
                | TREE
                      { approx.style            = miAPPROX_STYLE_TREE; }
                | GRID
                      { approx.style            = miAPPROX_STYLE_GRID; }
                | DELAUNAY
                      { approx.style            = miAPPROX_STYLE_DELAUNAY; }
                | LENGTH floating
                      { approx.method                  = miAPPROX_LDA;
                        approx.cnst[miCNST_LENGTH]     = $2; }
                | DISTANCE floating
                      { approx.method                  = miAPPROX_LDA;
                        approx.cnst[miCNST_DISTANCE]   = $2; }
                | ANGLE floating
                      { approx.method                  = miAPPROX_LDA;
                        approx.cnst[miCNST_ANGLE]      = $2; }
                | SPATIAL approx_view floating
                      { approx.method                  = miAPPROX_SPATIAL;
                        approx.cnst[miCNST_LENGTH]     = $3; }
                | CURVATURE approx_view floating floating
                      { approx.method                  = miAPPROX_CURVATURE;
                        approx.cnst[miCNST_DISTANCE]   = $3;
                        approx.cnst[miCNST_ANGLE]      = $4; }
                | GRADING floating
                      { approx.grading                 = $2; }
                ;

approx_view     :
                | VIEW
                      { approx.view_dep                = miTRUE; }
                ;

s_approx_names  : symbol
```

```
                        { mi_api_surface_approx($1, &approx); }
                | s_approx_names symbol
                        { mi_api_surface_approx($2, &approx); }
                ;

sds_approx_names: symbol
                        { mi_api_subdivsurf_approx($1, &approx); }
                | sds_approx_names symbol
                        { mi_api_subdivsurf_approx($2, &approx); }
                ;

d_approx_names  : symbol
                        { mi_api_surface_approx_displace($1, &approx); }
                | s_approx_names symbol
                        { mi_api_surface_approx_displace($2, &approx); }
                ;

c_approx_names  : symbol
                        { mi_api_curve_approx($1, &approx); }
                | c_approx_names symbol
                        { mi_api_curve_approx($2, &approx); }
                ;

spc_approx_names: symbol
                        { mi_api_spacecurve_approx($1, &approx); }
                | c_approx_names symbol
                        { mi_api_spacecurve_approx($2, &approx); }
                ;

t_approx_names  : symbol
                        { mi_api_surface_approx_trim($1, &approx); }
                | t_approx_names symbol
                        { mi_api_surface_approx_trim($2, &approx); }
                ;


/*-------------------------------------------------------------------------------
 * user-interface commands
 *-----------------------------------------------------------------------------*/

gui             : GUI opt_symbol
                        { mi_api_gui_begin($2); }
                  '(' gui_attr_list ')' '{' gui_controls '}'
                        { mi_api_gui_end(); }
                | GUI opt_symbol
                        { mi_api_gui_begin($2); }
                  '{' gui_controls '}'
                        { mi_api_gui_end(); }
                ;

gui_elems       :
                | gui_elem gui_elems
                ;
```

```
gui_elem        : '(' gui_attr_list ')'
                | '{'
                        { mi_api_gui_push(); }
                  gui_controls '}'
                        { mi_api_gui_pop(); }
                ;

gui_controls    :
                | gui_control gui_controls
                ;

gui_control     : CONTROL symbol opt_symbol
                        { mi_api_gui_control_begin($3?$2:0, $3?$3:$2); }
                  gui_elems
                        { mi_api_gui_control_end(); }
                ;

gui_attr_list   :
                | ','
                | gui_attr
                | gui_attr ',' gui_attr_list
                ;

gui_attr        : symbol
                        { mi_api_gui_attr($1, miNTYPES, 0); }
                | symbol boolean
                        { mi_api_gui_attr($1, miTYPE_BOOLEAN, 1, $2); }
                | symbol floating
                        { mi_api_gui_attr($1, miTYPE_SCALAR, 1, $2); }
                | symbol floating floating
                        { mi_api_gui_attr($1, miTYPE_SCALAR, 2, $2, $3); }
                | symbol floating floating floating
                        { mi_api_gui_attr($1, miTYPE_SCALAR, 3, $2, $3, $4); }
                | symbol floating floating floating floating
                        { mi_api_gui_attr($1, miTYPE_SCALAR, 4, $2,$3,$4,$5); }
                | symbol symbol
                        { mi_api_gui_attr($1, miTYPE_STRING, 1, $2); }
                ;
%%
```

[Driemeyer 99] T. Driemeyer, *Rendering with mental ray*, mental ray series Volume 1, Springer–Verlag, Berlin, Heidelberg, New York, Tokyo, 1999.

[Foley 90] J. D. Foley, A. van Dam, S. K. Feiner, J. F. Hughes, *Computer Graphics, Principles and Practice*, Second Edition, Addison-Wesley Publishing Company 1990.

[Hall 89] R. Hall, *Illumination and Color in Computer Generated Imagery*, Springer-Verlag, New York 1989.

[Herken 94] R. Herken, R. Hödicke, K. J. Schmidt, "High Image Quality, Interactive Rendering on Scalable Parallel Systems. An Interim Report on ESPRIT

Project 6173 (DESIRE)", *Proceedings of the 1994 EUROSIM Conference on Massively Parallel Processing*, J. C. Zuidervaart and L. Dekker (Ed.), Elsevier Science 1994.

[Niederreiter 92] H. Niederreiter, "Random Number Generation and Quasi-Monte Carlo Methods", *CBMS-NSF Regional Conference Series in Applied Mathematics*, volume 63, Society for Industrial and Applied Mathematics, Philadelphia 1992.

[Perlin 85] K. Perlin, "An Image Synthesizer", *SIGGRAPH '85 Proceedings*, pp. 287–296, ACM July 1985.

[RAY1 97] "mental ray 1.9 User's Manual", mental images 1997.

[Ward 92] G. Ward, "Measuring and Modeling Anisotropic Reflection", *SIGGRAPH '92 Proceedings*, pp. 265–272, ACM July 1992.

[Watt 92] A. Watt, M. Watt, "Advanced Animation and Rendering Techniques—Theory and Practice", Addison-Wesley Publishing Company, Wokingham 1992.

[Whitted 80] T. Whitted, "An Improved Illumination Model for Shaded Display", *Communications of the ACM*, Volume 23, number 6, ACM June 1980

Index

G

H

I

J

K

L

M

Springer-Verlag
and the Environment

WE AT SPRINGER-VERLAG FIRMLY BELIEVE THAT AN international science publisher has a special obligation to the environment, and our corporate policies consistently reflect this conviction.

WE ALSO EXPECT OUR BUSINESS PARTNERS – PRINTERS, paper mills, packaging manufacturers, etc. – to commit themselves to using environmentally friendly materials and production processes.

THE PAPER IN THIS BOOK IS MADE FROM NO-CHLORINE pulp and is acid free, in conformance with international standards for paper permanency.